Administering Health Systems

The Editors

MARY F. ARNOLD, Professor of Health Planning in the College of Human Development at Pennsylvania State University, received her B.A. from Smith College, her M.P.H. at the University of North Carolina, and her Dr.P.H. at the University of California, Berkeley. Dr. Arnold frequently lectures and serves as coordinator for government and voluntary-agency education programs given for professionals in the fields of health planning and evaluation. She has served as a consultant to various state and local health departments and voluntary health agencies. In addition to articles published in scholarly journals, Dr. Arnold has edited and written several works on the subject of health administration, including *Health Program Implementation through* PERT for the American Public Health Association.

L. VAUGHN BLANKENSHIP is Chairman of the Department of Political Science of the State University of New York at Buffalo. He was awarded his B.A. by the University of California, Riverside, and his Ph.D. by Cornell University. Dr. Blankenship has written widely for scholarly publications and has two other books scheduled for release.

JOHN M. HESS earned his B.A., M.A., and Ph.D. at the University of California, Berkeley. He has served as a consultant to various hospitals and hospital planning groups and has done extensive research in hospital administration practice.

Administering Health Systems

ISSUES AND PERSPECTIVES

Mary F. Arnold

L. Vaughn Blankenship

John M. Hess

Editors

ALDINE PUBLISHING COMPANY, *Chicago*

Address all inquiries to
Aldine Publishing Company
529 South Wabash Avenue
Chicago, Illinois 60605

Library of Congress Catalog Number 70-92060
ISBN 0-202-27002-5

Second printing, 1976

Printed in the United States of America

Designed by Andrea Clark

Contents

III. THE POLITICAL CONTEXT OF HEALTH ADMINISTRATION

IV. PLANNING AS A MEANS OF RATIONALIZING THE HEALTH SYSTEM

V. ORGANIZATIONAL PERSPECTIVES

Preface

During the years in which this volume was taking shape, our society entered a period of rapidly accelerating social change. Complacency that the vast scientific and technical capability of our society could find solutions to all problems is giving way as we find our organizational efforts unable to cope adequately with new developments. The physical environment is becoming despoiled with the wastes of our life style and our industrial technology. The human environment is becoming crowded, while at the same time communication by machine is replacing the satisfying personal relationships found previously at home, at work, and at play, and great ideological schisms are threatening to tear apart the social fabric that has held us together.

On the other hand, we are on the threshold of new scientific discoveries that will open new opportunities for man to control the population explosion; to heal in new ways and to extend life; and to expand man's cognitive capabilities. But we recognize that these new discoveries, just as in the past, will create new types of problems, and we must face the difficulty of keeping these new changes within bounds and under control even while we attempt to cope with past problems.

The ability to organize resources to meet these accelerating changes has not kept pace with technological and scientific expansion. We see things around us that we do not like, but we do not know how to set them right. We look ahead to alternative futures, but we do not know how to choose from among them nor how to achieve what we desire.

The health field, with its orientation toward the well-being of individuals, has felt the strong impact of these changes. No longer is the maldistribution of the rewards of our scientific quest in the health sciences tolerated. Health is now perceived as a right rather than as something to be earned, and many groups in this society and in other societies no longer tolerate deprivation of the life-saving and life-fulfilling opportunities afforded by present scientific capability. Recently the health field has become more cognizant of the broad implications of health activities and has begun to accept the challenge that this recognition brings. Health is no longer only a biological function—rather the quality of life is the concern.

In a period of rapid social change and uncertainty, it is difficult to identity those things that future historians will tell us were important. Today we can only partially understand what is happening to the world around us. However, from our meager knowledge of the past and our inadequate understanding of the present, we develop theories about what we might predict for the future. This book presents some intepretations of the forces and issues the editors believe to be significant for the administrator of health organizations in the changing health system. The authors come from a variety of disciplines, but all have a common interest: What is happening to the health system? Some of the authors have done research on various aspects of health systems; some have been or are now administrators of health agencies; and many are teachers of health personnel. It is hoped that the health systems approach of this book will provide the seasoned health administrator with a variety of perspectives for viewing the problems he faces in everyday administrative practice and will provide the student who is on his way to becoming a health administrator with an initial understanding of the breath of his newly developing occupation.

This book takes a health systems approach to the problems of administering health organizations. The appropriateness of such an approach is best illustrated by a description of the many varied contributions of individuals and agencies that helped develop the materials presented here.

Federal and state governmental agencies, private foundations, and voluntary health agencies are represented by the assistance they gave in the form of research and training grants. The research reported here, however, could not have been done without the interest and time-consuming participation of people in professional associations; in local, state, and federal governmental agencies; in voluntary health and welfare agencies; and in hospitals and of private physicians and patients. The people in the educational and other institutions in which the various authors have worked—colleagues, secretaries, and administrators—have all contributed greatly to this volume. This microcosmic systems outcome is the product of the work and participation of thousands of people, and we would like to be able to express our appreciation to each one. More particularly, we would like to acknowledge the specific research and training grants that have enabled the various authors to develop their material:

THE NATIONAL INSTITUTES OF HEALTH: Grant No. GM 12367 03–National Institute of General Medical Science (Chapter 5); Grant No. 5-SOl-FR 05441—General Research Support (Chapters 6 and 22); Grant No. I-SOl-FR 05441—General Research Support (Chapter 10); Grant No. W-127 (Chapter 11).

THE PUBLIC HEALTH SERVICE, U.S. DEPARTMENT OF HEALTH, EDUCATION, AND WELFARE: Grant No. CH-00232—Health Economics Branch, Division of Medical Care Administration (Chapter 20); Governmental Career Development Program, under P. L. 85–507 (Chapter 21).

THE ROCKEFELLER FOUNDATION (Chapter 8).

THE AMERICAN HEART ASSOCIATION, THE CALIFORNIA HEART ASSOCIATION, and the CALIFORNIA DEPARTMENT OF HEALTH, HEART DISEASE CONTROL PROGRAM (Chapter 17).

NATIONAL AERONAUTICS AND SPACE ADMINISTRATION: Grant No. NSG-243 (Chapter 23).

In addition to these particular grants that aided in the development of specific content in this volume, two other sources of assistance were of immeasurable help in the preparation of this volume: The editorial assistance of Mrs. Marcia Barnett was provided through a grant to the Hospital Administration Program, University of California, Berkeley, by the W. K. Kellogg Foundation, and many of the ideas were developed in a training program in Comprehensive Health Planning (Grant No. 95501–02–68) supported by the U.S. Public Health Service.

Several of the chapters have appeared elsewhere, and we appreciate permission to reprint the following material:

"Our Changing World," *Journal of the American Public Health Association*, 58:2 (February 1968), 238–245 (chapter 1).

"Professionalism and the New Concepts of Administration," *The Journal of Nursing Education*, 7:1 (January 1968), 5–10, 24–26. Copyright © 1968 McGraw-Hill, Inc. (chapter 3).

"Emerging Patterns of Federalism in Health," in part appeared in Murray S. Stedman, ed., *Modernizing American Government*, Englewood Cliffs, N.J.: Prentice-Hall, Inc. (chapter 8).

"Current Issues of Health Organization," *Journal of the American Public Health Association*," 58:7 (July 1968), 1192–1199 (chapter 9).

"Organizational Support and Community Power Structure," *Journal of Health and Human Behavior*, 3 (Winter 1962), 257–269 (chapter 11).

"Basic Concepts and Crucial Issues in Health Planning," *American Journal of Public Health*, 59 (1969) (chapter 13).

"Agency Problems in Planning for Community Health Needs," *Medical Care*, 6:6 (November-December 1968), 454–466 (chapter 17).

"Economies of Scale in Outpatient Medical Practice," *Group Practice*, 17:7 (July 1968), 24–33 (chapter 20).

Four of the papers (Chapters 10, 14, 15, and 16) were prepared in substantially similar form for a text on comprehensive health planning developed by the Comprehensive Health Planning Unit under the direction of Henrik L. Blum, M.D., of the Division of Public Health and Medical Administration of the School of Public Health, University of California, Berkeley. These papers also appear in Henrik L. Blum and Associates, *Notebook on Comprehensive Health Planning*, Western Regional Office, American Public Health Association, San Francisco, 1968.

There is another group to whom we owe a deep debt of gratitude. These are those, who as students in formal administration classes and seminars and as participants in health administration continuing education programs in various parts of the country, have made the development of this volume an exciting enterprise for the editors.

MARY F. ARNOLD
L. VAUGHN BLANKENSHIP
JOHN M. HESS

Contributors

JOSEPH A. ALUTTO, PH.D. Assistant Professor, Department of Organizations, School of Management, State University of New York at Buffalo

Teaching and research on socialization of professionals, especially nurses and teachers; and organizational analysis of professional associations

MARY F. ARNOLD, Dr.P.H. Professor of Health Planning, College of Human Development, Pennsylvania State University, College Park, Pennsylvania

Teaching and research in management, organization theory, and interorganizational analysis with emphasis on health planning

RICHARD M. BAILEY, D.B.A. Assistant Professor, Department of Business Administration and School of Public Health, University of California, Berkeley

Teaching and research in economics and business forecasting, in application of economic analyses to production and delivery of medical services, and in development of economic criteria for allocation of medical resources

L. VAUGHN BLANKENSHIP, PH.D. Associate Professor and Chairman, Department of Political Science, State University of New York at Buffalo

Teaching and research in organization theory and in science policy

EDWARD L. CAVENAUGH, Dr.P.H. Assistant Chief, Laboratory Consultation and Development Section, National Communicable Disease Center, Atlanta, Georgia

Experience in administration of communicable disease control and laboratory management in local, state, and federal programs; research in development of quantitative tools for use by health program administrators

RAY H. ELLING, PH.D. Professor of Sociology and Head, Social Sciences Unit, Department of Clinical Medicine and Health Care, Health Center, University of Connecticut

Teaching and research in medical sociology and the sociology of occupations with particular emphasis on work groups in the health field

EDNA M. GREXTON, Dr.P.H. Professor of Public Health Nursing, School of Nursing and School of Allied Health Sciences, State University of New York at Buffalo

Teaching and research in the education and socialization of the professions, with emphasis on interaction process and the development of professional work teams

JOHN M. HESS, PH.D. Lecturer in Public Health (Hospital Administration), School of Public Health, University of California, Berkeley

Teaching and research on the administrative organization, the patterns of hospital organization, and the professions and public policy

DOUGLAS L. HINK, PH.D. Assistant Professor, Florence Heller School of Social Work, Brandeis University, Waltham, Massachusetts

Teaching and research in social psychology, with emphasis on aging and on health service systems

ARNOLD I. KISCH, M.D. Assistant Professor of Preventive Medicine, School of Medicine, University of California, Los Angeles

Research and teaching in the area of modeling of health systems and health manpower utilization; author of a series of case studies on administrative decision-making in medical care

EDWARD S. ROGERS, M.D. Professor of Public Health and Medical Administration, School of Public Health, University of California, Berkeley

Teaching and research in public health organization and administration, medical care, and human ecology

MORRIS SCHAEFER, D.P.A. Professor and Head, Department of Health Administration, School of Public Health, Chapel Hill, North Carolina

Research and teaching in health planning evaluation and organization; application of the systems approach to health administration; health policy formulation

DAVID G. SMITH, PH.D. Professor of Political Science, Swarthmore College, Pennsylvania

Teaching and research on local government, public administration, and public policy; study of administration of social services in U.S. Department of Health, Education, and Welfare

DAVID B. STARKWEATHER, Dr.P.H. Assistant Professor of Hospital Administration, University of California, Berkeley

Teaching and consultation in hospital systems; research on health facilities planning and hospital mergers

DAVID H. STIMSON, PH.D. Associate Professor of Management, San Francisco State College; Lecturer in Social Policies Planning, Department of City and Regional Planning, University of California, Berkeley

Current research in the field of education and health, the administration of research on a university campus, and use of operations research and systems analysis in hospital administration

ISABEL M. WELSH, M.A. Research Assistant, School of Public Health, University of California, Berkeley

Doctoral candidate in political science; research on political decision-making at the community level

RODNEY F. WHITE, PH.D. Associate Professor and Program Coordinator, Sloan Institute of Hospital Administration, Graduate School of Business and Public Administration, Cornell University, Ithaca, New York

Teaching and research in medical sociology, in organization theory and behavior, and in sociology of occupations and professions; currently involved in a comparative study of health administrators in three medical care systems (United States, Canada, and United Kingdom)

I

THE HEALTH SYSTEM

1

Health in Our Changing World

Mary F. Arnold

The word "change" means "to alter by substituting something for, or by giving up for something else; put, or take another or others in place of . . . to make different, to turn, convert."[1] This is an active process, and what is exciting today are the opportunities we have at every turn to take an active part in our changing world.

Unless we fully understand, and tackle now, the health problems of the future, we cannot take a leadership role. Rather, we will be continuously reacting and adapting to the immediate situation. If one takes a Parsonian[2] viewpoint and assumes, therefore, that the major function of the medical or health system is social control—that is, controlling the deviant, who is socially defined as sick—then this adaptive and reactive pattern of behavior makes good sense. However, we do have other ways or modes of action available to us beyond just adaptive ones.

In public health a great deal of emphasis is given to the concept of planning. Every specialty group places emphasis on planning skills in its standards of training; program planning is one of the basic constructs of education for public health. However, planning involves projection into the future as well as analysis of what is now and, if we take this emphasis on planning seriously, we accept the challenge of determining what we believe the future should be like.

There are two postures one can take on planning. The first is to define planning as an intervention process to change current sets of behavior to new sets of behavior, in order to obtain a different set of outcomes from what would have happened if the plan had not been put into action. Emphasis here is on a desired state of the future, and this posture on planning assumes that we are capable of making decisions about desired outcomes as well as capable of setting the wheels in motion to get there.

A second posture on planning is to define it as "intelligent cooperation with the inevitable"—a posture that assumes that about all we can do is adapt and adjust gracefully to the myriad of complex interacting forces that move inexorably onward. Before bowing completely to this second posture, I would like to have a try at the first and at least test the assumption that we have the capabilities of rationally planning for the future.

One of the first steps in the planning process, no matter what expert one quotes, is that of identification of the problem around which one wishes to make plans. What is disturbing is the type of problem we are selecting for solution. We are in an unprecedented period, as far as history tells—a time of rapidly changing social, physical, and biological environment for man—yet there are very few attempts at projection to even a generation ahead, say 15–20 years. There is such a vast complexity of interacting forces that it is extremely difficult to forecast with any accuracy, but there are some things we could begin to think about at the same time that we are running to catch up with what has already happened.

This can be illustrated in more specific terms. We are in the midst of an epidemic of heart disease— we have some evidence that a better balance between our caloric intake and our exercise might reduce the risk of premature illness or death from this disease. We can reduce calories, increase exercise, or both; but we also know that, as the population increases and moves increasingly into metropolitan and urban areas, the kind of life that we lead in our society makes it almost impossible to increase exercise without making a fetish of it. So what do we do? We teach children physical fitness around the most boring sets of exercises one could devise. We think nothing of working with a community on a fluoridation project; but how much have we done to try to find socially interesting exercise patterns that would fit into the life style of the community? Recently, in a study of the nonmedical needs of patients with coronary occlusion, a major problem was found to be the lack of social and recreational outlets.[3] To build in the opportunity for exercise in community and regional planning seems to me to be a perfectly valid public health education activity. We can preach all we want, and the doctors can prescribe all they want, but until the social opportunities are made accessible, exercise as a desirable health behavior will not be performed.

To extend this idea further: I have a young friend named Mike who in just 15 years will be twenty-one. What is Mike's world going to be like 15 years from now? What health programs can be planned now so that we can honestly say that at least some of Mike's potential health problems will have been prevented? Mike is lucky, because he has already started out with great advantages. He is a bright, happy child, with a history of longevity on both sides of his family. He has had the best of pediatric care available up to now. His mother and father are well informed about health matters (she is a bacteriologist; he, a physiologist). Mike is growing up in a warm family, with two younger sisters. From all the things one can see, Mike has a healthy start in life—or does he? Are not his chances of accidental injury and/or death increasing? Is he learning a risky way of life in terms of his coronary arteries? Is the world that he will face in 15 years the one we are preparing him for now? Have we seriously tried to think what his life will be like and what he will need to live that kind of life to his best advantage? Can we really teach Mike what healthful living should be, when we have not really assessed what his life will be like? In assessing what Mike's world will be like, we should take a global view.

THE IMMEDIATE FUTURE

It seems to me that there are three irreversible trends, or changes, that are of particular importance:

1. The people of this earth are increasing in numbers at an ever expanding rate. These people need, minimally, land, food, and water to survive.

2. We have a knowledge explosion that is producing revolutionary changes in our technology and in its demands on education, energy, and cooperative effort.

3. Along with more people and more knowledge has come an expanding awareness of inequality of opportunity, of human potential, and of our world-wide interdependence.

In turn, these forces are creating some profound social changes that are now affecting, and will affect even more in the future, the everyday lives of each of us.

Let us look, first, at these major forces and see what is happening. Barbara Ward's provocative book *Spaceship Earth* provides an image of the world that puts all these massive changes into context.

> The most rational way of considering the whole human race today is to see it as the ship's crew of a single spaceship on which all of us, with a remarkable combination of security and vulnerability, are

> making our pilgrimage through infinity. Our planet is not much more than the capsule within which we have to live as human beings if we are to survive the vast space voyage upon which we have been engaged for hundreds of millennia—but without yet noticing our condition. This space voyage is totally precarious. We depend upon a little envelope of soil and a rather larger envelope of atmosphere for life itself. And both can be contaminated and destroyed.... This is how we have to think of ourselves. We are a ship's company on a small ship. Rational behavior is the condition of survival.[4]

What is actually happening to this spaceship? What will it be like in less than 20 years? My information has been taken from two volumes edited by Calder, *The World in 1984*,[5] which is the report of a conference of world-wide experts held in 1964 by the *New Scientist*, a British journal. These experts' predictions were based on 1964 knowledge and therefore are very conservative, because the consequences of new information and technology compound and accelerate change.

Crew of the Future: Our Population Trends

For every seven crew members on our spaceship in 1944, by 1964 there were 10 and by 1984 there will be 16. Even with successful family planning programs, we can expect a larger and larger crew. To feed this expanding crew in 1984, we will have to increase food production from the 1964 level by 57 per cent in the world as a whole and, in the less developed areas, by 68 per cent. If we wish to minimally improve the diets of this crew, there will have to be a 275 per cent increase in food production in the less developed areas. Assuming that our technical abilities will enable us to increase production, we still have two very basic problems: (1) all these people need space, and there will be less and less land to be cultivated, and (2) because of the scarcity of land and the fact that people are also congregating in urban areas, distribution of this food becomes more and more complex, requiring more processing and giving us problems in maintaining the food's nutritive value.

In addition to food, water is necessary for life. Batisse of UNESCO estimated that we will have to at least double the domestic requirements for water by 1984. For industrial use, at least 150 per cent of current needs will be required and at least double the current requirements for agricultural use. In the near future the supply will not be the problem, it will be distribution. We are already seeing large-scale, long-term regional, interstate, intercountry, and even continental-wide planning getting under way. Water in the next few years will no longer be so freely used, and it will become increasingly costly. We may find that, within our lifetime, we ourselves will have separate distribution systems, separating our drinking water and waste disposal water. Just as milk is bought, our drinking and cooking water will probably be bought. In some parts of the United States, this has started. To increase the supply of arable land, even more water will be necessary. To maintain and develop the required food and water distribution, increasingly larger economic resources will be needed. These are not far distant problems. They are with us now. In 15 years will we worry as much about dietary patterns, or will this be as much a matter of individual choice? My hunch is that we had better start educational programs aimed at the distribution system level. Should not these be the concerns of health education or public health?

Expanding Knowledge and Technology

The second major change is in our knowledge and technology. Perhaps the most important technical change is the development of the computer and the use of cybernetic theory—enabling us to deal in very different ways with the increasing knowledge becoming available. The computer and cybernetic theory can be likened to the invention of the wheel. They have created for us totally new ways of dealing with problems. An article from a series on the computer in *Fortune* magazine perhaps summarizes best what the computer has done for us:

> A man cannot instruct the computer to perform usefully until he has arduously thought through what he is up to in the first place and where he wants to go from there... the rethinking process gets more difficult as the computer gets better. Wherever the computer is used, it is improving enormously the quantity and quality of human cognition, and it is rapidly becoming a kind of Universal Disciplinarian.[6]

The computer has provided facilities for storing and using information in very different ways. It is possible to simulate consequences of actions and policies, to ascertain consequences for future planning. The computer is used to run plants, to plan farm crop yields, to plot and plan inventory, to estimate flow of traffic, for teaching, for medical diagnostic purposes, for laboratory analysis, for record-keeping and processing, for patient surveillance, and in innumerable other ways.

Our technology has provided the means to communicate rapidly around the world, to phone in data from the West Coast to a computer on the East Coast and get the answer within seconds. Newsprinting and other printing is automated, and the use of space and television enables us to see and hear an occurrence around the world at the time it is occurring. The computer enables us to have data banks; counties, states, and even the federal government are studying how to put such systems into effect. It is quite probable that all babies will be given a social security number at birth, and Mike's total record will be available on tape at the touch of a button anywhere he goes. Obviously there are some knotty problems involved in this. How do we protect privileged information? What should be considered privileged information? What is private and what is public? Can the computer help us solve our organizational problems in providing health services, or will it just compound old problems?

Ideological Trends

The third major force is partly due to this expanding technology and partly due to the expanding population, but there is a growing awareness of inequality—of opportunity and of the potentialities of human beings. Margaret Mead, in a television interview, summed up this trend when she said in response to a question about the world-wide unrest: "Until people see a glimmer of light, there is nothing to fight for." Our world is industrializing rapidly; and there is a pressing urgency of peoples everywhere demanding freedom from want, demanding human dignity and the right of self-determination. These demands create great ideological and political schisms; but if we look behind the protests, the wars, the political maneuverings of newly created states, we see a great striving and anxiety to reach new human values and to create new utopias.

These, then, are the ferments and changes that are occurring around us. As mentioned earlier, they in turn are creating some profound social changes that are affecting, and will affect, our everyday lives. Several of these changes have particular implications for those in the health field.

EFFECTS OF CHANGE

All these changes must be thought of as dynamic, of building one upon the other. No longer can we simplify our thinking to assume direct cause and effect or that one problem can be tackled and nothing else will be affected. One of the consequences of our population, knowledge, and ideology explosions is that *organizational relationships are changing and will change quite drastically.*

Continously, in the literature, in the newspapers and in conferences we hear that we must find new social arrangements and organizational patterns to deal with new complexities. But we should first look at what is actually happening.

The use of the computer and cybernetics has resulted in major changes in the administrative managerial process. Complete and partial automation of industrial process is creating the paradox of acute manpower shortages among technical specialists, professionals, and highly skilled workers and greater unemployment for people with out-of-date skills or minimal skills. Decision-making in the managerial process depends more and more upon coordination of technical specialty skills and knowledge. Technical decision tools in the form of various mathematical and decision models are now available. Our strongly held beliefs about the authority of the hierarchy of position, as seen in organizational charts, is no longer functional, and we are being forced to find newer and more functional ways of structuring and organizing work. Task-force administration or problem-centered administration is taking over the old ideas of hierarchical administration. PPBS (program budgeting) and cost-effectiveness analysis are thrust upon us; systems analysis and operations research bring a new look to the study of governmental processes as well as of industrial processes. As soon as one starts to think in terms of the problem of the flow of information or people (as in systems analysis), old organizational structures have to be bypassed because they become barriers to thinking and acting. We have the opportunity today to be creative in our planning, but only in so far as we make explicit what we want the future to be like and the choices that are available to us.

Urbanization and the need to plan on a region-wide basis for environmental protection (air pollution and water pollution, for example), for transportation, for population expansion, for civil rights, and so on, mean that governmental jurisdictions, as we have known them, are no longer functional and that either their functions will have to change or boundaries will have to change. Our generation has little or no experience in experimentation with governmental structure. The textbooks in public health administration, for many years, were written normatively, e.g., every country should have a local health department and every health department should have a board of health. These "shoulds" have put blinders on us as to other ways of accomplishing the same goals. If we stay wedded to structure we shut ourselves off from finding alternative ways of reaching our goals.

Changing Concepts of Education

A second consequence of our population, knowledge, and ideology changes is a shift in our thinking about education. To be able to function well in this rapidly changing world, agencies, industry, medicine, and most services will need people who not only are very highly skilled but, because skills go out of date so rapidly, also have the additional qualities of (1) mental flexibility, (2) logical thinking, (3) ability to think creatively, as well as logically, and (4) a high receptivity to new ideas. We can no longer think of education as being essentially completed by finishing a particular level of schooling. My friend Mike will not only have to have the kind of education that provides him with a technical competence, but he will also have to have an education that prepares him continually to learn new and even different skills and technics. As health educators, should we not feel concern about his physical and psychological ability to cope with this kind of life?

As a society we need to provide access to this continual education. We are going to have to provide new kinds of educational institutions, and the old ones need drastic revisions. The person who would like to return to school for three or six months or even a year to retool is not provided for in our educational system. Most continuing education is short term or tacked on as in-service education to an agency. It seldom provides adequately for retooling in depth. This means a major change in our thinking about professional growth, about in-service training, and about provision of educational opportunities. In particular, it means a complete change in our society's assumptions about education. I have a twelve-year-old neighbor who, when introduced to two of our doctoral students, asked, "Are you really going to school? What do you plan to be when you grow up?" In our culture, going to school means you have not yet become a productive adult.

Another force affecting our educational system is the political recognition that too much of our population is out of the economic, occupational, and social mainstream of the society and that the problem is becoming worse, not better. Operation Head Start, Upward Bound, and other poverty programs are attempts to do something about this. But these programs and the problems of offsetting de facto segregation are forcing us to question some of our sacred assumptions about education and how education should be organized. In a sense we have combined problems or the solutions to problems. This need to provide equal opportunity has a positive value in itself, but it also is tied closely to the expanding problem of unemployment for persons with a poor educational background. With the growing unemployment of those minimally educated, those semiskilled, and those in late middle age (many middle-management people in their forties and fifties are losing high-salaried positions), we find a paradox, because we have terrible manpower shortages in the highly skilled and professional occupations. This situation, too, is a challenge to our educational system. Will not solutions to these educational problems influence our health programs of the future?

Changing Work Patterns

This leads me to the third consequence of social changes that are around us. Here there is an unequally distributed and dysfunctional division of labor, and it is becoming necessary to rethink job functions, professional functions, and our patterns of work to meet these challenges. Nursing, in some ways, has been in the forefront in the health field, with the development of the LVN and the aide, but professional and specialty domains that have been carved out and often jealously guarded are in the process of change. As each of us learns new skills and takes on new functions, we have to share functions with someone else, with others who have different kinds of skills. Carefully guarded domains of influence, of necessity, are breaking down rapidly. There is a propensity in the health field to characterize and stereotype people by their profession rather than by their particular and individual mix of skills. A professional affiliation does give an anchor and support, but it also pummels us into a mold from which it becomes hard to escape. This problem of professional domains and values leads to the fourth effect of our changing world.

Necessity of Making Explicit Value Choices

Technology and expanding knowledge are creating a conscious awareness that our world is a dynamic ecosystem. We are faced with making choices — choices between the immediate and the long range — about the kind of community we want and about the kind of life we want for the future. What concerns me is that the opportunity for having a dialogue about these choices is so slim. Communication media are area-wide, or politically or geographically oriented, and the public at large has little opportunity to learn much about the alternatives available and the consequences of each alternative. Adjusting to immediate political interests and group interests as we have always done in the past may set us in a different direction from that in which the majority would really like to go in the future if they had the choice. With new predictive tools of our technology, there is a new opportunity to make choices about the kind of society we want in the future. Certainly one leadership function we can perform is to consider and bring up for discussion the alternatives available to us as a society in terms of health.

IMPLICATIONS

This, then, is our changing world — our spaceship. We can no longer think only about our local area or our state or even the world. We have to begin to think as space citizens. This may seem overwhelmingly complex to us, but to my friend Mike it does not need to be. In the year 1984 he will be starting out to make his way, making decisions as to what kind of world he wants for his children. He will have to cope with a quite different world than we know today. If we take on the responsibility for planning for his health, what do we know today that can help him meet that world of tomorrow? Even without a detailed analysis, we know that he will have to learn to cope with ambiguity better than we have. Some of the Mikes of this new world will have to learn how to use leisure time in a more creative way; others will have to learn to pace themselves under heavy pressures of work. He will probably have to be more future-oriented and more inner-directed if he is to live comfortably with crowding and comfortably with crowding and complexity. He will need to think clearly, creatively, and rationally to cope with technology of the future. His stability cannot be dependent upon a traditional society or community, but rather it will have to come from the creative potentialities of all people and upon continual learning and change. He will need the physical and psychological foundations to learn this way of life. He will have to take much more responsibility for maintaining his own health, for understanding his own capabilities, and for developing a healthful life style.

This is a pretty large order, and even if we agreed that these things were what were needed, we do not know too well how to help him become such a person.

But how do we set the wheels in motion to at least attempt to deal with Mike's world of tomorrow? One way is to begin to spell out our goals in more comprehensive, yet explicit, terms. We are coming to recognize that health per se may not have the overriding value we have given it. James put it his way:

> There is an increased willingness to consider health not as a pure and uncontestable human good but as a generally desirable element in active competition with other human needs such as economic gain, recreation, or just plain pleasurable living.[7]

The National Center for Health Statistics provides us with some interesting conceptual problems on the development of an index of health, indicating that perhaps the best definition of morbidity is in terms of disruption of social activities.

Today much of our health education activity is focused on rather isolated health practices—stop smoking, lose weight, get your child immunized, get your Pap smear, and so on. We talk about the need for providing comprehensive care, but we certainly do not think in comprehensive total-system terms in our own health agency activities. Medicine, because of its expanding technology, has divided the patient up into organ systems. And for all the current emphasis on the whole patient, the expanding technology and knowledge almost preclude the possibility of developing this approach to medicine, unless there are major changes in the occupational structure of the health system.

Perhaps the way in which public health and public health education can make the greatest contribution is to move out of disease system orientation and take a comprehensive approach to the social world in which Mike and his friends will be living. More attention should be focused on ability than on disability, on the definition of the "good" life than on a diseaseless one. We may not agree on what we want, but let us at least begin to define what choices we have.

Our man-made spaceships are guided to their destination by locking onto a distant target star, and then the pitch and yaw are adjusted to keep a constant fix on that distant star. The condition of our spaceship earth is becoming apparent to us. We are in the space age: We must learn to use space-age concepts and look for the guiding star upon which we want to fix.

References

1. *Webster's Collegiate Dictionary*, 4th ed., Springfield, Mass.: G. & C. Merriam Co., 1931, p. 168.
2. Talcott Parsons, *The Social System*, New York: The Free Press, 1951.
3. Mary F. Arnold and Douglas L. Hink, "A Study of the Adjustment Techniques of Patients and their Families to the Nonmedical Needs Resulting from Chronic Illness," mimeographed.
4. Barbara Ward, *Spaceship Earth*, New York: Columbia University Press, 1966, p. 15.
5. Nigel Calder, *The World in 1984*, Vols. I and II, Baltimore, Md.: Penguin Books, 1965.
6. Gilbert Burke, "The Boundless Age of the Computer," *Fortune*, LXIX: 3 (March 1964), 101–103.
7. George James, "Emerging Trends in Public Health and Possible Reactions," *Public Health Reports*, 80: 7 (July 1965), 580.

~ 2 ~

A Social Systems View of Health Action

Mary F. Arnold

Over the centuries man has evolved complex ways of trying to solve the problems of illness, of accidents, of survival, and even of death. Depending upon his perception of the world around him and his place in the cosmos, as well as upon his beliefs about what causes what, hé has developed ways of attempting to protect himself from those things he believed he could control. Even in very primitive societies, elaborate ways are found by which men deal with, what we call today, the health needs of their society. Birth, death, illness, and disability are disruptive to the routine of daily living and, where man has been unable to control his environment physically or intellectually, he has provided for himself prescriptive social norms, often religiously based, to aid in reducing his uncertainties about the environment in which he lives.

In looking back to ancient times, for example, we find that the early Greek states with their hostile environment required a highly cooperative society in order to cope with needs for food, water, shelter, and protection from marauders. Consequently, their mythology and religion emphasized interpersonal relations and methods of dealing with different kinds of personalities. Human heroes were deified, and the gods were given human qualities. In contrast, the mythology that grew up around the highly centralized agricultural system of the rich Nile delta, with its periodic disastrous floods, depicted the gods as operating at whim, and emphasis was placed on problems of death rather than on those of everyday living. Thus we find that a great deal of a society's pattern of behavior is part of an integrated system of response to its physical and social environment.

A THEORETICAL OVERVIEW OF THE HEALTH SYSTEM

The Health System as a Construct

It is difficult to differentiate the "health system" from other systems of the society because health action is interrelated with all other aspects of the society: its physical environment, its religious and philosophical assumptions, its economy, and its political organization. We shall consider the health system to include all activities carried out within a society that have as an expressed purpose the maintenance of a positive biological relationship to the environment and the prevention of those disruptive behaviors the society attributes to ill health.* The notion of a health system derives from the analytic construct of a social system wherein it is assumed that there are aggregates or patterns of action connected each to the other in a nonrandom or ordered way and that from these interconnected systems of action particular social outcomes emerge.† The study of a system, whether it be a social or a transportation system, requires an analysis of the input, transactions, and output of interacting component parts.[2] In the case of the social system, or any of its subsystems, this analysis entails what is done by individuals and institutions (the actors), how these actions are interrelated, and how the outcomes affect and are affected by all parts of the total system and its environment. When we define the health system by certain consequences of social action, however, it is necessary to recognize that we are only analyzing causality relations retrospectively and the actual reality of present patterns of action may result in different social outcomes.

If it is assumed that the outcome of the general health system of any society is that society's health and illness experience, it must also

* These purposes represent partial fulfillment of two of Marion J. Levy's ten functional requirements for any society.[1]

† The arguments against this functional approach to social outcomes for the most part are that it calls upon an assumption of a static equilibrium in the system and that it is teleological. Obviously, when we define and describe a system by its consequences we are working with a teleological construct. However, when one starts with a concern for a particular social outcome such as "health," it is analytically useful to take a functional approach in order to delimit and set parameters for what data will be considered. Nor is it necessary to assume a static equilibrium when considering a social system, because in many ways the very idea of a system assumes a dynamic quality.

be recognized that the society's health and illness experience helps to shape what is done within the society in regard to "health." It is therefore necessary to review some of the factors that help to shape what is done in our society about health before setting a framework for viewing the health system.

Definitional Problems in Dealing with the Concept of Health

Concepts of wellness or of illness and disease are highly dependent upon the belief systems in the society and the meaning put on their experiences by the people of the society. Polgar suggests that in order to decide a course of action an actor must deal with both etiological notions and incidence notions; thus, what is considered to require health action is dependent upon what is observed and perceived to be a problem and upon beliefs about its causality.[3] Variations of patterns of behavior in seeking professional help for health problems among highly educated persons of the upper income group have been documented by Blackwell.[4] These variations depend upon the meaning placed on the symptoms presented and the beliefs held about what should be done about those problems of which the symptoms are indicative. In a recent study of beliefs about severity and seriousness of tuberculosis among Anglos, Latinos, and Negroes in a Florida community, it was noted that the different beliefs and attitudes reflected very closely the actual morbidity and mortality experiences of the different groups.[5]

The ways of describing or defining health differ within our society. Since the classic study *Health in Regionville*,[6] it has been demonstrated time and again that persons with different life experiences in our society act from different beliefs about the meaning of "health." Baumann has shown that the younger, more highly educated persons (including health professionals) tend to take a symptom orientation when defining health, whereas the older, less well-educated persons tended to define health in terms of an activity (or disability) orientation. Those who were least well-educated seemed to define health in terms of a feeling state rather than with a more specific orientation.[7] It would be logical to expect that those who are most knowledgeable and comfortable with Western scientific thought would think in terms of indicators of specific disease processes (symptoms), while those who are not as knowledgeable of these etiologic possibilities would be unable to identify specific symptoms. In addition, salience is an important factor in one's view of health. Disability is more salient for older people and for those with a low income and, of course, older people are more aware of a high incidence of disability in their age group. Thus etiological and incidence notions can color one's definition of health.

There is a large and growing literature on sociocultural notions about illness and its alleviation with emphasis on the differing perceptions of patients and professionals.[8] One generalization that can be made from this literature is that the definition of health needs and the demands made on the society for health action depend upon who in the society is making the judgment, and that the allocation of resources and the institutionalization of health action depend upon the beliefs and notions of what should and can be done about things perceived to be "health" problems.

The Interrelationship of Scientific Thought and Health Action

The somewhat atomistic and mechanistic approach of Western scientific thought[9] exemplified by the germ theory of disease and the mind-body dichotomy has provided the prevailing general theory about the etiology of health and illness in our society. Illness is generally assumed to occur because of a malfunction in a particular organ or organ system of the body. Of necessity, this leads to mechanistic solutions to health problems, even to the extreme of the current emphasis on organ transplants and the development of artificial organs. Although there is recognition and lip service being given to the idea of the whole man, we still tend to isolate and treat symptoms of illness on an atomistic basis. For example, the tremendous growth in number and kinds of medical specialties is based on a highly skilled application of specific technologies to solve problems of health and illness. Even our social institutions that have developed for dealing with health problems are kept quite separate from one another. The separation of mental health agencies from general public health agencies, the use of the medical model in dealing with mental retardation, and an educational model in dealing with vocational rehabilitation are cases in point.

This is not to say that the mechanistic approach of Western scientific thought has not been successful. In recent years the effects of the application of a rapidly growing scientific technology to problems of health are becoming highly visible. Communicable diseases that were killers of the very young have been controlled relatively easily in our society through specific measures applied to the water and milk supply and waste disposal and through specific immunization. Application of antisepsis techniques, immunization, and the antibacterial drugs have reduced mortalities from maternity, from the pneumonias, and from other diseases amenable to these measures.

However, there have been other social effects of these singular successes in reducing mortality. We have an accelerating population growth and an increase in the numbers of persons disabled by the degenerative diseases for which we have no simple measures of control. One of the prices of increased longevity is long-term and costly chronic illness at the end of the life-span. Heroic and costly methods of medical treatment become necessary, and this in turn affects not only the costs of medical care but also what is considered important as a research problem, what direction the training of health professionals should take, and so on. The rapid developments in medical science have provided new expectations for diagnosis and treatment of illnesses for which only supportive therapy or no therapy previously was available. This accelerated expansion of medical knowledge and technology also has led to a proliferation of medical specialties and their support services, which in turn has led to increased fragmentation of the care of the ill as well as to a perceived crisis in medical and health manpower. Thus our society's emphasis on the application of Western scientific technology to problems of health has had consequences that are now creating strains in the system, and effects can be observed in the economic, educational, political, and other systems of the society.

The Effect of Political, Economic, and Social Values on Health

Another set of values and ideas that affects the health system is related to questions about the role of government and the criteria to be used by the society for the allocation of resources. If government is seen as an instrument of community growth, the basis of decision-making will be economic; if it is seen as a provider of amenities, the allocation decisions will depend on beliefs about basic rights and privileges. On the other hand, if government is perceived as limited only to certain care-taking functions or only to arbitrate conflicting interests, then the criteria for resource allocation would be more limited. The prevailing political ideology and the structure of the government have an effect on the ways in which health services can be organized, as well as on what health actions will be assumed to be the responsibility of the public sector, the private sector, and finally the individual.

During the past several decades there has been a gradual shift in the United States in the political and social values regarding health and health services. The generally accepted norms that previously separated clearly those health functions expected to be performed through the public sector from those expected to be performed through the private sector of the society have been the subject of much political controversy, and a new philosophy seems to be emerging that values health as a basic human right rather than as a privilege to be earned. With rising expectations, due to the expanding medical and scientific technology, new demands have been placed on the health system, in terms both of service needs and demands and of the allocation of resources to provide these services. These demands are making it necessary to change past patterns of action regarding health in both the public and private sectors of the society. The dynamics of these changes additionally affect and are affected by changes in all other subsystems of the society.

A FUNCTIONAL VIEW OF THE HEALTH SYSTEM

It has been indicated that actions perceived as related to health and to what a society does about health are not only tied closely with the meaning and experiences of health and disease in the society but also are tied to the prevailing theories about etiology and to the way in which action is organized in the society and resources are allocated. If we make the assumption that the health system is that system of activities in our society that serves two needs for the society—maintenance of a positive biological relationship to the environment and prevention of disruptive behaviors attributed by the society to ill health—it becomes possible to identify the components of the health system in relation to these functions. Obviously, activities categorized as belonging to the health system will not be the only pattern of action that serves these functions and, conversely, activities classified as components of the health system will have outcomes other than health. For analytic purposes, however, it is helpful to classify those activities that have the expressed purpose of serving these two functions as components of the health system.

MAINTENANCE OF A POSITIVE BIOLOGICAL RELATIONSHIP TO THE ENVIRONMENT

In designating which activities have the express purpose of serving the function of maintaining a positive biological relationship to the environment, it is recognized that notions and beliefs about etiology and incidence color what is assumed to be health-related and what is, therefore, assigned to the health system. A good example is found in the rather ambiguous boundary between the health system and the economic system in relation to agriculture. Is food more importantly perceived as an economic commodity or as an essential biological element? It is interesting to trace the shifts in assignment of milk control in the United States from one of private concern to the public sector and then from governmental agencies primarily responsible for health (e.g., health departments) to those concerned with the economics of agriculture (departments of agriculture) as the milk-borne diseases decreased in prevalence. Thus an activity may decrease in its importance for health and increase in its importance for some other subsystem of the society. Activities considered to be part of the health system and actions considered to be outside of the health system are in a constant state of dynamic change. One way of designating a pattern of action as a component of the health system is to distinguish the value basis upon which decisions are made regarding the action. Even though a variety of values may enter into the action decision, an assumption of rationality would suggest that one has primacy. To illustrate: The handling of nuisance complaints is more often than not assigned to the health department in local communities. Although there is little scientific evidence of a specific health hazard involved, such activities are often justified by the professionals as preventive measures for accidents or as a means of delimiting rat harborage. However, if one looks at popular or folk beliefs as to etiology of disease, value in our society has been placed on relating aesthetics to health.

There are many areas for ambiguity in deciding whether or not to assign an activity to the health system. One is safety. The prevention of fire hazards, or other accidental hazards, has both life-saving and economic implications. We often find, at both the state and local levels, combinations of governmental agencies such as health and safety or health and welfare. For purposes of identifying the components of the health system, we will claim those activities, therefore, where the primary value used in decision-making is that of maintaining a favorable biological status. There is some evidence that this too may be inadequate. The World Health Organization defines health as including mental and social well-being, as well as physical well-being[10]; and although today physical, mental, and social health are still used as separate constructs, there is an eager search for a new construct that overrides these. Perhaps the current growing concern about the quality of life is the beginning of a new theory of health.

Recent efforts to make our governmental allocation of resources more rational, as in the effort to apply planning–programing–budgeting systems to governmental operations, are creating an awareness that there are times when we will find conflict even within the health system regarding which value should have primacy. Across the nation today we see dilemmas about the definition of life: for example, in the question of availability of a donor for heart transplants, the issues around abortion and contraception, and the test-tube reproduction of cellular matter. As decision techniques become more sophisticated, we are becoming aware that value choices are continually made in our allocation of resources between programs for the young and those for the older person, between life-enhancing and life-saving, and the value issue of the quality of life is rapidly becoming an explicit problem for the society.

Prevention of Disruptive Behaviors Attributed by the Society to Ill Health

In this chapter two functional requisites for the society are considered to be health-system related. As discussed above, mere biological maintenance is recognized as inadequate. But when we start to identify patterns of action that are related to the prevention of disruptive behaviors that are attributed to ill health, we are once again faced with shifting assumptions about etiology. An interesting illustration is that of mental health. In general the behavior exhibited by the mentally ill is socially disruptive behavior, either for the individual himself, for his primary group, or for the community in which he lives. Historically, the methods used to deal with this type of behavior have differed from those dealing with obvious biological illness. But as Western scientism has proceeded, the notions about etiology of mental illness have been changing. However, because of past theories of behavior, an almost separate system has developed around the treatment of behavioral disorders.

Philosophically the mind–body issue in the history of science has affected the notions about etiology of mental illness. Today we find ambiguous boundaries between what is defined as a health problem and what is defined as a problem of social deviance. Are alcoholism and drug addiction health problems or problems of criminal behavior? Another example is that of poverty. This condition is becoming an unacceptable one in our society, but we are faced with various conflicting notions about its etiology. We have known for some time that poverty and ill health are positively correlated, but varying programs of action will depend upon the assumptions about the causal relationships between poverty and health. Because of these unresolved problems of etiology of poverty we find health activities in programs such as the Head Start program of the Office of Economic Opportunity and in the Department of Housing and Urban Development's Model Cities program.

The Functional Model

It is extremely difficult to classify activities as belonging to the health system, and it is recognized that assignments always will be arbitrary. However, if we return to the two basic functions of the society served by the health system and consider what actually has to occur to fulfill these functions, given Western scientific assumptions about etiology, we find four general sets of activities that are performed:

1. Activities required to treat and care for the individual defined as ill or as potentially ill. These are the direct care services often discussed as the "laying on of hands." We shall identify these as *personal care activities*.

2. Activities directed toward the maintenance of a protective environment for living. These include control of environmental hazards, including preventable disease. These will be identified in this model as the *protective activities*.

3. Activities designed to educate and socialize individuals to norms of behavior that are believed to maintain a healthful state. These shall be identified as the *educational and promotional activities*.

4. Planning activities that are expected to create the social and institutional patterns of action that affect the total state of the health of the society or of smaller segments of the society. These shall be designated as *social policy planning activities*.

Behind these activities are the subsystems that support these functions, and provide the inputs of manpower, technology, scientific knowledge, facilities, and organizational and economic support needed. Figure 1 shows this system as a model.

If the health system is said to include these sets of activities or components, then for each of these functional elements the following questions should be asked: Who are the actors? What is their relevant organizational environment? What factors have a major effect on decisions for action within each functional sector? How are these functional sectors interrelated?

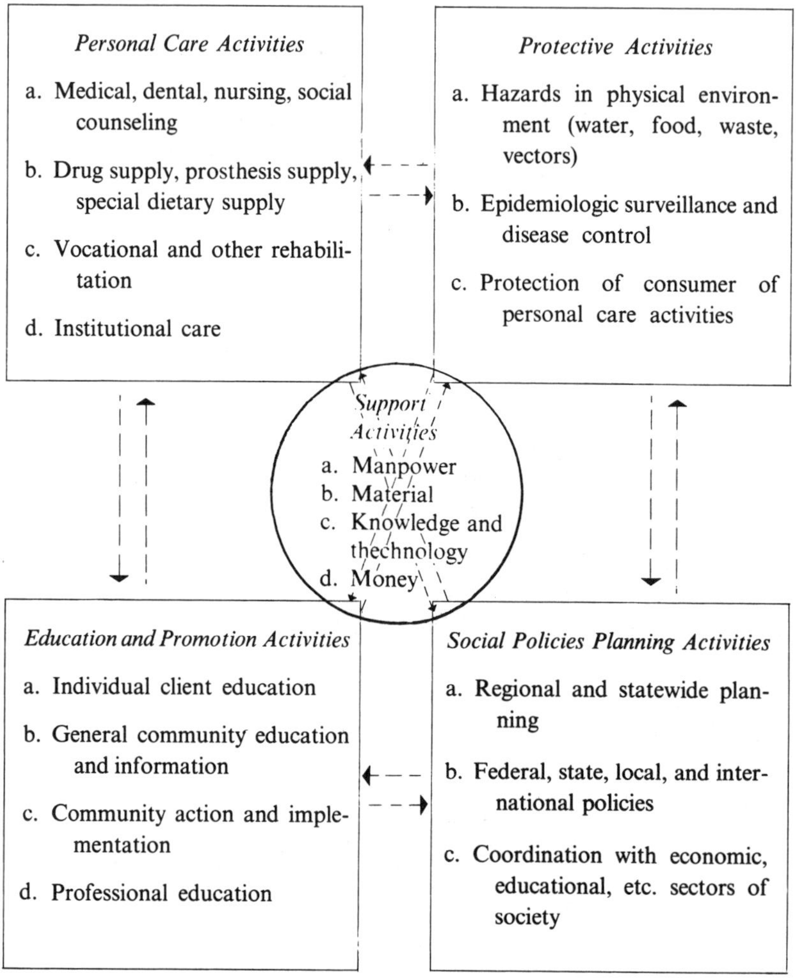

FIGURE 1. *A Functional Model of the Health System*

THE HEALTH SYSTEM IN ACTION

There are several ways of characterizing the actors in the health system: At times we may be concerned with the characteristics of those persons who actually carry out the activities performed, such as physicians, nurses, therapists, and aides; for other purposes the actors may be considered to be the institutions and organizations that have the expressed mission of providing health activities and within which the individual health actors works. Examples are hospitals, nursing homes, voluntary health agencies, and health departments.

Individuals as Actors of the Health System

There are many ways of classifying individual health actors. One is to categorize them as being professional, subprofessional, and lay or folk practitioners. In general the professional health actor can be considered to be the person from whom the client requests a health service and who is legitimized by the society as a specialist in health matters. In our society the health professional is expected to be trained in the Western scientific tradition. This training is generally beyond high-school level and is controlled by the professional peer group and the society through such mechanisms as accreditation, licensure, or registration. However, ideas about what is and what is not professional vary[11] and, although there are differences in meaning attached to the term professional, the criterion most often used to differentiate between a professional and a subprofessional is that of higher education. To further differentiate between those who are specially trained in health matters and those who are not, the term lay or folk practitioner is used.

Which activities each of these types of actors is permitted legally to perform varies in this country from state to state. In addition to the legitimation at the societal level, there is a wide variation among individuals in different segments of the society in their beliefs about who is a legitimate health professional. Among all the health actors the physician enjoys the highest status, but he also has the greatest responsibility for life and death matters for the individual. His work requires the most intimate contact with the patient when rendering personal health care, and he undergoes the longest period of training and socialization into the profession.

However, today more than 300 types of "health manpower" categories are currently recognized in the United States[12] and, as technology expands and our ways of delivering health services change, new categories are continually developing. The provision of an adequate supply of manpower to the health system is dependent upon the numbers and quality of training institutions as well as upon the economics of the health system and the role each specialist is expected to perform. If the educational system does not provide an adequate output of health manpower there is, in turn, an effect on the functioning of the health system.

The complexity of supplying health manpower can be seen in recent efforts to increase the manpower supply. One finds an upsurge in the development of new training programs in universities, colleges, and junior colleges, and service agencies are beginning to develop their own specialized training programs. One finds demonstration programs and innovations, such as the training of physician helpers, of aides of all kinds, and of the nurse-practitioner. Also, there are strong pressures for the reduction and revision of the length and character of medical education that will eventually result in changes in the sets of skills and knowledges the physician will bring to the health system. The supply of manpower can be increased by increasing the capacity of the educational system, restructuring the role functions of the various actors in the system, and organizing the work in a more efficient manner.

Thus the supply of the professional actors that enter the health system is in a continual dynamic change process. This change in input, in turn, is affected by the educational and economic values of the society as well as by the development and expansion of the scientific knowledge and technology to be applied for health purposes. The changes that occur in turn will feed back into our notions about what we define as a health problem.

Institutions as Actors in the Health System

At another level of analysis, administrative organizations and agencies can be considered as actors in the health system. Here one thinks of institutions such as hospitals, nursing homes, health departments, home health agencies, and the disease and organ voluntary health agencies. There is no simple way to classify the tremendously complex and varied organizational structure within which health action takes place. Many typologies have been suggested: One can distinguish between public and private ownership, although we find quasi-public organizations such as the Red Cross; one might classify organizations by the type of membership as being predominantly volunteer or paid; or one might distinguish between a product or a service output. Other classifications might be made by the major system of the society that is served, such as educational or political; by the general structure of the organization, such as corporate, partnership, or statutory; by the primary source of funds, such as taxes, stock, or dues; or by the primary beneficiary, such as members, owners, clients, or public at large.[13]

It is useful, however, to separate two major sectors of the society in attempting to understand the complexity of the organizational base of the health system. Figures 2 and 3 list some of the more important dimensions for classifying these organizations.

In our society certain functions may be carried out primarily by public (governmental) agencies, as one finds with the military functions,

Dimension	*Types of Categories*				
Governmental level	International	Federal	Regional	State	Local
Source of administrative power	Election	Political appointment		Civil service	
Source of legal power	Legislation	Constitution		Rules and regulations	
Fiscal (tax) base	Personal property	Personal income	Corporate income	Sales	Excise
Type of governmental function	Executive	Administrative	Legislative	Judicial	Combinations
Primary action	Funding	Regulatory	Direct service		Information

FIGURE 2. *Important Dimensions for Classifying Agencies in the Public Sector*

Dimension	*Types of Categories*				
Breadth of constituency	International	National	Regional	State	Local
Major control of administrative power	Membership	Stockholders	Partnership	Board of trustees	
Primary beneficiary	Public at large	Clients	Members		Owners
Sources of fiscal support	Gifts and Donations	Dues	Grants		Earnings and fees
Major work done by	Volunteers	Members			Paid staff
Activity output	Product				Service

FIGURE 3. *Important Dimensions for Classifying Organizations in the Private Sector*

or by other agencies, primarily through the private sector, as found with religious functions. These will differ in different societies, however. In the United States, education, for example, is primarily the responsibility of the public sector of the society, although we find competing institutions in the private sector. Until relatively recently the norms for health functions of our society were relatively clear. Personal health care services were expected to be the province of the private sector, although exceptions to this included the military, Indians, the other wards of the government, and persons with illnesses that threatened harm to others or to disrupt normal community life. Functions that required application of legal sanctions or were necessary for public safety were also assigned to government—for example, environmental control and control of communicable disease.

A recent major change in the health system is an adjustment of the norms for the roles of the private and public sectors. Since the passage of the Social Security Act in 1935 a certain amount of governmental responsibility has been taken for the poor, the aged, and the disabled. This responsibility has been extended with the passage of Titles 18 and 19 (Medicare and Medicaid) in 1965. But over the past several decades the role of the public sector has been extended in other areas: in supporting certain health functions through grants-in-aid and contracts to lower levels of government and community agencies; in the massive support given through the National Institutes of Health for biomedical research; and in the aid to training institutions and the provision of fellowship monies. It is important to note that these major changes have come primarily in the supporting environment of the health system. Changes, however, in the supporting base will result in changing organizational structures in the health system itself. The passage of the Economic Opportunity Act, of the Department of Housing and Urban Development's Model Cities program, and of Public Laws 89–749 (comprehensive health planning) and 89–239 (regional medical programs) are initiating a new departure for the federal government wherein local community action and planning are being actively supported.

Mode of Action in the Health System

After one identifies the actors in the system, the next question is: What is their general mode of action? The output of administrative organizations can be goods or services. For the most part health agencies, with the exception of those supporting industries that manufacture drugs and equipment, provide services, but these services are of a wide variety. In some cases the mode of action is the provision of a direct service to an individual, and this ranges from actually doing something to him, as in surgery, to counseling him about a problem or providing him with a specific learning situation. Another type of direct service is the actual physical treatment of some part of the environment, as in spraying for mosquitoes or the handling and disposal of wastes. These types of direct services are primary in that they require direct action on a client or a part of the environment.

A second kind of service is that of facilitating the primary actions of others through the provision of funds, as in the case of governmental grants or provision of insurance. Other facilitating services are those that provide the social milieu in which other actions can take place. Here we find community organization efforts, or coordinating efforts.

A third mode of action is that of control of the action of other actors through the setting of standards, the control of performance, and the control of access to the occupation or the administration of rules and regulations by application of legal sanctions. Sanctions may be legally applied, as through court procedures, or they may be legitimated voluntary sanctions, as one finds in the accreditation of hospitals.

A fourth type of service is that of intelligence. Although every organization requires information in order to operate, there is a general need in our society for certain kinds of information.[14, 15] The collection, compilation, and provision of information such as vital data, communicable disease intelligence, demographic data, and mortality and morbidity rates are necessary in order for both general and specialized organizations to serve their missions. A major portion of this surveillance and intelligence service, particularly where legally sanctioned, is carried on by governmental agencies; however, in many cases we find special interest groups and coordinating groups of agencies that primarily provide this kind of service. For example, a major role of most councils of social agencies is that of providing information.

Figure 4 gives examples of some of the more important agencies that are actors in the health system and suggests their relative modes of action. Levine and White have suggested that community agencies provide seven services: education, prevention, treatment, rehabilitation, resource-giving, research, and coordination.[16] This classification, however, does not take into account the broad spectrum of actions actually carried out both within and beyond the community level and, more specifically, it does not include the specific social control services nor the intelligence services rendered in the health system.

Figure 4 is only suggestive of the kinds of action typically performed. For example, some state health departments provide biologicals whereas

Type of Organization	Mode of Action				
	Product	Primary Services	Facilitating Services	Controlling Services	Intelligence
U.S. Department HEW	±	XX	XXX	XX	XXX
State health department	±	X	XXX	XXX	XXX
State mental health department	—	XXX	XXX	XXX	X
State welfare department	—	±	XXX	XX	X
Local health department	—	X	XX	XXX	XXX
Local welfare department	—	XX	XXX	XX	—
County hospital	—	XXX	X	X	±
Voluntary hospital	—	XXX	X	—	±
Private medical group	—	XXX	—	—	±
Insurance agency	—	—	XXX	X	X
Drug manufacturer	XXX	—	X	—	—

FIGURE 4. *Organizations Performing Functions in the Health System and Estimates of Their Relative Modes of Action*

others do not, and some voluntary health agencies provide primary care services while others have an explicit policy against such a service. But a tentative chart such as this indicates that the primary modes of action in the public sector are facilitating, control, and intelligence, while the major mode of action in the private sector is that of the provision of primary care services.

Interrelationships of the Functional Sectors

The society's beliefs about etiology and incidence, its values regarding the salience of health matters, and the prevailing attitudes about the roles of the public and private sectors of the society affect the distribution of resources for action among a variety of individual and institutional health actors. Furthermore, this distribution is in a continual dynamic change, and the boundaries of the health system itself are constantly shifting.

In the same manner the boundaries between the functional sectors of the health system are diffuse. If we assume by definition that health action is purposeful, then each of the functional sectors is tied to etiological assumptions about how to maintain a positive biological relationship to the environment and how to prevent disruptive behavior attributed to ill health.

There are some obvious interrelationships among these functional activities in the health system. For example, treatment of an individual suffering from a communicable disease such as tuberculosis also serves a protective function for other persons in the society, and we find specific mechanisms of information exchange and control that have developed between actors primarily concerned with primary care and those concerned with the protective function. Laboratories are required to report positive laboratory tests for certain conditions, and physicians are required to report certain diseases. In certain cases where the protective function takes precedence, personal care may be given by the legitimate agent of control such as the health department.

In some ways one can say that the personal care and the protective functions are the least random subsystems of health action while the educational and promotional and the social policy-planning functions are not as ordered systematically in our society. However, it is through these latter functional sectors that change in the health action system is facilitated. The support activities are a major part of input environment of the institutional actors within the health system, and the health system must compete with other subsystems of the society for these resources and, as such, also play a part in change of the system.

Recently there has been an interest in the role that environments play in relation to organizational systems. Emery and Trist's suggestion that the environment of organizations provides a determining condition for the interrelationships within a system has important implications for the health system.[17] There is some evidence in our society that the organizational environment is moving toward Emery and Trist's "turbulent field" "both the theoretical and case study literature on organizations suggests that these systems are increasingly finding themselves in environments where the complexity and rapidity of change in external interconnectedness gives rise to increasingly unpredictable change in their transactional interdependencies."[18]

How the organizational actors in the health system cope with the uncertainties of their transactional environment is important to an understanding of the interrelationships among the functional sectors. Thompson suggests that "organizations cope with uncertainty by creating certain parts specifically to deal with it, specializing other parts in operating under conditions of certainty or near certainty."[19] An organization is dependent upon its environment in that it needs resources to perform its mission, and the distribution and availability of such resources can increase or decrease the organization's dependence on its transactional partners. On the other hand, an organization can be said to have more or less power if it provides scarce resources on which others are dependent. Thus it is to the advantage of each organization in the system to seek a situation in which it has the maximal resource alternatives and minimal output competition. The organization must develop strategies for reducing its uncertainty regarding input resources as well as strategies for dealing with its output exchange. Thus, on an assumption of rationality it should be expected that the actors within the health system would attempt to carve out domains of action in which their resource boundaries are expanded and their output boundaries are restricted. In the area of the personal care activities there are constraints on the supply of manpower (e.g., standards of training) as well as on the distribution of money to support the care services, since the need for care is not dependent upon the ability to finance the care. Because of these and other constraints on the transactional possibilities, it would be expected that this sector would have more ordered patterns of action. The same argument holds true for the protective area, but the constraints are on the modes of action available. In the sectors of education and promotion and social planning, however, there is much more opportunity for transactional relationships with other subsystems of the society, leading to a more random pattern of action.

Just as the changes in the salience of health in relation to other social values create a fluctuating boundary for the health system, so there is a changing social emphasis on different functions in the health system. During the early part of this century the problems of epidemic communicable diseases held primacy. Once a technology was made available for the solution to these problems, primacy was placed on the protective function. As this became less of a public problem, emphasis shifted to that of promotion and education for individual action. This emphasis in turn has been displaced with a concern for the provision of care services first with the expression of need for facilities and for research and later with the establishment of financial supporting mechanisms. Then came the recognition that care services were unevenly distributed, and financial support was extended to include medical care for the aged and for certain groups on public assistance.

Today major societal concern is focused on the functional problem of providing care services, but we are seeing the strains created by the increasing specialization and differentiation of functions that are reflected in recent efforts to stimulate planning. Planning is being initiated in all areas of the health system, with an implicit expectation that uncertainty in the turbulent transactional environment of the health system will be reduced.

SUMMARY

If we think of the health system as a dynamic open subsystem of the society that serves the function of maintaining a positive biological relationship to the society's environment and preventing disruptive behaviors attributed to ill health, we also can assume that the patterns of action will reflect the society's beliefs about etiology, its definition of what constitutes a health problem, as well as the relative values that health (as defined by the society) has in relation to other concerns. Furthermore, we should be able to better understand the dynamic ways in which patterns of health action emerge and change and are allocated among the health actors of the system. It is at this point of understanding that we should be able to develop the predictive capacity to better understand the transactional relationships of the health system and estimate potential outcomes from the ways in which health action could be structured. Although the complexity and the dynamic quality of this health system model are almost beyond our total comprehension, a beginning understanding is the first step toward enhancing the rational control of social change.

References

1. Marion J. Levy, Jr., *The Structure of Society*, Princeton, N.J.: Princeton University Press, 1952, pp. 149–197.

2. For a discussion of the underlying logic of a systems approach, see C. West Churchman, *Systems Approach*, New York: Delacorte Press, 1968.
3. Steven Polgar, "Health Action in Cross-Cultural Perspective," in Howard E. Freeman, Sol Levine, and Leo G. Reeder (eds.), *Handbook of Medical Sociology*, Englewood Cliffs, N.J.: Prentice-Hall, 1963, pp. 397–419.
4. Barbara Louise Blackwell, "Upper Middle Class Adult Expectations About Entering the Sick Role for Physical and Psychiatric Dysfunctions," *Journal of Health and Social Behavior*, 8:2 (June 1967), 83–95.
5. David C. Jenkins, "Group Differences in Perception: A Study of Community Beliefs and Feelings About Tuberculosis," *American Journal of Sociology*, LXXI:4 (January 1966), 417–429.
6. Earl L. Koos, *The Health in Regionville*, New York: Columbia University Press, 1954.
7. Barbara Baumann, "Diversities in Conceptions of Health and Physical Fitness," *Journal of Health and Human Behavior*, 2:1 (Spring, 1961), 39–46.
8. See, for example, Benjamin D. Paul (ed.), *Health, Culture and Community*, New York: Russell Sage Foundation, 1955; Dorrian Apple (ed.), *Sociological Studies of Health and Sickness*, New York: Blakiston Div., McGraw-Hill, 1960; David Mechanic, *Medical Sociology*, New York: The Free Press, 1968.
9. The effects of Western scientism are discussed in Ernest Becker, *The Structure of Evil*, New York: George Braziller, 1968, and Susanne K. Langer, *Mind: An Essay on Human Feeling*, Vol. I, Baltimore: Johns Hopkins Press, 1967.
10. Constitution, World Health Organization.
11. Mary F. Arnold, "Professionalism and New Concepts of Administration," *Journal of Nursing Education*, 7:1 (January 1968), and reprinted in this book, see Chapter 3.
12. U.S. Department of Health, Education, and Welfare, Public Health Service, National Center for Health Statistics, *Health Resources Statistics*, 1965, Appendix II, pp. 171–177.
13. Peter Blau and W. Richard Scott, *Formal Organizations*, San Francisco: Chandler, 1962, pp. 40–58.
14. Harold L. Wilensky, *Organizational Intelligence*, New York: Basic Books, 1967.
15. Karl W. Deutsch, *The Nerves of Government*, New York: The Free Press, 1966.
16. Sol Levine and Paul E. White, "The Community of Health Organizations," in *Handbook of Medical Sociology*, pp. 321–347.
17. F. E. Emery and E. L. Trist, "The Causal Texture of Organizational Environments," *Human Relations*, 18:1 (February 1965), 21–31.
18. Shirley Terreberry, "The Evolution of Organizational Environments," *Administrative Science Quarterly*, 12:4 (March 1968), 590–613.
19. James D. Thompson, *Organizations in Action*, New York: McGraw-Hill, 1967, p. 13.

II

THE ACTORS IN THE HEALTH SYSTEM

THE "ACTORS" IN THE HEALTH SYSTEM ARE INDIVIDUALS whose function is, collectively, to produce health services. The chapters in this part deal with selected dimensions of these functions. A crucial problem in understanding the health system is to recognize what ties these actors together. The articles that follow focus on selected aspects of the relationship of these individuals to each other and to the body of rational knowledge on which their skills are based or to the organization in which they work and to the larger community. A common theme is emphasis on dynamic change.

The health system is not standing still, and the actors in it are being subjected to numerous and almost continuous pressure for experimentation and change. They are being challenged to justify themselves and the resources they use in the name of health and their right to call themselves professionals and to define "health." They are finding that some of the old beliefs by which they lived — that it is impossible (if not immoral) to attach economic and social values to a human life; that the doctor (or the professional) always knows best what the patient (or community) *really* needs; and that health problems can be solved by discovering a single causal agent — are decreasingly tenable. There are many sources of these pressures.

To begin, some of the basic biological assumptions and models about things like disease, life, death, and cause and effect — models that have provided the rational underpinning for our conceptions and the "practice" of health — are being altered as a result of new research and theories in both the physical and life sciences. Many of the social sciences — economics, political science, sociology, and social psychology — are beginning to come into their own in the sense that they are offering alternative models for viewing and defining health problems. The boundaries between policies relating to unemployment, poverty, medical care, education, and welfare as well as between organizations with some degree of formal responsibility for them become increasingly difficult to draw. Problems require multiorganizational, multidisciplinary attention. We have begun to realize that the states of living and nonliving systems are interrelated in a number of highly complicated and little understood ways. Consequently, more often than not the apparent "solution" to one problem — for example, developing a means of controlling one disease — leads to a host of new, unanticipated problems and attempts to solve them are not only time-consuming but usually generate still a third generation of issues to be dealt with.

Decisions which will affect individual as well as community health levels are becoming politicized and rationalized. Decisions about such things as research strategies and targets, the allocation of funds and training programs, and the distribution of facilities — decisions that were once relatively private affairs* involving more modest commitments and individual researchers, practitioners, communities, hospitals, and universities — have become the subject of attention for the national political system. This situation occurred in some instances because problems seemed beyond the political or economic capacity of local or private arrangements to handle and in others because certain groups, most recently and notably Black Americans, could only begin to get attention and satisfaction by end-running the local

* "Private" in the dual sense that it was believed that government, at least at the national level, had no "right" to be interested in them or play a significant role and that the consequences of these decisions were circumscribed — they affected very limited numbers of people.

power structure. The population as a whole has come to expect more from the federal government.

Once national responsibility for such decisions was institutionalized in the form of ever expanding budgets, programs, bureaucracies, advisory bodies, study councils, pressure groups, and the like, the process of politicization became increasingly self-generating. Change bred still further change. When more and more areas of activity are subject to some form of conscious planning and administrative control, those which remain unrationalized become intolerable anachronisms that seem to stand in the way of efficient solutions to health problems. As budgets for health as well as for other things — education, defense, welfare, the space program — get larger, each area is under additional pressure to rationalize its offerings and to justify its expenditure of limited national resources in economic terms. Activities that can be most concretely operationalized in terms of payoffs for important values will receive the greatest level of support.

The professional model which has dominated the health-related occupations is that of the medical practitioner. He was and is a private entrepreneur, a small businessman. As befits a small businessman, he was appropriately conservative in his political and economic views and individualistic in terms of his beliefs about how society should be arranged. Today this model is an anachronism. By far the largest number of "actors" in the health system are salaried employees of some bureaucracy. Even significant numbers of physicians are part of the broad white-collar strata that cuts across large organizations in every sector of society. They receive salaries rather than fees; their careers involve promotion up an administrative hierarchy rather than success (or failure) in the marketplace; their identifications are with those above them in the hierarchy rather than with their peers or those below them, yet this identification has not been very satisfactory. They think of themselves as professionals and surround themselves with the trappings of professionalism, though for many the claim to professionalism is tenuous at best. They are faced by increasingly militant, organized groups of unskilled and semiskilled service workers on whom they depend in important ways, groups which in the past were underpaid and without status or power in the health system. In some instances they are faced by an increasingly militant, organized community that is demanding a significant say in what has traditionally been their professional prerogative.

These, then, are some of the sources of pressure for change experienced by the "actors" in the health system; it is against this background that the essays in this section, dealing with their relationships with each other and with the community, must be viewed.

3

Effects of Professionalism on Health Systems

Mary F. Arnold

Our modern world, with its ever-expanding technology, its explosive population growth, and amplification of complexity is rapidly forcing us to realize the inadequacy of our organizational skills, whether at the international level or at the level of the bedside care of the patient. Recognition that there is a need for new organizational forms has come about not only because of the frustrations of our times but, more importantly, because the need is becoming explicit with the development of the systematic study of social action and social organization. New knowledge suggests new ways of examining what we do; in turn, new concepts lead us to seek additional information.

The health worker in the United States is currently in the center of some major social changes, rapid scientific and technical developments, increasing expectations and public demand for health services, and a diminishing manpower potential. Already the health field is experiencing organizational change, e.g., Medicare, and there is every likelihood that other changes will be accelerated. There are two conceptual barriers, however, that may inhibit effective adaptation to the coming changes. These barriers are (1) the strongly held beliefs about professionalism and (2) the normative assumptions about how organizations should be structured and administered.

PROFESSIONALISM

Definitions of a Profession

The term *professional* is an ambiguous one. Popularly its meaning ranges from implying the existence of a "unique body of knowledge," from which stems a particular mode of practice, to a status symbol for certain occupational groups seeking upward mobility, as may be seen, for example, in the substitution of the term "maintenance engineer" for custodian or janitor. In this country particularly, as occupational groups become self-conscious and begin to organize for mutual protection, two directions for development are open to them—unionization or professionalization. When the group begins to set standards for education, ethics, and practice and to emphasize the application of scientific knowledge in the interest of the client, the group is said to be professionalizing. Glaser defines a profession as "a cohesive and autonomous body of trained persons who perform work for the benefit of the public on the basis of applied scientific knowledge."[1]

The word "profession" stems from root words expressing the idea of being bound by a vow, as a priest is bound by vows to serve the church or as the physician is bound to serve the sick by the Hippocratic oath. Up to the present time, the literature on the professions* has emphasized the assumption that the professional provides a service to his client (an individual or an organization) and that, in providing the service, judgments are made based on the special knowledge of the professional, knowledge that can be assessed only by the professional's peers. Additionally, the professional is expected to act in behalf of his client regardless of his own self-interests. One of the functions, therefore, of the institutionalization† of the profession is to protect the unknowledgeable client from inappropriate or irresponsible action on the part of the professional. At the same time, the professional needs protection from inappropriate public demands. In every professionalizing group the problems of ethics and commitment to the needs of the client, as well as the development of mechanisms for membership control, become major issues.

Goode defines a profession as analogous to a community in that it has the following characteristics: a sense of identity; shared values and

* In particular, Parsons' discussion of the professions has been the major influence.[2]

† The formation of a professional association and the development of mechanisms for accreditation of training are typical of professionalizing groups.

common role definitions, as well as a common language; the status remains constant once it is achieved; power over its members; identifiable social limits to the action of its members; and a reproductive function that operates through recruitment, selection, and training.[3]

With our expanding scientific knowledge and the development of highly technical areas of specialization, these definitions of the professional become less useful in distinguishing between activities that might be considered professional and activities that might be considered nonprofessional. In highly technical specialized occupations the welfare of the client, or the public, is dependent upon the technical judgment and competence of the specialist. There has been a proliferation of technically specialized occupational groups whose work is based on applied scientific knowledge and whose work is vital to the public or clients' welfare. Yet, can we say these specialized occupations are professions? Is the airline pilot a professional? Is the computer programmer a professional?

Profession as a Folk Concept

In his discussion of the nature of a profession, Becker suggests that the meaning of "profession" is best used in the sense of a folk concept rather than as a definitive scientific concept and that the term calls forth, or is symbolic of, a set of ideas or beliefs which in themselves perform certain functions in society.[4] Thus, if an occupational group considers itself a professional group and if, in general, the members are expected by the public to act in a professional way, it is a profession. An occupational group, therefore, as it becomes self-conscious, attempts to form itself in a way that meets this professional image.*

Today the popular concept of a professional includes a belief in the monopolistic character of the body of knowledge that is basic to the practice of the occupation—often called the "scientific base"—and a strong belief in the uniqueness of the related set of technical skills that can be acquired only by supervised practice and experience. The belief assumes that access to the profession should be controlled by its membership and implies that the professional should be autonomous in his work situation. Thus one of the manifestations of having achieved the honored status of professional is the control of one's own work.

* There are also those who believe that only the "learned professions" can be called truly professional. These are sometimes listed as theology, law, and medicine; sometimes a fourth is added, education.

PROBLEMS OF PROFESSIONALISM

The difficulty in defining what type of work or activity is professional and what type is not leads us to some knotty problems. Is control by the professional, or occupational group itself, an adequate social control to protect the public's welfare? What acceptable alternatives are available? Traditionally, the professional–client relationship has been a unique, contractual one protected by the standards developed by the profession but, as society becomes increasingly complex and as the expanding scientific knowledge forces intensive specialization, the traditional professional–client relationship is mediated by the need for organizational coordination.

Problems in the Hospital Setting

In the health field the honor and the high status accorded the physician has served to legitimate and cement an extremely complex organization of professional and technical specialists. In the area of patient care the nurse has served as the mediator or coordinator between the individual physician and the organized services of the hospital.[5] As social and technical forces increase the complexity of health organizations, and the practice of medicine becomes more and more specialized, this legitimating force becomes increasingly unrealistic. Magraw suggests that "the hospital (with its assembly of necessary ancillary personnel and equipment) has emerged as a rival entrepreneur (to the physician) able to undertake some of the things doctors cannot do, either as individuals or as a group."[6] How, then, do we reconcile the strong values of professionalism—the idea that the profession alone is responsible for the management and control of the work of the professional—with the need to coordinate *and integrate* the rapidly increasing numbers and types of technical specialists?

In addition, how do we reconcile our old ideas of organizational coordination through a hierarchical authority structure with the obvious reality of the authority of knowledge that each professional and technical specialist brings to the organization? In a study made some time ago, the activities that elicited the greatest disagreement between three professional groups as to which group properly should carry out the activity were those for which decisions would affect the specific work of other individuals.[7] Certainly coordination and integration under these circumstances would be difficult and conducive to intraorganizational conflict.

Professionalism in the Health Department

Most health departments are organized today on a specialty basis. Subunits are specialized in terms of specific health problems such as disease control, maternal and child health, or environmental control. This structure reflects the growth of public health activities as a result of the Emerson Report of 1945, which established minimal "basic six" functions of local health units.[8] Clients receiving health services, however, are spread throughout the community. To provide a specialized public health nurse from each of these specialized units to serve clients created duplication and confusion at the point of delivery of the service. It was not unusual in the days of "specialized nursing services" to find the nurse in the tuberculosis unit, the nurse in the acute communicable disease unit, the nurse in the school health unit, and the nurse in the maternal and child health unit each serving the same family. This confusion led to a concept of the generalized family health nursing service, and the generalized service is now to be found in almost all local health departments. This shift has been justified on two premises: (1) preservation of the professional image that only a peer can evaluate or supervise the work of a professional (only nurses should manage nurses and only doctors can supervise doctors) and (2) prevention of duplication of service. This structural pattern, however, leaves much to be desired. The Director of Nursing is placed in an adjudicative position since she controls the personnel resource (nurses) for delivery of services to the client, and much programming of specialized health activities depends upon the nursing time available. In the usual organizational structure the Director of Nursing functions at the same administrative level as the Director of Maternal and Child Health, the Director of Disease Control, etc., and these positions usually are filled by physicians. Thus, in addition to having to allocate resources for her administrative peers, the nurse has the added difficult problem posed by the traditional status of the physician and the carry-over of attitudes and expectations about nurse–physician relationships from the hospital setting. It follows, therefore, that in most health departments today these built-in structural conflicts take on interprofessional connotations.

In addition to the built-in strain cited, there is an unintended consequence to this normative structural pattern. Simon has indicated that subunits of any organization develop strong subunit loyalties, norms, and goals and a tendency to compete with other subunits of the organization.[9] The mode of specialization in public health agencies has followed the orientation to specialized health problems in much the same manner as medical specialties have focused on specific biological systems. Specialized curricula in schools of public health are found in maternal and child health, in industrial health, in school health, in chronic diseases, in nutrition, in health education, and in many other areas. The way in which these specialties have developed, and the specialized training provided, further reinforce the separate specialized structure pattern found in most health departments. From the administrative standpoint, the structure by specialty tends to subvert the over-all goals or output of the organization to the enhancement of the professional or specialized group. This reinforcing cycle of structure patterning the specialization, and the specialization in turn reinforcing the structure, enhances the stereotyping of professional roles and the expectations and interprofessional conflict.*

CHANGING CONCEPTS OF ADMINISTRATION

It has been noted that ideas around professionalism lead to difficulties in the organizational setting. Solutions for these problems lie not so much in the area of professionalism as in the kinds of ideas one has about what constitutes "proper" organization. The study of the administrative organization has been eclectic, and concepts from sociology, political science, psychology, economics, and mathematics have been interchanged in the process. Such study is characterized by the lack of a common theory, but this eclecticism has provided a rich source of data and concepts for adding to our understanding of organizational behavior. During the past several decades certain identifiable themes or conceptual modes have patterned the development of our organizational skills.

The Structural Approach

The modern approach to administrative organization started with a focus on how work should be divided and how this division of labor could be made more rational. The bureaucratic model of Max Weber,[11] the scientific management approaches of Gulick and Urwick,[12] the so-called "principles of administration" of Mooney and Reiley,[13] and the human engineering model of Frederick Taylor[14] all emphasized

* To some extent this follows the pattern described by Selznick,[10] although in this case, the struggle for professional status adds an important dimension.

structural rationality. The underlying assumption was that all tasks could be separated into discrete parts and that job functions could be delineated by clear-cut boundaries between positions. These separate tasks were to be coordinated through a hierarchical structure of authority. The superior in the scalar hierarchy had authority over the subordinate, but in a legitimate sense by reason of position rather than because of personal qualities. Thus the smooth functioning of the organization was dependent upon how well the jobs were defined to prevent overlapping of function, and coordination was effected through the authority of the superior. This mechanistic model with historical antecedents from an era prior to the industrial revolution has acquired a normative value in our society.

The Process Approach

As the scientific management model was gaining popular acceptance, we began to learn, through works such as those of Mary Parker Follett[15] and the Hawthorne studies,[16, 17] that the social process within an organization must be taken into account. In the literature on organization, references to the informal structure as separate from the formal structure became popular. A great rash of studies on social process appeared, and concepts such as human relations, participative management, and interpersonal communications became popular. On the basis of some very broad generalizations from a few studies, we centered our attention on the problems of motivation. Underlying most of this emphasis on motivation was the assumption that there is conflict between the individual and the organization, and the social process movement remained an attempt to fit people into a mechanistic structure. For example, Likert's linking-pin model[18] still assumes that work must be functionally divided into discrete units. Many writers who emphasize social process assume that the needs of the individual should have primacy over the needs of the organization.* The problem of reconciling the structural orientation and the social process orientation has been difficult and has not been solved.

The Decision-Making Approach

Simon, in focusing on the administrative process as a decision-making process, opened a new way of looking at the organization.[20]

* Chris Argyris probably represented the extreme in this point of view, although his current work does not take such an extreme position.[19]

On the assumption first suggested by Barnard[21] that one could look at the organization as a cooperative system, Simon developed the concept of the "principle of bounded rationality" and outlined different kinds of objective rationality, arguing *that the central core of administration* was the decision-making process. The literature on organizational decision-making is extensive, but the major issues evolved around the economic model of rationality, with arguments about whether it is an effective model in considering organizational behavior. Braybrooke and Lindblom's "disjointed incrementalism,"[22] Simon's "satisficing" model,[23] and Cyert and March's behavioral theory of the firm[24] are examples of decision models that are suggested as adaptations or substitutions for the rational economic model.

The Systems Approach

In the late 1940's some new concepts began to emerge from mathematics, physics, and engineering and generated new ways of thinking about the administrative organization. Cybernetics, information theory, mathematical decision-making, and particularly the idea of systems brought two completely new conceptual orientations to the world of management. During World War II teams of scientists, in attempting to solve certain operational problems, began to look at these problems as created by a system of interacting variables rather than discrete causative relationships. The techniques of "operations research," or the systems approach, are based on the underlying assumption that the whole consists of interacting systems that are in dynamic equilibrium. An organization is therefore a dynamic system, and rationality is focused on the process of *guiding* the organizational output. With these conceptual developments of system, of feedback, and of control, the individual is incorporated as a dynamic subsystem in the organization or, depending on the problem or subsystem under study, the individual might be viewed as a decision-maker, as an information-processing unit, as a constraint, etc. Most important, this new dynamic model focuses attention on the output of the system rather than on a rational structure or a social process. We are no longer tied to an attempt to reconcile the inconsistencies of the old, so-called "principles of administration" with conflicting theories of individual needs.

The change in conceptual orientation does not eliminate the problem of administrative integration, coordination, and control. It does, however, open the way for learning a great deal about organizational behavior and for finding new and more effective organizational forms. With the focus of attention on output, we can become less dependent on prescribed structures and on the definition of prescribed work roles and functions. However, such a change in conceptual orientation to concern with output should profoundly affect our assumptions and ideas about the functions and roles of the professions, especially in the situations in which the professional is a member of an administrative organization.

We are currently in a transition period. The characteristic beliefs about professionalism emphasize the differences between professions, divisiveness in organizational structure, and autonomy in the form of peer-sanctioned activity on the part of the professional. However, while our concepts about administration are shifting away from ideas about discrete roles and positions to a new focus on dynamic interchange within a system, our beliefs about professionalism are still focused on ideas of discrete bodies of knowledge and boundaries separating the professions. Actually, these beliefs are much more compatible with the structural approach to administration than with the systems approach. The systems approach requires a focus on the output, the benefit, or service to be derived from the professional's activity in concert with others rather than a focus on the professional's discrete or unique contribution.

SOLUTIONS TO THE DILEMMA

It would seem there are at least two ways to make the coming functional and organizational changes less traumatic. One way is to provide transitional structures that give persons in the organization an opportunity to experience different patterns of organization. Another way is through educational and socialization experiences for young people coming into the professions.

Organizational Solutions

With the recent legislation requiring a focus on planning in the health field* there is an opportunity to experiment with a variety of

* Public Law 89–794 ("comprehensive health planning") and Public Law 89–239 ("regional medical programs") require and provide funding for planning at the regional, state, and areawide levels.

structural innovations. For example, the use of task forces with flexible structures organized around problem-solving rather than around specific kinds of activities. Variations of team nursing might be developed. There is some evidence, from certain innovative patterns that have been developing,* that new specialties within the professions might be going through an evolutionary process. The formation of new types of organizations permits innovation since old patterns of work are not present. For example, the rapid development of home health services and the use of the aide lend themselves to innovative organizational structures without completely disrupting strongly held current patterns of work.

Educational Solutions

We are experiencing, during this period of rapid proliferation of technical specialization, a blurring of boundaries between specialized bodies of knowledge. What differentiates the "unique body of knowledge" of each profession is, in reality, a particular mix of knowledge and skill, and along with this comes a sense of group identification that provides a unique perceptual orientation to the world. One point of attack, therefore, is in professional education where the individual is socialized into his profession. Emphasis on the contribution the particular professional practice makes to the *organized* attainment of certain social goals should, hopefully, focus more attention on the social goals rather than on particular means.

Additionally, increasing emphasis could be placed on commonalities among professional groups rather than continuing the current emphasis on differences. For example, the study of theories and concepts of social change is not unique to nursing, to social work, to psychiatry, or to health education. If educators for the professions would diligently explore and experiment with ways of integrating the different commonalities among professional groups and include the more specific focus on the particular professional practice in a different setting, these attempts at least would call the attention of the neophyte to the need for integration. One innovation in professional education is that of joint curricula. This is rarely found in professional schools, but mechanisms should be developed for providing all with the common concepts and yet allow for individual professional integration.

* The use of electronic data processing in hospital communications, the development of the multipurpose worker, and the nurse-practitioner demonstration in Colorado are all innovative structural patterns for organized health services.

These solutions do not require world-shaking changes, nor may they lead to a great deal of change. Essentially, to adapt effectively to the changes of the near future, health professionals will have to (1) reduce their dependence on organizational structure to maintain their professionalism and (2) begin to accept the idea that the hallmark of professionalism will be a commitment to broad social goals and not to a "unique body of knowledge."

References

1. William A. Glaser, "Nursing Leadership and Policy: Some Cross-national Comparisons" in Fred Davis (ed.), *The Nursing Profession: Five Sociological Essays*, New York; John Wiley, 1966, p. 7.
2. Talcott Parsons, "The Professions and Social Structure," *Social Forces*, 17 (1939), 457.
3. William J. Goode, "Community Within a Community: The Professions," *American Sociological Review*, 22 (1957), 178.
4. Howard S. Becker, "The Nature of a Profession," in Nelson B. Henry (ed.), *Education for the Professions*, The Sixty-First Yearbook of the National Society for the Study of Education, Chicago: University of Chicago Press, 1962, pp. 27–46.
5. H. O. Mauksch, "The Organizational Context of Nursing Practice," in Fred Davis (ed.), *The Nursing Profession: Five Sociological Essays*, New York: John Wiley, 1966, pp. 109–137.
6. Richard M. Magraw, *Ferment in Medicine*, Philadelphia: W. B. Saunders, 1966, p. 106.
7. Mary F. Arnold, "Perception of Professional Role Activities in the Local Health Department," *Public Health Reports*, 77 (1962), 1.
8. Haven Emerson, *Local Health Units for the Nation*, New York: Commonwealth Fund, 1945.
9. James G. March and Herbert A. Simon, *Organizations,* New York: John Wiley, 1958, pp. 112–139.
10. Philip Selznick, *TVA and the Grass Roots*, Berkeley: University of California Press, 1949.
11. Max Weber, *The Theory of Social and Economic Organization*, New York: The Free Press, 1957.
12. Luther H. Gulick and L. Urwick (eds.), *Papers on the Science of Administration*, New York: Institute of Public Administration, 1937.

13. J. D. Mooney and A. C. Reiley, *The Principles of Organization*, New York: Harper & Row, 1939.
14. Frederick W. Taylor, *Scientific Management*, New York, Harper & Row, 1947.
15. H. C. Metcalf and L. Urwick (eds.), *Dynamic Administration: The Collected Papers of Mary Parker Follett*, New York, Harper & Row, 1939.
16. Elton Mayo, *The Human Problems of an Industrial Civilization*, New York: Macmillan, 1933.
17. F. J. Roethlisberger and W. J. Dickson, *Management and the Worker*, Cambridge: Harvard University Press, 1939.
18. Rensis Likert, *New Patterns of Management*, New York: McGraw-Hill, 1961.
19. Chris Argyris, *Personality and Organization*, New York, Harper & Row, 1957.
20. Herbert A. Simon, *Administrative Behavior*, New York, Macmillan, 1947.
21. Chester I. Barnard, *The Functions of the Executive*, Cambridge: Harvard University Press, 1938.
22. David Braybrooke and Charles E. Lindblom, *A Strategy of Decision*, New York: The Free Press, 1963.
23. Herbert A. Simon, *Models of Men*, New York, John Wiley, 1957, pp. 241–260.
24. Richard M. Cyert and James G. March, *A Behavioral Theory of the Firm*, Englewood Cliffs, N.J.: Prentice-Hall, 1963.

~ 4 ~

The Hospital Administrator's Emerging Professional Role

Rodney F. White

Like many other aspects of modern society, the character of administration in hospitals has become significantly altered in the period following World War II. This shift is related to changes in medical technology, the increasing demand for health services, and other social factors. The aspect of the administrative process most affected is the role of the hospital administrator. The changing nature of this role is making new demands on the present occupants of administrative posts, and this in turn is reflected in changes that are occurring in the recruitment and training of people to fill these positions. In addition, the nature of the role as it exists in the field today can be expected to be importantly different again in five or ten years because of further changes in the larger medical care system.

When one examines the ways in which the role of the hospital administrator has been changing, two separate but overlapping developments can be discerned. The first is the emergence and expansion of the administrator's executive function as the hospital has grown in size and complexity. This function must be distinguished from the medical supervision and control functions performed by members of the clinical organization. In fact it is the growth of the former that has produced and then accentuated the increasingly familiar dual authority pattern that now characterizes hospital and other medical care administration.[1]

The other and more recent development is that of hospital administration away from a narrowly institutional focus toward a concern with providing a range of medical care services to the community as a whole. This latter has resulted from the changing function of the hospital from that of basically providing doctors' workshops to that of serving as health care centers for a region.

The fact that neither of these developments has been completed is evidenced in current controversies about the proper role and preparation of hospital administrators and in some of the ongoing debates as to whether hospital administration is a profession. As a consequence, there is a growing amount of research and study which is seeking to assess the current state of the occupation, and professional associations in the field are actively organizing programs aimed at its over-all advancement.

The purpose of this chapter is to sketch the evolution of the hospital administrator's role up to the present, to describe what it is like currently, and to indicate some of the further directions it may take. In doing this the changing relationship between the different groups responsible for the administration of the hospital are examined, and a number of the more crucial factors influencing the changes in these relationships are noted. Finally, suggestions are made regarding the import of these developments for the general administration of hospitals.

AN HISTORICAL OVERVIEW

As hospitals in Western society, in response to changing social conditions, have changed their function from almshouses to community medical care centers, the job of administering them has grown in importance and complexity. To understand the changing nature of the hospital administrator's role, one first must look at how hospitals as institutions have altered and then examine the changing division of labor among the four groups which share the major burden of administering the hospital — the board, the administrative staff, the medical staff, and the nursing staff.

Before attempting to generalize about these relationships, two points should be made. First, there are important variations in American hospitals, depending on their size, ownership, services, and average length of patient stay. Although there are trends toward the consolidation of institutions and the integration of different medical services within a single institution, there are still significant differences in the ways in which these different types of hospitals are organized and administered. Second, the relationships between the four occupational groups mentioned above are extremely complex, and so generalizations about these relationships at any point in time necessarily must be an oversimplification of the situation in a particular hospital.

For the purpose of analyzing changes in the administration of hospitals it is useful to consider three broad phases of their institutional development, all of which continue to be reflected in the current situation:[2] an early phase in which the hospital was largely a refuge for the sick poor and served more social than medical functions; a more modern phase when the developments in medical science and technology converted the hospital into a medical workshop to serve the sick of all classes and care became subordinated to cure; and finally a phase still in its developmental stages in which the hospital is extending its concern over the full spectrum of health services from prevention to rehabilitation and is taking as its target the medical care of the population as a whole.

Using a relatively simple analytical framework, one can focus on three major activities involved in the administrative process as it operates in a hospital and examine which groups performed these activities in the past and which ones do now. These activities are making hospital policy, coordinating the treatment and care of the patient, and evaluating the performance of the institution from the standpoint of both effectiveness and efficiency.

Starting with policy-making, which is an extremely complex process, it currently involves all four groups in different degrees depending on the nature of the hospital.[3] In the early phase of hospital development, to the extent that it was consciously performed by anyone, it probably emanated from the board or its equivalent, with religious and secular authorities influencing the outcome. As progress in medical science and technology permitted the hospital to concern itself more with providing medical care, the hospital tended to become more physician-dominated, and policy-making was done largely by key members of the medical staff working through the board and administration. Finally, as hospitals have grown in complexity and their operations have involved more and more relationships with government and other institutions outside the hospital, policy-making and particularly long-range planning have become more political and administrative in character, and the policy process is demanding an increasing involvement of the administrative staff.

Moving now to the coordination of the treatment of patients, it is clear that this was hardly needed at all in the first phase, since hospitals served largely as places where people went to die and the doctor's contribution to the patient was more supportive than medically therapeutic. With the growth and continuing development of medical science that led to the second phase, the doctor's role in the hospital became more and more important and the other groups combined their talents and resources to provide the medical staff with a place to work and care for their patients. Thus the medical staff was the coordinator of treatment and the administrator focused his attention on the business side of the institution. In the current phase, however, medicine has become increasingly specialized, and a number of other occupations are contributing to the treatment of the patient. Thus the task of coordinating the various services the patient receives has shifted increasingly to the hospital administrator. Also, as a number of the medical specialties are requiring more complex and more costly equipment, the doctors in these specialties are becoming increasingly dependent on the hospital for the provision and maintenance of this machinery. These and other trends, particularly in the large hospitals and medical centers, have accentuated the need for a central executive function to be performed and have involved the administrator more and more in the provision of medical care.

As regards the coordination of the care of the patient, the group which has always been responsible for both the continuing administration and provision of care is the nursing staff. Of course the character of nursing has improved markedly from one phase to another, and the knowledge and sophistication they have brought to the task of caring for the patient has increased significantly over the period under consideration and continues to rise. In the first phase they were virtually on their own, but when doctor's role in the treatment area increased during the second phase, he became the authority over the medically determined aspects of patient care. However, the nursing staff, by virtue of being the one group in direct contact with the patient 24 hours a day, remained the effective administrators of the patient-care unit.[4] During both these phases the board and administration were mainly concerned with the business side of the organization and had little to do with patient care as such. In the third phase the doctor's role remains much the same except that any one doctor often shares his authority with other doctors. The major change has been in greater concern with patient care on the part of the administrator, whose increased responsibilities in personnel management, purchasing, building design, and other areas have taken him into almost every corner of the hospital. While relatively fewer directors of nursing in America were in the position of virtually running their hospitals in the way that the matron in Britain did, the growing complexity of hospital administration has meant that nursing has relinquished some management functions to the administrative staff. In fact, as hospitals continue to introduce innovations such as computer scheduling, hospital information systems, and ward clerks, the nurse's role is likely to become even more clinical and less administrative in the future.

Finally, in the area of evaluating the performance of the institution, the administrator's role is again taking on important new dimensions. This aspect of administration was hardly even a consideration in earlier times, when hospitals provided care on a rather random basis. Although a few nursing pioneers like Florence Nightingale were concerned with improving the design and operation of hospitals, they were very much in the minority. At a later period, when voluntary hospitals were financed largely through charitable contributions and wealthy board members made substantial gifts to the hospital, the administrator functioned largely as a bookkeeper or business manager and financial decisions were made at the board level, with relatively little attention being given to efficiency. The evaluation of effectiveness was the province of the medical staff, and it based its determinations on the level of care provided to the patients.

Now the situation has changed again, and a large part of even the voluntary hospital's support is derived from so-called "third parties." This development in combination with the rapidly rising costs of hospital care and the resulting outside pressures for controlling these costs has encouraged the administrator to develop programs of cost analysis, budgeting, work study, job analysis, and various other approaches that have been used for some time in industry, and these have expanded his role considerably. In addition, as the goal of the hospital shifts to providing medical care programs to meet the health needs of the community, its effectiveness must be assessed in the broadest terms, with the board, medical staff, and administrative staff all participating. In fact, as national and regional planning for health services continues to expand, more evaluation of hospitals is likely to be made at these higher levels and communicated to the hospital through the administration.

THE ADMINISTRATOR'S PRESENT ROLE

The major result of the historical trends outlined above has been the expansion and increasing professionalization of the hospital administrator's role. The current situation has produced a growing demand for professionally trained administrators in at least the larger hospitals—individuals who can play a full-time executive role in an organization characterized by a pattern of "dual authority." This is a difficult role to perform because it calls for sensitivity to the needs of both the medical staff and the community, as mediated by the board, and the maintenance of what has been aptly described as a "negotiated order."[5] This role is continuing to change so rapidly that this author's description of it a few years back already is somewhat out of date.[6] However, it is by no means unique, since administration in a hospital has many parallels to that in a university, and administration in other organizations is rapidly moving in the professional direction.[7]

In the health field in general, demographic changes and rising expectations have led to greatly increased demands for medical care services and pressure for more and better hospitals. As a consequence there has been increased activity in the field of health planning at federal and state governmental levels and a rapid growth of organizations concerned with hospital and medical care planning at regional and local levels. These developments, with their resulting pressures for more coordination and cooperation between medical care organizations, coupled with the increased dependence of hospitals on financing from "third parties" have forced a greater looking outward on the part of hospital administration. In response to this need for an expanded orientation some larger hospitals have appointed "outside men" to their administrative staffs to deal with these "extra hospital" concerns—or at least have increased the size of their existing administrative staff in recognition of the fact that these outside activities would demand an increasing amount of time.

These additional responsibilities have meant a larger part of the average administrator's time is taken up with filling out forms, making reports, and generally dealing with the demands of outside organizations. Also, it usually has resulted in greater participation of hospital staff in meetings outside the hospital and brought increased pressures to keep up to date with changes in the total health field through reading and visits outside the hospital. Finally, the pressure for coordination of their activities with other medical care agencies and the rising costs of hospitalization have led a number of hospitals to experiment with less costly methods of care such as hospital-affiliated nursing homes, home care programs, and increased ambulatory care facilities. All of these developments have tended to shift the administrator's attention more out into the community and stimulate him to a broader consideration of medical care problems.

Another change in hospital administration is one which it shares with other complex organizations. This is the growth in size of the administrative establishment, particularly in the large institutions. For example, some hospitals have promoted their administrators to the position of executive director or president and appointed vice presidents or associate directors below them. Others have brought in assistant administrators, administrative assistants, and other junior staff to take over the burgeoning administrative duties in the institution. This latter has the additional advantages of enabling hospitals to bring in younger men with professional education and train them for higher posts in the organization. With the growth in administrative personnel some hospitals have decided that there is a need for a division of function within the administrative staff and have created separate administrative posts reporting to the director with responsibility for broad areas such as management of operations, financial control, and long-range planning, in a pattern similar to that found in industry. All this means that there are, in fact, a growing number of different roles within hospital administration with differing activities and levels of responsibility.

Internally the hospital administrator's role is encompassing a growing level of expertise in a variety of areas. Since most hospitals are faced with rising costs, shortages of professional staff, increasing obsolescence of personnel and equipment, and pressures for expansion of plant, the administrator is expected to be a semiexpert in industrial engineering, personnel management, cost control, and hospital design or at least be able to make effective use of outside experts in these fields to solve his current problems. Although some larger hospitals are beginning to establish separate departments in personnel, data processing, and industrial engineering, many others are looking to their new administrative personnel to double up in several of these developing fields.

As expansion and renovation of hospital plants is becoming a normal occurrence, members of the administrative staff of many hospitals are being assigned the full-time job of planning and supervising new construction projects. In fact, some administrators who have become expert in this relatively new role in one hospital will move from it to another as the first hospital's expansion is completed and another is waiting to begin.

Finally, the political nature of the administrator's role has expanded in several respects. For example, as his status and importance in the hospital has increased, he inevitably is in greater danger of conflict with either the medical staff or the board, particularly in areas where the decisions of these latter groups were previously unchallenged.[8] To avoid direct confrontations he must be able to convince the medical staff that the administration shares their objective of an increasingly high level of medical care to each patient while making the board aware of his concern for the needs of the community in general. If he is successful he may avoid direct clashes unless a major principle is at stake and he cannot reach agreement without one.

Similarly, as greater shortages of personnel have developed and unions have become more active in hospitals, the administrator is often in the position of trying to balance the needs of the patients against those of the staff without sacrificing either. Also, as the number of different occupations and professional groups in the hospital continues to increase with each one having its own special needs and problems and many having subdivisions within them, he is faced with discovering some effective combination of "programed" and "non-programed" coordination if he is to steer the organization toward a common set of goals.[9] Finally, as outside constraints on the hospital's activities grow in number and strength he has the problem of reconciling the needs and objectives of his organization with those of the larger community. All these developments call for a political astuteness not demanded of most earlier administrators.

In summary, the role of the hospital administrator is continuing to change fairly rapidly and has grown in complexity and challenge. The type of position he fills is becoming better known, and the occupation is rising in prestige. People already in the field are increasingly well paid and are generally satisfied with their career possibilities.[10] The occupation is becoming more professionalized, and there are efforts on the part of the professional associations and educational programs in the field to upgrade it further. For example, both the American College of Hospital Administrators and the Association of University Programs in Hospital Administration have expanded their educational programs recently in recognition of the development of needs of the modern administrator, and a committee on program for the American Hospital Association has recommended changes in that organization.[11] However, it has not yet attained the status of a profession in the estimate of a number of observers and may never do so, since administration is essentially a generalist function and probably will continue to attract persons with a wide range of educational preparation and experience.[12]

CHANGES IN PREPARATION FOR ADMINISTRATION

Given the changes discussed above, both in the hospital as an institution and in the role of the administrator, it is not surprising that the ways in which administrators are being prepared for their jobs are undergoing significant changes. The major shift in method of preparation has been from something approaching apprenticeship to the development of formal training programs in hospital administration as such. Although there were moves in this latter direction in the twenties in this country and the first university-based program was established in the midthirties, the move to postgraduate programs in hospital administration is largely a post-World War II phenomenon. It is interesting to note that this trend has recently been evident in Europe with formal programs being set up in Britain during the fifties and later being developed in Belgium and other countries in western Europe.[13] In fact, there is now an association of western European programs in hospital administration, which was formed at a recent international conference and resembles the AUPHA in this country.

It is important to realize that these changes in methods of preparation that have come about largely in response to the changing roles in the field are themselves contributing to further changes in these roles. Professionally trained administrators have risen to positions of influence in hospitals and elsewhere and are making a significant impact on the institutions in which they are employed and on the health field in general. There is a trend toward boards of trustees giving preference to program graduates in filling their administrative vacancies, particularly in the larger hospitals. In addition, the growth of programs in the field has affected the development of the professional associations, and these in turn are increasing their efforts to upgrade the profession.

Another indication of change is that the original format in the training programs with its one year on campus and a second one out in a residency has now become a two-year academic program in a number of cases, and lately an increasing number of doctoral programs are being established to train planners, researchers, and teachers in this expanding area. All of these highly trained people entering the hospitals, regional organizations, and governmental posts cannot fail to influence both the expectations others have of administrators and the developing patterns of behavior in the field.

The actual content of the graduate programs in hospital administration again reflects the changing role of the hospital administrator as outlined previously. The length of the program, the subjects covered, and the over-all emphasis all vary between schools—particularly depending on the part of the university in which they are located—but all programs aim at providing their students with both an advanced training in administration and a broad understanding of the field of health and medical care. There are differences of opinion among the programs regarding the desirable length and positioning of the residency period, but there has been general agreement on the need to increase both the academic content of the courses in areas like economics and the behavioral sciences and to include more instruction in the new techniques of general management such as accounting, quantitative analysis, and operations research.[14]

Another change in the content of educational programs also reflects the direction in which the health field is going. This is the increased emphasis on planning in the curricula of many schools and, in some cases, the development of programs to prepare people for positions in health planning. These changes have come about in recognition of the demands that recent legislation such as P.L. 89–749 is placing on administration at various levels in the medical care system.[15]

Surveys of people currently in the field have indicated a general recognition of the need for more advanced training if administrators are expected to handle the increasingly complex problems of the modern hospital. This need is partly being met by the offering of more extramural courses by universities and by the revised program of regional educational assemblies conducted by the ACHA. In addition, regional extension centers have been established to provide training in administration and other fields to a variety of occupational groups within the hospital who feel the need to supplement their original preparation.

It is also interesting to examine the changing educational background of people now entering the field of hospital administration. On the one hand there is an increasing number of persons with specialized training in hospital administration and on the other a decreasing number with medical and nursing backgrounds. Not only is this the trend historically, but the majority of administrators now in the field appear to favor this change. For example, the results of a recent survey of top administrators conducted by the writer and a number of colleagues indicated that a majority of those questioned would prefer that their successors be graduates of a program in hospital administration; only a minority would prefer someone trained in either medicine or nursing. This is not to suggest that they believe administrators should not be knowledgeable about medicine and medical care, since most programs in hospital administration include courses of orientation to public health or clinical medicine or both. However, it does indicate general acceptance of the position that clinical training is not a necessary preparation for the administration of hospitals and that advanced training in management is highly desirable.

IMPACT ON THE ADMINISTRATION OF THE HOSPITAL

The previously noted changes in the hospital as an institution and the associated changes in the role of the administrator have had important effects on the organization and administration of the hospital. One of the major effects has been the greater institutionalization of the hospital and the resulting increased power of the administrator vis-à-vis the medical staff.[16] This should not be interpreted to mean that the dual authority pattern in the hospital is disappearing nor that the administrator is moving into a position where he will be directing the activities of the medical staff. It does mean that as the hospital has grown in size and complexity and as medical technology has advanced, procedures in the hospital are becoming more regularized and systems of monitoring and control developed to the point where operating the hospital as an administrative system is becoming an increasingly important task.

The growing responsibility of the administration for the performance of the hospital has been highlighted by recent court decisions that have held the hospital liable for the quality of care it provides to patients. The board has always been the ultimate authority in the hospital from a legal standpoint, but the medical staff has been considered as bearing the major responsibility for the quality of care rendered. Now that the patients are being treated by a wide range of medical and ancilliary specialists and many hospitals are providing emergency as well as regular care on a 24-hour-a-day basis, the adequate equipping and staffing of the hospital and the coordination of the services provided play an increasingly important part in determining the quality of care that the patient receives. The responsibility for the above functions is as much administrative as clinical, and until most hospitals are employing full-time medical staff the majority of this burden will fall on the nursing and administrative personnel.

Other developments in the medical care field are making for more involvement of the administrator in the patient care side of the hospital. The fact that accreditation or nonaccreditation by the Joint Commission may be used by third parties, including government agencies, to determine the eligibility of the hospital for payment and that it also may be an important factor in attracting or discouraging the applications of new staff has meant that the administration gets heavily involved in the accreditation procedure and in doing what they can to ensure that the hospital receives a good rating. This not only stimulates the administrator to keep a constant watch for failure in the hospital that might prejudice its case for accreditation, but it can give him an effective weapon to use in convincing the medical staff to improve their committee system, raise the completion rate on medical records, or otherwise upgrade medical procedures in the hospital.

In addition to its involvement in the accreditation process, the hospital may be a participant in a program like the Professional Activities Study, which provides them with a statistical analysis of their medical records plus comparative data from other hospitals. The administration then may use this to compare their hospital's performance with that of other similar institutions. Again this does not allow the administrator to control the medical staff, but it does enable them to raise questions that may spur the doctors to closer self-examination and improve the quality of care given in the hospital.

As hospitals extend their activities into the community they require a much broader base of knowledge for the purposes of decision-making and policy formulation. Also, as the trend toward greater regionalization of health facilities continues, there is growing pressure for a more community-wide orientation. Hospitals have been obliged to develop more extensive information systems in order to keep themselves up to date with developments at regional and national levels and to provide them with comparative data that allows them to compare their performance with other institutions in the same region. Some hospitals have conducted studies to analyze the demographic changes in their service areas so as to plan their expansion of services in a way that will best meet the changing health needs of their community. In most cases hospitals are making more use of the services available to them at regional councils and hospital associations, and administrators are in the habit of employing the services of consultants in a wide variety of fields, from fund-raising to food services.

With hospital costs continuing to rise, particularly in the wake of recent successes in bargaining by both unions and professional associations, administrators are under pressure to raise the efficiency and productivity of the hospital. Internally, the growth in size and complexity of hospital organizations has stimulated the development of better costing and budgeting procedures and there is a trend toward the installation of more data processing and computing machinery to speed up office procedures and record-keeping.

With the need for better budgetary controls and a belief in the desirability of greater decentralization of operating decisions, some hospitals are moving in the direction of what Peter Drucker and others have referred to as "management by objectives."[17] Through the use of a system whereby department heads make proposals regarding their own programs, which are related to objectives that they themselves have helped to establish, and later receive periodic feedback on their progress, these institutions can both improve the administrative ability of their staff members and increase the confidence of their boards in the efficiency and effectiveness of the management of the hospital.

Finally, with the pressures on hospitals continually to extend their plants and expand the range of services they provide to the community, the role of the board in the voluntary hospitals has tended to grow in importance. Their focus of attention is moving away from an almost exclusive concern with financial matters, and they are developing greater interests in both internal operations and the relationships of the hospital to the surrounding community. As health care and its rising costs continue to be in the spotlight of national concern, trustees are becoming increasingly aware of the broader public responsibilities of hospitals and the need for greater cooperation with other health agencies through some form of comprehensive health planning. Also, as the hospital has become more complex and the problems of operating it grow more difficult, the board must depend to a greater extent on the professional guidance of the administrator. However, depending in large part on the strength of the board chairman and the relative sophistication of the administrator, boards will run the gamut from making most of the important decisions themselves to merely rubber-stamping those of the administrator.

A VISION OF THE FUTURE

The task that now remains is to look into the future and to speculate on the shape of things to come. Here it is important to separate promotion from prediction—to distinguish between what is believed to be desirable from the standpoint of effectiveness and efficiency and what is thought of as likely to result from the interplay of the various forces at work in the system. In making any forecast one needs to recognize that all changes can be viewed as either a challenge or a threat. The changes that are taking place and those that seem likely to occur in the future offer great opportunities, but they also threaten to affect further the status and power of persons and groups and to increase the obsolescence of some individuals and organizations. It is a combination of the inventiveness and determination of those seeking changes and the nature and strength of the reactions of the individuals and groups affected that will determine the extent to which the developments that are forecasted in the following paragraphs actually will happen.

As was suggested in the introduction to this chapter, the one thing that appears almost certain to take place is further change in the medical care system—not only in America but in all other countries as well. This is partly a result of the changing role of public health from a concern with the traditional functions of sanitation, disease control, and other narrow activities to the development of broad programs of medical care. There is planning activity evident at all levels, and the reports, recommendations, and legislation that have appeared or are in preparation presage continuing developments in all areas of the system. Also, medical care and hospitals, as major institutions involved in the provision of care, will continue to be major issues in the arena of public policy for some time to come.[18]

In fact, what appears to underlie many of the changes that are occurring and can be expected to continue is the expansion of the boundaries of the system within which hospital and medical care administration take place. This is in line with the recent legislation in the field and the growing acceptance of the concept of "creative federalism." Decisions are no longer taken in the splendid isolation of the individual hospital or health department but in the context of regional, national, or even international constraints. This will place a greater burden on those administering medical care institutions to know and understand the larger health system in which they are operating.[19]

Focusing now on the hospital itself, it also seems reasonable to predict that the function of administration in these medical care systems will continue to grow in importance and scope, particularly in the larger units. Hospitals can be expected to grow even more in size and complexity and to both develop new services and establish closer relationships with other medical care agencies in the community. Greater regionalization of services seems likely in the future, and the coordination of the units involved, particularly the central facilities, will be a substantial administrative task. In part these developments will depend on a continued demand on the part of the public for an expanded scope of medical care services and greater accessibility to them; but again this is to be expected.

The most difficult question to answer is what part the various groups and institutions who are now participating in the medical care system will play in the more complicated system of the future. One can assume that, in a highly developed democratic society, the major elements needed are public involvement, medical expertise, and administrative know-how. However, it is by no means certain what type of organization and combination of talents can best supply these elements. In order to assess the different possibilities let us examine how the various requirements of the system might be met.

The growing sophistication of the public concerning the potentials of medical care and the greater public demand for services due to the growth of insurance and supplementary governmental programs have led to increased desire to influence what type of care is provided and how it is administered. To the degree that local influence and control are desired, the roles of hospital boards and regional councils with local representation can be expected to become more important. In fact, it has been proposed in some quarters that educational programs should be developed for voluntary members of boards so that they can carry out their responsibilities more effectively. In addition, it has been argued that influential trustees are needed in the administration of hospitals to mediate between the administrators and the medical staff.

It has also been pointed out that the need for planning and coordination on a regional or national basis will mean that more decisions affecting the hospital will be made at these higher administrative levels in the future. If this is the case, public involvement will have to occur either by means of influence on legislation and government activity generally through the exercise of the franchise or through the influence that can he exerted on voluntary bodies which will be operating or advising at these levels.

If we then consider the elements of medical and nursing expertise, the question arises as to whether these can be provided by some form of technical advisory committees or whether persons with clinical training should fill the top administrative posts. If a regional system of hospitals develops that is based on the medical teaching centers, as some predict will happen, then medical school personnel will be in a strong position to affect administrative decisions.

Regarding administration at the hospital level, there is still considerable opinion that hospitals should not have chief executives in the future or, if they do, these should be medically trained people, since the hospital's product is medical care.[20] In part this would seem to depend on the extent to which American hospitals move in the direction of the European pattern and appoint more full-time medical staff in their organizations. Also, it will depend on the future supply of physicians in the country as the increasing demands for them in research and clinical practice threatens to reduce the numbers in administration even more than has been occurring up to now. Basically, however, the argument appears to hinge on the question of qualifications for an executive position in the hospital. Some have argued that the administrator who is not medically trained is a layman because he is a "nonexpert."[21] But why should clinical training and experience in medicine be the only recognized basis for expertise in hospital administration? Surely the major criteria for appointing an executive should be administrative ability and knowledge of the system he is coordinating, not his particular disciplinary preparation.

With regard to the role of the medical staff in hospital management, it should be recognized that all doctors associated with the hospital must perform a range of administrative functions as part of their normal activities running from influencing the deployment of resources through managing the care of their patients to the more extensive responsibilities of department heads and chiefs of staff.[22] There is the increasing conviction, therefore, that they should be more involved in the budgetary process, along with the administration, and that they both should be aided in this endeavor by information-reporting systems at state and national levels. This is one of the recommendations of the recently published Barr Committee report on hospital effectiveness.[23]

If the administrator's role does continue to expand, one can predict some increased conflicts between the administrators and their boards and medical staffs. Although it is possible to conceive of a division of administrative responsibility within the hospital that would maximize both efficiency and effectiveness under the conditions that have been set out, it is not realistic to assume that this can be brought about without some resistance from those whose power would be reduced as a result. The transition is likely to occur more smoothly if the professionally trained administrators are able to demonstrate clearly their growing importance in the hospital to the satisfaction of the medical staff.

Part of the emerging role of the hospital administrator is this increasing involvement in research in his institution, both clinical and administrative. As the need to involve health institutions in the developmental phases of administrative and organizational research becomes more widely recognized, administrators should be prepared to play a key role in demonstration projects and other research aimed at improving the delivery of health services.

Finally, as the public's expectations for health and other services continue to rise, the administrator is likely to find himself involved in several sets of conflicting demands. Of these, the most difficult one to resolve will be that between the increased community demands for care and the needs of the providers of care for higher levels of education, opportunities for research, etc. This could include such decisions as whether to locate services closer to the consumers in institutions like the newly established neighborhood health centers or to concentrate them in a central location that is part of a medical teaching complex. The administrator also may be called upon to help assess the community's relative needs for extended health services versus those for improvements in education or welfare services.

SUMMARY

Changes in the over-all health care system are forcing significant changes in the traditional role of the hospital administrator and in the relationship between him and other key groups involved in the operation of the hospital. He is becoming more of a chief executive in the hospital and also more concerned with the provision of health services to the community. His role is increasingly that of a systems manager whose major concern is the improvement of the process whereby medical care services are delivered to the public.

Increasing professionalization in hospital administration and other health occupations suggests that there will be continuing pressure for more and higher levels of education in most, if not all, of these fields. With closer relationships being established between hospitals and other medical care organizations a greater degree of mobility of personnel between these organizations should be anticipated, particularly between planning organizations and the various operating units.

It follows from what has been said that the field of administration in hospitals and other medical care institutions of the future is an extremely challenging one. The more developed a society becomes, the more demands it makes for higher levels of medical care. Science and technology are producing increasingly effective methods and machinery for promoting health and combating disease. The problems of developing and operating the administrative systems that will optimize the mobilization of this medical care potential to serve the health needs of the public are both substantial and largely common to all highly developed countries. This task calls for as many energetic, intelligent, and dedicated administrators at all levels in these systems as are capable of being developed. The effective administrator of the future must be a person who combines individual sophistication and creativity with a strong feeling of the need for collective responsibility. The solutions adopted in any one health system will benefit from a comparative approach that will draw on the experiences of all nations in administering their health services.

References

1. For an early discussion of this, see Harvey L. Smith, "Two Lines of Authority Are One Too Many," *The Modern Hospital* (March 1955).
2. A sociological analysis of the historical development of hospitals from medieval times to the present has been written by George Rosen. See his "The Hospital: Historical Sociology of a Community Institution" in Eliot Freidson (ed.), *The Hospital in Modern Society*, New York: The Free Press, 1963. For a summary of the recent developments up to 1960 see Herman Somers and Anne Somers, *Doctors, Patients, and Health Insurance*, Washington, D.C.: The Brookings Institution, 1961.
3. A series of case studies of the policy-making process in hospitals can be found in A. B. Moss, et al., *Hospital Policy Decisions*, New York: Putnam, 1966.
4. For an analysis of the nurse's role see Hans Mauksch, "The Nurse: Coordinator of Patient Care," in James K. Skipper and Robert C. Leonard (eds.), *Social Interaction and Patient Care*, Philadelphia: Lippincott, 1965.
5. See Anselm Strauss *et al.*, "The Hospital and Its Negotiated Order" in E. Freidson (ed.), *The Hospital in Modern Society*.
6. Rodney F. White, "Current Trends in Administration," in J. K. Owen (ed.), *Modern Concepts of Hospital Administration*, Philadelphia: W. B. Saunders, 1962.
7. Analyses of the current changes in organizations have been made by Victor Thompson. See his "Bureaucracy and Innovation," *Administrative Science Quarterly* (June 1965).
8. Some of the conflicts in hospital decision-making are discussed in Frederick Bates and Rodney F. White, "Differential Perceptions of Authority in Hospitals," *Journal of Health and Human Behavior* (Winter 1961).
9. These terms were developed in Basil Georgopoulos and Floyd Mann, *The Community General Hospital*, New York: Macmillan, 1962.
10. A preliminary report of findings can be found in Miriam T. Dolson, Rodney F. White, and Paul P. Van Riper, "Study Reveals What Administrators Earn," *The Modern Hospital* (April 1966).
11. See "Report of the Committee on American Hospital Association Program," Chicago: *American Hospital Association*, 1967.
12. Recent analyses of the problems faced by hospital administrators in striving for professional status are contained in Harold Wilensky, "The Dynamics of Professionalism: The Case of Hospital Administration," *Hospital Administration*, 7:2 (Spring 1962); and Charles V. Letourneau, "Hospital Administration: A True Profession," *Hospital Administration*, 13:1 (Winter 1968).

13. An analysis of developments in this field internationally can be found in T. E. Chester, "Hospital Administration, an International Survey," *International Review of Administrative Sciences*, XXIX (1963).
14. A series of articles on the present situation with regard to graduate education for hospital administration is contained in a special issue of *Hospital Administration* (Fall 1967).
15. For a discussion of the increasing role of comprehensive health planning see "Symposium on Comprehensive Health Planning," *American Journal of Public Health* (June 1968).
16. For some interesting discussions of the recent changes in the administration of hospitals, see the Proceedings of the Sixth Annual National Symposium on Hospital Affairs in Chicago, in *The Impact of Changing Medical Practice on Hospital Administration*, Chicago: Health Information Foundation, 1964.
17. For a description of how this operates in one hospital, see Robert E. Toomey, "Setting Objectives: A Guide to Efficient Management," *Hospitals, Journal of the American Hospital Association* (August 1963).
18. For an analysis of some of the continuing issues following the beginning of Medicare see Herman Somers and Anne Somers, *Medicare and the Hospitals: Issues and Prospects*, Washington, D.C.: The Brookings Institution. 1967.
19. This is now a subject of research both in this country and on a comparative international basis. See, for example, Kerr L. White, "Research in Medical Care and Health Services Systems," *Medical Care*, VI:2 (March-April 1968).
20. For a recent American statement on this question see Richard L. Johnson, "Do Hospitals Need a Chief Executive?" *The Modern Hospital* (September 1964). A discussion of it as it applies in Britain is presented by Geoffrey Hutton in "Who Runs A Hospital?" *New Society* (February 27, 1964).
21. See John H. Knowles, "Medical Care: Its Social and Organizational Aspects —The Balanced Biology of the Teaching Hospital," *New England Journal of Medicine* (August 22 and 29, 1963).
22. For a discussion of this topic as it applies in Britain see "Management Functions of Hospital Doctors," a paper of the Advisory Committee for Management Efficiency in the National Health Service, London, October 1966.
23. Compare the *Report of the Secretary's Advisory Committee on Hospital Effectiveness*, Washington, D.C.: Department of Health, Education and Welfare, 1968.

5

Occupational Group Striving in Public Health

Ray H. Elling

The context of this essay relates to some of the general problems dealt with in the sociology of work that are more adequately covered elsewhere.[1] One concern is with the basic division of labor in society both as a determinant of and as a result of the form of the society.[2] The individual's life chances and his course through life, including educational as well as work experiences, have been examined in studies of careers. Closely associated with this last concern has been the study of the values and orientations of members of different work groups and socialization to these.[3] The public's view of the relative prestige of different occupational positions and the role of occupation in determining social class status and political behavior have been major topics of concern.[4] Another somewhat controversial problem (identical in my opinion to the question of prestige and "standing" generally of a work group in society) is the matter of distinguishing so-called "professional" groups from other work groups and observing movements toward "professional status" on the parts of those not yet deserving of this approbatory label.[5] Recently interest has been aroused among social scientists about problems devolving from the articulation of occupational groups and complex organizations.

This chapter, which draws upon concepts dealing with occupational group "establishment," was stimulated by a study of occupational groups in public health.[6] The term "establishment" is general and includes considerations of rewards, power, and prestige, which determine the life chances of members of a work group and the group's ability to control its destiny.

As far as the individual and his occupational group are concerned, a field of work like public health presents two primary problems: (1) the range or set of functions that are to be covered, e.g., the content of the work, and (2) how the work is to be arranged. In this latter problem, relationships to other men are involved and the question of who is going to do what arises. This question is particularly salient today in the field of public health since it is undergoing vast and rapid change. The acquisition of new tasks and the sloughing of old ones always means a new cut of the work pie with consequent concerns on everyone's part for where he and his group stand.

THE DOMAIN OF PUBLIC HEALTH

In the health field alone in this country there are more than 150 occupational groups in any large hospital and health center complex.[7] Within the once relatively unified profession of medicine there are now numerous specialties that in effect operate as independent occupational groups.[8] From 1931 to 1959 the number of full-time specialists in medicine more than tripled (from 22,158 to 78,635) while general practitioners (including part-time specialists) declined by one quarter (from 112,116 to 81,957).[9] The patient's experience of this development is clear from the work of Dochez, who examined records of two similar cases of heart disease in the same hospital—the first occurred in 1908, the second thirty years later. While the first case took up $2\frac{1}{2}$ pages of written record and involved three professionals, the second took up 29 pages and drew the attention of 32 professionals.[10]

With this degree of complexity and change in the division of labor, every occupational group with pretentions of being accorded professional standing becomes, as one investigator put it, "nervous in the status."[11] There are high personal stakes to be won or lost, domains to be conquered or relinquished for a whole work group, more or less attractive work conditions to be attained, better or poorer recruits to renew the ranks. In short, the conditions and consequences of occupational group establishment are at play.

Depending on how one defines its boundaries, public health may include the total spectrum of health occupations. Most narrowly, it can be said to embrace the groups working in local health departments and in state health departments and the U.S. Public Health Service.

A fair estimate is given by the fact that some members of well over 30 special groups have identified themselves with the field enough to have joined the American Public Health Association or one of its regional or state affiliates.[12]

WHO IS GOING TO DO WHAT?

For the field of public health the struggle of occupational groups over who is going to do what has both an internal and an external aspect. This no doubt is true of any field, but again it seems particularly noticeable in public health because of the changing substratum of health problems that the society faces and because vague but identifiable and powerful but competing interest clusters in health—among them private practice medicine (organized medicine), medical education, hovered close to 32 years in the recent periods for which data are health institutions undergo continual, increasing change toward a more encompassing and controlled form of organization.[13]

Internal Problems

The question of leadership offers one example of a point of internal contention. Historically we see a shift in leadership. Prior to the nineteenth century it was generally the lay social reformer, the man of some standing in the community, who concerned himself with general sanitary reform and the health of the public. Very early, engineers and chemists took leading positions in the field. Indeed, physicians were equipped to do little until the advent of the "germ theory," as it was called. Only after physicians began to apply the biochemical discoveries of a French chemist (Pasteur) did they begin to take an ascendant position in the field.[14] More recently the leadership of physicians in this field has been challenged on grounds of the inadequacy of their preparation in the study of administration and planning of community health services and the inadequate numbers of M.D.'s who enter the field as a speciality.[15]

Another internal issue is the cohesiveness of the field. This can be thought of primarily as a question of relations of specialty groups within public health to the field as a whole.

In connection with the Joint Committee Study of Education for Public Health, students in the 14 schools of public health in the United

States and Canada were administered a confidential mail questionnaire as they were finishing their first year of study in the spring of 1962. In answer to the question: "Do you consider public health as a profession or as a collection of separate professions?" the majority of respondents (58%) considered the field to be a collection of separate professions. As one student of the field put it, "Every person in public health is professionally bisubcultural."[16] This is the case because, almost without exception, workers in the field first receive preparation and the identity of a discipline (chemistry, physics, sociology) or another profession (medicine, engineering, nursing) and only then enter public health as a secondary profession. This is substantiated by the fact that the mean age of students in schools of public health has hovered close to 32 years in the recent periods for which data are available.[17] Partly in response to this lack of cohesiveness and partly to improve recruitment and to free an overcrowded curriculum, schools of public health are moving toward two-year master's degree programs with direct entrance from college in place of the one-year program for those with prior professional degrees and experience.

External Problems

This internal dialectic of fractionation and integration of public health is directly related to the external dialectic of expanding and contracting work boundaries. The domain of "health" in the broadest sense changes. For example, as some old problem such as pollution appears in new guises, the individual engineer, physicist, or chemist may take up work on the problem, but do so in an organizational context not traditionally considered as public health (e.g., industry or agriculture).

Within "health" various interest clusters nibble away at or relinquish to public health. Physicians interested in medical care organization, community mental health, or mental retardation may well pursue their work in settings that they and others would not identify with public health. Mental health efforts, while remaining firmly within public health at the federal level, are often in separate departments at the state level. Medicare has gone to the Social Security Administration and is administered by agencies headed largely by social workers.

Even education for public health itself is not entirely under the control of the accrediting arm of the APHA as it would be under the counterpart organization in other professional fields. Nurses train and accredit for public health work, so do engineers, hospital administrators, and physicians—the latter in departments of preventive medicine in some medical schools and in residencies accredited by the AMA.

PROFESSIONS AS INTEREST GROUPS

In the extensive literature that attempts to analyze and define professions as distinct from other work groups, a number of characteristics have been identified as crucial for a group to achieve before it can be thought of as "truly professional." There is a degree of control over entry, socialization, and practice implied by the traditional use of the term "professional," and it is assumed that members will follow well-recognized, orderly career patterns. As Everett Hughes has put it, "A profession is a work group which assumes the right to judge its own mistakes."[18] The professional is not supposed to be influenced by the referral and economic needs of his colleagues, the demands of the organization he works in, or other factors; and, with stringent entrance and educational requirements, the popular notion is that any member of the profession should be able to offer the core services of the group.

While the term profession may carry this connotation of pursuit of high ideals and moral behavior, it also serves as one of several means by which occupational groups seek to establish themselves. Certainly almost every work group with any degree of self-consciousness and organization is in pursuit of having the term applied to its members. The suggestion is made here that this striving is really for power and prestige worked out in terms of a rewarding work domain and other concomitants of establishment in the social order.[19] It appears that the structure and function of work groups in an hierarchized order is involved.

It therefore becomes theoretically important, and empirically interesting, as well as vital for practical administration and planning to know the characteristics of groups that do have the term profession applied to them by closely associated work colleagues[20] and others. This is a matter for continuing investigation. But it appears that there is a hierarchy of professionalism in public health, as shown by data available from the Study of Public Health Careers. In Table 1 we see a ranking of special work groups according to "how professional" their fellow members of the APHA or one of its affiliates judged them to be.[21]

One of the interesting facets of Table 1 is that it shows the bosses of major health organizations (health officers, hospital administrators,

TABLE 1. *Rank Ordering of Occupational Groups*[a] *in Public Health by Professional Status and Median Income*

Self-Identified[a] *Basic Discipline*	*Ranking of Professional Status Assigned by Total Sample*[b]	*Median Income (1964), in dollars*	*Income Ranking*	*Total Respondents (8691), in per cent*
Physicians[c]	1	17,849.50	1	5.3
Public health dentist	2	10,699.50	4	0.6
Veterinarian	3	11,249.50	3	0.8
Laboratory scientist	4	8,199.50	9	4.1
Health officer	5	12,849.50	2	2.7
Public health engineer	6	9,549.50	6	3.4
Biostatistician	7	7,099.50	11–13	1.4
Public health nurse	8	4,201.00	16	14.8
Other nurses	9	4,401.00	15	1.5
Hospital administrator	10	10,499.00	5	5.0
Other public health administrators	11	8,899.50	8	5.9
Health educator	12	7,099.50	11–13	2.2
Nutritionist	13	7,099.50	11–13	1.2
Public health social worker	14	7,599.50	10	1.2
Sanitarian	15	5,099.50	14	6.4
Occupational hygienist	16	9,149.50	7	2.4
Other		8,249.50		40.2

[a] Subjects indicated their identified discipline from a list presented to them.
[b] Each respondent ranked each presented discipline on a five-point scale from "highly professional" to "not professional at all." "Don't know" answers were not included in the ranking scores.
[c] These are largely clinical M.D.'s in public health and occupational health M.D.'s. Excludes M.D.'s who identified themselves elsewhere, e.g., Health Officer.

and other public health administrators) as standing lower in prestige and income than some of the people whose efforts they must coordinate. Of course this is not unique to public health but highlights in another way the problem of specialty group autonomy and varying lines of authority identified by others.[22]

The determinant conditions of professional standing need further exploration, but it seems a reasonable hypothesis at this point, supported in part by these data, that as in other hierarchical systems a differential distribution of autonomy, rewards, and power generally are associated with one's position in the hierarchy. I suspect that the struggle among groups in the field of public health and between the field and outside groups has as much or more to do with this aspect of "Who's going to do what?" than it has to do with the most efficient and effective division of labor for the solution to the community's health problems.

To understand the positions of groups in Table 1, the sociological regularities of striving for work group establishment must be elucidated. This task cannot be completed here, because it includes study of the conscious and unconscious but nevertheless patterned aspects of recruitment whereby persons with great talent are channeled more into certain work groups. The task reaches as far as studying the details of organized lobbying before legislatures and other supporting and controlling bodies and includes better understanding of "negotiation" vis-à-vis the school and the work organization.

The Strategies and Means of Work Group Establishment

The health professions here are being discussed as group units (occupational groups) *as if* they acted in some corporate, but not necessarily conscious, fashion to achieve the autonomy, rewarding domain, and power that go with an established professional position. It should be clear that while examples are drawn from the health field, the following analysis is hopefully applicable to any field of work. The intermixture of points regarding strategies and citing of examples otherwise will be confusing.

Students of occupations have examined some of the general means, strategies, and barriers of establishment. Summarizing briefly from the work of Oswald Hall and Harold L. Wilensky[23] and from my observations, the steps toward establishment (some overlapping in time with others) would include the following:

1. A self-conscious recognition that others are performing similar tasks and face similar "life chances" and risks. For example, Oswald Hall described these beginnings of work group organization in a presentation on a new occupation, the inhalation therapists.[24]

2. Establishment of an association to (a) promote the development of new knowledge relevant to solving problems within the work domain, (b) exchange this knowledge among members, (c) communicate other information of mutual interest such as job conditions, job openings, public reactions to the group's activities, etc., (d) act politically through lobbying and other means for the protection of the work

domain and other conditions of establishment, (e) establish a code of ethics and police publicly exposed members who violate it as well as combat nonmembers ("quacks" and "charlatans") working what the group considers to be its territory, and (f) set up legitimating bodies to accredit the training schools and programs and sometimes the work organization. (For example, the approval of hospitals by the Joint Commission on Accreditation of the AMA and the AHA.)

In some groups, as for example in nursing and pathology,[25] rival associations develop with different ideologies. This is confusing both to the insider and the outsider and may represent differences inherent in the group from the start or new specialization and a breaking apart of the groups. Competition among such associations is seen by their meeting at different places at the same time. Other examples are the Health Officer's Section of the APHA and the Association for Public Health Management or the American School Health Association, the Society of Public Health Educators and the Health Education Section of the APHA.

On occasion different but related associations hold joint meetings and thereby attempt to support each other's influence and possibly coopt each other's members. The danger is that consensus will exist only in a vague, undefinable way and the field will be unable to project an attractive image.[26]

3. Performance of the work as a full-time, specialized occupation. For example, administration of larger health organizations has only been identified and "pulled out" as a special occupation in the last thirty years or so. This still has not occurred in many European hospitals.[27]

4. Restriction of supply by means of control over entry and socialization of new members through the founding of training schools. As the degree of establishment increases, these training programs will move from 3-week, independent affairs to association with a college and then a university as a major status-giving instrument of our society. Finally, the programs will become longer in length and move toward higher and higher degrees. The schools themselves will form a mutual interest association such as the American Association of Medical Colleges or the Association of Schools of Public Health. This association allows a limited exchange of competitive information among the deans or heads and facilitates a common front vis-à-vis specialty groups that want a greater share of the curriculum and unreasonable practitioners who want students prepared to go to work their first day on the job.

5. The less challenging, exciting, and rewarding tasks are sloughed off. This may occur by simply leaving certain things undone until other groups take them up. Or there may be a conscious effort to develop

and "shove a new group under" (for example, the case of the licensed vocational nurse).

At the same time that unpleasant tasks are discarded, attempts are made to move in on higher level tasks and new domains. This may be accomplished by filling gaps left by a shortage of manpower in other fields, fulfillment of demands by disillusioned or uncaptured clients or by acquisition of special knowledge or schooling not available to the traditional practitioner, by administrative fiat, by manufacture of more believable myths, or by other means. For example, the nurse may finally get general acceptance of her performance of intravenous procedures or, frustrated in this general line of establishment, she may take up the social-psychological management of the patient situation as a new area of exotic expertise, and overworked psychiatrists are not likely to complain but social workers may become anxious.[28] The public health nurse may seek to replace the now largely mythical family doctor, at least among low-income families, by becoming a "family health counselor" who would link the home and neighborhood to the complex health center.

6. A sometimes wonderous effort at domain maintenance and expansion deserves mention as a special point. This we could call myth-making. It is characteristic of every group to present an all-knowing façade in the face of unsolved and possibly unsolvable problems. In public health various examples could be chosen.[29]

7. A special language is developed to serve both technical communication and protect the special knowledge of the field from use by the uninitiated. It is clear to all in public health, for example, that a person is not "a public healther" if he does not understand the difference between incidence and prevalence.

8. A more potent protective measure is to convince the state legislature and governor through political action that the correct performance of the group's functions are so vital that licensure or certification is required. This is the ultimate lockout of some unauthorized person.

The criteria for licensure may include a degree of a certain kind from an accredited school; and this may reinforce the school's position. Licensure or civil service requirements may be employed to pressure the school into admitting a new group to receipt of the core degree. Examples of the strategy of political pressure include such activities as the health educators in California getting the state civil service to write the M.P.H. in as a requirement for certain health education positions. The case of the registered sanitarian provides another.

9. Recruitment and esprit de corps must be maintained lest the

ablest members or potential members drift elsewhere in our complex world of work opportunities. Thus successes of the field are publicized, meetings are held in alluring settings, awards are given, and hero stories are told.[30] Other inducements to recruitment also may be offered in the form of fellowships, exemption from active military duty, etc.

10. Finally, conflicts between ideologies and realities must be resolved. One strategy has been the formation of authoritative study commissions. Their reports may end up denying the existence of some new reality, or they may recognize but denounce new departures too evident to be denied. The more daring commissions, usually composed of outsiders as well as insiders (though not too many outsiders), may even provide a set of sophisticated rationalizations for behavior that already is taking place and in which a new leadership recognized as inevitable or desirable or both. This process has been examined for the American society as a whole.[31] However, I am not aware of any systematic examination of study commissions as a strategy and means of occupational group establishment.[32] Yet practically all mature and some not-so-mature fields have become self-conscious and uneasy enough about new undertakings and demands or losses of old functions to launch a major self-examination.

Although a systematic examination of this strategy cannot be offered here, it appears to me that the traditional core leadership first becomes uneasy about its position and directions of the field. The major sources of power are then gathered together through representation on a joint study commission. (In the Study of Education for Public Health it was the professional association, the association of schools, and the Association of State and Territorial Health Officers, with unofficial representation from major governmental agencies through which an important share of the field's finances are channeled.) A certain broad-mindedness is achieved by adding a limited number of members who specifically do not represent the traditional leadership. Depending on how autonomous and courageous they are, these members can have a sharp effect. The study staff also may be chosen with some such balance in mind and again can have a telling effect.

The commission's investigation involves hearing leaders of all the groups with vested interests in the field and some who it is felt should be interested but are not. External groups that must be counted on in one way or another are consulted. Information is gathered on the composition and function of training institutions in the field and competing schools outside the field on organizations, job vacancies, recruitment efforts, and the control of new functions and problem areas. This systematic coverage of factual and opinion information is presented to the committee and digested until a significant degree of consensus develops. The more radical the points and interpretations, the longer it will take for the commission to feel at all comfortable about reporting back to its constituting bodies. These bodies, being somewhat anxious, will arrange for periodic presentations from the commission staff to see what is going on. If mutual suspicion grows too great, the commission, depending on its integrity and original terms of reference, may declare or reaffirm its independence. The report then inevitably is a mixture of caution and boldness. If adequate, it will succeed in reformulating the ideology of the field to correspond more with the realities it faces. If truly successful, it may define a great leap forward.

The above is hardly an exhaustive list of strategies and means of occupational group establishment. Further, it gives too static an impression. The reader must realize that striving for establishment in public health goes on in the midst of striking dynamic features—a shifting groundwork of problems, changing technologies, uncovered areas between domains, overlaps in other areas, manpower shortages, and increasing public appreciation of health care. Nevertheless, this framework may serve as a backdrop for considering the articulation of occupational groups and complex organizations in the health field.

At some level, almost without regard for how fractionated a field of work or a particular work organization may be, there is a commonly accepted goal statement that provides the semblance of a common universe of discourse. This is usually so general that people can talk at and past each other, but it is never concrete enough to unfailingly indicate specific directions. It must be this way, or violent splits would replace many an apparent but unfounded consensus.[33] In public health the overarching goal is to guard against disability and, if possible, to enhance the level of ability in the populations of our communities. No one in the field will fundamentally disagree with this, though nuances of phrasing may become terribly important since they suggest greater or lesser degrees of breadth and other characteristics to the field.[34]

In view of the problems of occupational group striving outlined above, with ever-higher degrees, restriction of manpower supply, struggle over work domains, etc., all taking place in a fast-changing environment where problems, demands, and challenges loom large, the answer to the question "How is the work to get done?" will not be a simple one.

Throughout this chapter I have emphasized the general view of public health. Each specialty group has problems and requirements of its own. But the study of occupational group striving leads one to suspect that these special interest groups may be better able to take care of themselves than will the field as a whole.

References

1. Everett C. Hughes, *Men and Their Work*, New York: The Free Press, 1958; T. Caplow, *The Sociology of Work*, Minneapolis: University of Minnesota Press, 1954.
2. Emile Durkheim, *The Division of Labor in Society,* trans. G. Simpson, New York: The Free Press, 1947; A. Inkeles and P. Rossi, "National Comparisons of Occupational Prestige," *American Journal of Sociology*, 61 (January 1956), 329–339.
3. Vernon K. Dibble, "Occupations and Ideologies," *American Journal of Sociology*, 68 (September 1962), 229–241. Anne Roe, *The Psychology of Occupations*, New York: John Wiley, 1956; M. Rosenberg with the assistance of E. A. Suchman and R. K. Goldsen, *Occupations and Values*, New York: The Free Press, 1957. Examples of studies of socialization to the medical profession are Howard S. Becker *et al.*, *Boys in White: Student Cultures in Medical School*, Chicago: University of Chicago Press, 1961; Robert K. Merton, George Reader, and Patricia Kendall (eds.), *The Student–Physician*, Cambridge, Mass.: Harvard University Press, 1957. The study of leisure might be thought of as a special problem area but also can be viewed as a matter of orientations of different work groups. Erwin Smigel (ed.), *Work and Leisure, A Contemporary Social Problem*, New Haven: College and University Press, 1963; A. C. Clarke, "Leisure and Occupational Prestige," in E. Larrabee and R. Meyersohn (eds.), *Mass Leisure*, New York: The Free Press, 1958, pp. 205–214.
4. A. J. Reiss *et al.*, *Occupations and Social Status*, New York: The Free Press, 1961; National Opinion Research Center, "Jobs and Occupations: A Popular Evaluation," in R. Bendix and S. M. Lipset (eds.), *Class, Status and Power*, New York: The Free Press, 1953, pp. 411–426.
5. Howard S. Becker, "The Nature of a Profession," Sixty-First Yearbook of the National Society for the Study of Education, Part II, *Education for the Professions*, Chicago: University of Chicago Press, 1962. The writer is indebted to this important work for much of the brief summary of professional characteristics presented above. For a similarly critical analysis of the concept "profession" see R. W. Habenstein, "Critique of Profession

as a Sociological Category," *Sociological Quarterly*, 4 (Autumn 1963), 291–300. For a more traditional conception of the term that focuses on the consensus and control aspects of work groups, see William J. Goode, "Community Within a Community: The Professions," *American Sociological Review*, 20 (April 1957), 194–200.

6. Data stem from two primary sources. First, the writer had the privilege of serving for three years as Field Director of the Joint Committee Study of Education for Public Health under the direction of his respected colleague, Dr. William P. Shepard. The methodology for this extensive effort is reported in Hilary Fry, with the collaboration of William Shepard and Ray H. Elling, *Education and Manpower for Community Health*, Pittsburgh: University of Pittsburgh Press, 1968. Second, with Drs. Shepard and Charles W. Dean and others the writer has been engaged in a study of careers in the field of public health, involving a mail questionnaire survey of some 10,000 public health workers sampled from a nonduplicative membership list of the American Public Health Association and its regional and state affiliates.
7. The last count by the National Health Council referred to here is now outdated. See A. R. Rivin, "Your Hospital, A Center for Community Services," Chicago: Blue Cross Commission, 1960.
8. R. Bucher and A. Strauss, "Professions in Process," *American Journal of Sociology*, 66 (January 1961), 325–334.
9. W. H. Stewart and M. Y. Pennell, "Physicians' Age, Type of Practice, and Location," *Health Manpower Source Book No. 10*, Washington, D.C.: Public Health Service Publication No. 263, Section 10, 1960, p. 4.
10. As cited by George Rosen, "The Hospital: Historical Sociology of a Community Institution," in Eliot Freidson (ed.), *The Hospital in Modern Society*, New York: The Free Press, 1964, p. 27.
11. "Almost every profession nowadays feels 'nervous in the status.' Over the past year, half a dozen committees and commissions from as many professional associations have come to my office at the National Opinion Research Center to talk about programs of research designed to help improve their status (or the Madison Avenue equivalent, 'image'). Veterinarians, engineers, pharmacologists, oral surgeons, professors, morticians, and even the highest and mightiest of professions, the medicine men, all show signs of being uncertain of where they stand in the eyes of the American public and in the regard of their next-door neighbors. Even businessmen are apprehensive that America has not accorded them their proper place." Remarks by Peter Rossi on a paper by Harold Lancour, "The Librarians' Search for Status," in P. H. Ennis and H. W. Winger (eds.), *Seven Questions About the Profession of Librarianship*, Chicago: University of Chicago Press, 1961, p. 82.
12. The author and coresearchers in the Study of Public Health Careers found it necessary, following a pretest, to elaborate our mail questionnaire to 33 categories. We still found that 6.8% or 448 of employed professionals

in the sample of the APHA and its affiliated associations fell in an "other" category. For further detail as to methods, see W. P. Shepard, R. H. Elling, and W. F. Grimes, in *Education and Manpower in Public Health.*

13. This trend is analyzed and its continued development predicted in Milton I. Roemer, "The Future of Social Medicine in the United States," presented at the Annual Meeting of the Medical Sociology Section of the American Sociological Association, Miami Beach, August 30, 1966.
14. C. E. A. Winslow, "Public Health," in the *Encyclopedia of the Social Sciences*, New York: Macmillan, 1933, Vol. 12, p. 647. Also George Rosen, *A History of Public Health*, pp. 224–225.
15. The Joint Committee Report, *Education and Manpower in Public Health*, raises this question of current leadership. At one of the conferences held by the Joint Committee (The Ithaca Conference, an unpublished, mimeographed report, September 1961) one of the truly great physician figures of the field said, "The leaders of public health today lack fire in their bellies." Winslow raised this question of leadership at an earlier conference. See *The Changing Front of Health*, New York: Milbank Memorial Fund, 1940. On problems of recruiting physicians to the field, see Kurt W. Back, Robert Coker, and Thomas Donnelly, "Public Health as a Career of Medicine: Secondary Choice Within a Profession," *American Sociological Review*, 23 (October 1958).
16. A "jargony" but accurate observation by a noted social scientist who attended the Joint Committee Workship on Social Science and Public Health, November 21, 1962, Manger-Vanderbilt Hotel, New York City.
17. Annual reports prepared for the staff of the Committee on Professional Education of the American Public Health Association by each school of public health, Dr. James L. Troupin, Executive Secretary of the CPE.
18. Everett C. Hughes, "Mistakes at Work," *The Canadian Journal of Economics and Political Science*, 17 (August 1951), 320–327.
19. The fact that one author rejects the notion that many groups are in fact achieving professional status does not gainsay the fact which he recognizes that "many occupations engage in heroic struggles for professional identification"—Harold L. Wilensky, "The Professionalization of Everyone?" *The American Journal of Sociology*, 70 (September 1964), 137–158. For an analysis which suggests that every group can try and "make it," see Nelson Foote, "The Professionalization of Labor in Detroit," *The American Journal of Sociology*, 58 (January 1953), 371–380. The suggestion here is that all may pursue this fata morgana, but there is little substance to it other than power and prestige.
20. For the suggestion that this radically sociological view be empirically explored by examining what groups "have been fortunate enough in the politics of today's work world to gain and maintain possession of that honorific title," see Howard S. Becker, "The Nature of a Profession," Sixty-First Yearbook

of the National Society for the Study of Education, Part II, *Education for the Professions*, Chicago: The University of Chicago Press, 1962. Also, by the same author, "Some Problems of Professionalization," *Adult Education* 6 (Winter 1956), 101–105.

21. This ranking is based on usable replies to the question: "People differ in their opinion with regard to the professional status of various occupational groups. In your own judgment, how professional is each of the following groups?" With approximately 80% return from a 3 in 10 sample (9,954) of members of the APHA or one of its regional, state, or local affiliates, 7,976 generally complete questionnaires were in hand. From this number we subtracted 1,282 cases including so-called "nonprofessionals" (secretaries, file clerks, animal caretakers, etc.) and those unemployed or not in the labor force. In addition, since we wanted the "insider's" estimate of professional standing, the question itself was directed only toward those who said their work was "in public health," thus eliminating another 1,402 cases. The resulting base of relevant respondents for this question was 5,292. The number of responses to this question vary insofar as some occupational groups received more replies than did others. The usable replies ranged from 4,771 to 4,911 for the 20 groups (see the table in the text) with an average of 4,867.

    A rank was obtained for each group by scoring responses as follows and obtaining an average: "highly professional," 4; "professional," 3; "somewhat professional," 2; "not professional at all," 1. "Don't know" responses were fairly evenly distributed and were not scored. On the average 234 cases responded "don't know" to the question of professional ranking. Since other ways of manipulating the scoring system are possible and since different samples might give different results, this hierarchization cannot be viewed as final. Further, it is supposed here that change may occur in the position of any of these groups over time.

22. H. L. Smith, "Two Lines of Authority: The Hospital's Dilemma," in E. G. Jaco (ed.), *Patients, Physicians and Illness*, New York: The Free Press, 1958, pp. 468–477; O. Hall, "Half Medical Man, Half Administrator: An Occupational Dilemma," *Canadian Public Administration*, 2 (December 1959), 185–194; M. Goss, "Influence and Authority Among Physicians in an Outpatient Clinic," *American Sociological Review*, 26 (February 1961), 39–50; R. N. Wilson, "The Physician's Changing Hospital Role," in W. R. Scott and E. H. Volkart, *Medical Care, Readings in the Sociology of Medical Institutions*, New York: John Wiley, 1966, pp. 406–420.

23. Oswald Hall, "The Place of the Professions in the Urban Community," in S. D. Clark (ed.), *The Changing Canadian Community*, Toronto: University of Toronto Press, 1960. Also Harold L. Wilensky, The "Professionalization of Everyone?" *The American Journal of Sociology*, 70 (September 1964), 137–158.

24. Delivered in the Hospital Administrator's Development Program, Cornell University, Ithaca, New York, Summer 1961.

25. The NLN and ANA in nursing. For the case in pathology see Rue Bucher, "Pathology: A Study of Social Movements Within a Profession," *Social Problems*, 10 (Summer 1962), 40–51.
26. K. E. Boulding, *The Image*, Ann Arbor: University of Michigan Press, 1966.
27. William A. Glaser, "American and Foreign Hospitals: Some Sociological Comparisons," in Eliot Freidson (ed.), *The Hospital in Modern Society*, New York: The Free Press, 1963.
28. Some of these incipient shifts in the division of labor and the general problem are discussed in Cecil G. Sheps and Meriam E. Bachar, "Nursing and Medicine, Emerging Patterns of Practice," *The American Journal of Nursing*, 64 (September 1964).
29. Specialty groups within the field each develop their own supporting myths. "The epidemiologic method," for example, which is nothing more than the scientific method applied to the occurrence of disability in populations, is discussed and sometimes taught as if it were unique. See Vernon K. Dibble, "Occupations and Ideologies," *American Journal of Sociology*, 68 (September 1962), 229–241.
30. Hero stories also serve to uphold the best traditions of the field, but some persons are heroes who have been so successful they have moved out of the field in being called to higher things—one man, now a college president, is often cited in public health.
31. Thurmond Arnold, *The Folklore of Capitalism*, New Haven: Yale University Press, 1937.
32. For a suggestive piece see C. Wright Mills, "What Research Can Do For Labor," *Labor and Nation*, 2 (June–July, 1946), 17–20. Also, "On Knowledge and Power," in *Power, Politics and People*, The Collected Essays of C. Wright Mills, edited by Irving L. Horowitz, New York: Oxford University Press, 1963.
33. The head of a major hospital and the head of the American College of Radiologists both professed to a primary interest in "good patient care" even though they were in violent disagreement over payment schemes and other means of achieving this good care. See the Albert W. Snoke and Vincent W. Archer exchange, "Financial Relationships Between Radiologists and Hospitals," *Hospitals*, 34 (January 16, 1960), 38–68ff, and 34 (February 1, 1960), 43–107ff.
34. Our phrasing here is admittedly very broad. A more traditional statement would be that public health seeks to prevent disease through organized community efforts. We have chosen the broader formulation, since this traditional conception is not without problems when it comes to the establishment of public health: "One broad feature which forms a background to the whole fifty years may be mentioned at this point—everyone says that prevention is better than cure, and hardly anyone acts as if he believes it, whether he is attached to Parliament, central or local government, or the commonalty of citizens. Palliatives nearly always take precedence over pre-

vention, and our health services today are too heavily loaded with salvage. Treatment — the attempt to heal the sick — is more tangible, more exciting, and more immediately rewarding, than prevention" — J. M. Mackintosh, *Trends of Opinion about the Public Health*, 1901–51, London: Oxford University Press, 1953, p. 5. To make the subject compelling is one of the main problems in teaching preventive medicine: W. P. Shepard and J. G. Roney, Jr., "The Teaching of Preventive Medicine in the United States," special issue, *Milbank Memorial Fund Quarterly* (October 1964).

6

Organizational Control and the Public Health Nurse

Edna M. Grexton

An interesting problem in the study of the administrative organization is that of the management of conflicting role expectations by the members of the organization. One type of role is that in which the members of the organization have face-to-face relationships with the clientele of the organization. The salesman in the business firm, the teller in the bank, the policeman, and the schoolteacher all have to face the problems of adjusting organizational expectations with those of the client. How these role adjustments are managed is a problem for the administrator in that the work of the organization is dependent upon how these roles are enacted.

One general way in which these role difficulties are managed in our society has been through the professionalization of the work group whose behavior is patterned according to a general professional ethic, as well as through rules of judgment accorded to a specific body of knowledge the profession claims. Stemming from this is the belief that only a person from the particular profession can supervise the work of his professional colleagues. In this way, also, the professional ideology is incorporated within the authority structure of the organization.

Other means of managing such role relationships may be through control of the setting and rules by which the interactions take place. Symbols and trappings such as the white coat or uniform, the use of formal titles, and designation of a special meeting place such as the office or clinic operate to limit and control the interaction.

When the mission of the organization is diffuse and general there is often a wide range of behavior that must be left to the judgment of the organizational members in these boundary roles. This becomes a rather difficult problem for the person in such a role when the organization's mission is one of social control. The policeman or the probation officer, for example, must use his judgment as to when he should act with legal authority, when he should use an educational approach, or when he can overlook the unacceptable behavior of his client.

A case in point is the situation faced by many staff members of the local health department. The sanitarian, for example, must use judgment in his work with restaurant operators when administering food service sanitation laws. The public health nurse is faced with judgment problems of setting priorities in relation to the health needs of her clients; yet each is also expected to follow organizational policies. Even the physician faces the problem of managing the medical needs of the client within the framework of the agency's goals. The health agency, however, is of special interest, because the persons enacting these boundary roles are health professionals.

As part of a study of nurse-client interactions, information was gathered on how such role dilemmas are managed within a nursing division of a local health department. The ways in which these management problems of face-to-face relationships with clients were handled by the agency and by the nurses can provide clues for understanding the coping mechanisms used by professionals in the administrative organization. Nineteen public health nurses from one official public health agency were observed in 403 interactions* in a variety of settings, for example, in the homes of clients, in clinics, and in hospitals. The nurses were selected from three categories of experience, and an effort was made to match as closely as possible for cultural characteristics, i.e., geographical origin by region and density of population, education, and age. The clients represented different races, ethnic groups, educational levels, socioeconomic backgrounds, ages, and sex; and the types of visits represented the agency's 21 classifications of nursing visits: those that were regulated by clearly defined policies and procedures and those that were not.

Personal observation was the primary tool for collecting data. However, data were also collected from family records of the nurses, personnel records, interviews with each nurse, a one-way window in the setting of a child health conference, and the evaluations of six supervisors.

* Edna M. Grexton, "Interactions Patterns in Professional–Client Relationships," unpublished doctoral dissertation, Berkeley: University of California, 1968.

Public health nursing services in a health department are usually administered by a nurse who is responsible to the health officer, usually a physician. The nursing services, due partly to funding mechanisms in the agency, are administered in relation to specific programs (e.g., mental health, maternal and child health, and tuberculosis control), and the nurses' visits to clients are categorized according to such programs. In general the public health nurse, unless the agency operates what is known as a bedside care program, does not carry out the functions traditionally and popularly attributed to nursing. Rather her agency role is to facilitate the client's ability to cope with those health problems in which the agency has concern. Additionally, she is expected by the agency, and expects in terms of her professional ideal, to assist the client in coping with all the health problems of the family. Often, for example, the nursing division in a health department will state that it provides a "generalized family health service."

Thus the public health nurse has to manage the problems of adapting the expectations of the agency to the realities of the client's needs as she perceives them and as the client defines them.

THE MANAGEMENT OF AGENCY PRIORITIES

The relative emphasis placed on the various programs of the department varies from time to time. What the agency does is defined operationally by what the community is willing to purchase. What programs are supported are the outcome of professionally (and legally) determined priorities adapted to political realities, and public financial support may shift in sympathy with interests or concerns about specific diseases or defects. For example, if the legislative body provides for programs designed to assist individuals with orthopedic defects or cancer, rather than venereal disease or dental caries, the nursing administrator is obliged to set priorities of the nursing services in terms of visits to clients with these diseases.* Additionally, the mechanism by which the program is carried out will affect agency priorities. For example, some health programs have police power implications, as in the control of certain communicable diseases (e.g., tuberculosis); other programs may provide some kind of financial assistance for specific health problems (e.g., orthopedic defects in children) that is regulated through fiscal and quality controls.

When the nursing administrator sets program priorities, she may not

* It was stated by one of the supervisors of an agency studied by this author that 60% of the visits made by the nurses in her area were Crippled Childrens' Services visits.

always be aware herself of the various rationales for the priority decisions she makes, or she may not communicate the rationale to the staff nurse. Although, in essence, the final outcome of the intentions of the nursing administrator is determined by the actual work of the nurses at the operational level, in the process of translation of values, goals, objectives, and priorities a gap is created. As a consequence, the end product is frequently different from that intended by the administrator.

Therefore, it is not surprising to find that the public health nurses in the study did not understand or accept the reason for some of the policies and stated that many of their visits seemed unnecessary. And as one nurse said, "I've learned from experience just to do it right the first time. Never mind how illogical it is." (She was filling out Crippled Childrens' Service forms at the time.) The nurses faced the problem of trying to determine the priorities of the agency and meet its requirements while attempting to set priorities for assessing and meeting the needs of the families.

Much of the time of public health nurses studied was spent making home visits to mothers for purposes of either reminding them of child health conference* appointments or to discover the reasons for not attending the clinic. Emphasis on such activities is valued by society and was rationalized by the nurses themselves on the basis of the inherent good for the health of the children, for example immunization.

It is difficult at times for the administrators of nursing services of health departments to operationalize values in terms of health. The professional ethic infers that positive health is good and that human life should be saved with no exceptions. However, it is not clear what "good," "better," or "community" health is and how much ill health a community should tolerate. Health is not an absolute and permanent value but is a relative concept. Therefore, in facing the difficulties of operationalizing public health values, and lacking other criteria of measurement, nursing administrators manage this problem by putting emphasis on programs given budgetary support. This emphasis, in the study, was often at variance with the problems encountered by the nurse as she visited the homes of the clients.

In the effort to compete with other community organizations (as well as with other units of the department) for the allocation of funds and resources, the expenditure of money on the nursing program and its personnel,† needs to be justified, and nursing administrators are

* The term applied to a clinic for well children where "preventive" services are emphasized.

† Fifty per cent of the public health budget is spent on the nursing program. The greatest proportion of the public health professional personnel is the nursing staff.

likely to emphasize those aspects of the existing programs that are most easily documented quantitatively. Therefore, the collection and recording of statistical data, such as morbidity, attendance at clinics, and numbers of home visits by program categories made by the public health nurses, are emphasized. This emphasis is reinforced by rewards administered for such activities as how well the nurse organizes her work or keeps records current and shows efficiency in her activities. In this way the staff nurse learns where priorities are placed in her line of work.

Adapting Professional Behavior to Agency Priorities

Where the public health agency prescribed priorities of activities and patterns of behavior for the nurses it placed restrictions on the behavior of the public health nurses. The nurses recognized these restrictions and altered their behavior to fit the circumstances. Some of this behavior they learned by being sensitive to cues and by maneuvering on the spot in a trial-and-error manner. Some they learned from their peers. They learned how to approach delicate situations with a minimum of embarrassment to the clients and themselves. For example, when making a visit regarding the health supervision of an illegitimate child, they learned to ask the person who answered the door if Baby Jones lived at that address. By doing this they avoided asking for "Miss" or "Mrs." Jones, whichever name the client was using. Also, nurses gained information from their peers regarding "good" or "uncooperative clients," which clients may be believed or ignored, and which homes were "just not right."

Some of the values of our society appear at times to be in conflict when examined within the framework of the health system. For example, individuals in the community are expected to be "good" mothers or clients, to take advantage of existing health facilities when advised, to cooperate with health professionals by following the suggestions of physicians, nurses, social workers, etc., and to change and improve their attitudes and practices when health workers believe it is necessary. Moreover, although as professional members of the health team public health nurses are expected to be impartial and to give equal services to everyone, their personal beliefs influence to some degree their professional behavior.

The public health nurses in the sample expressed appreciation, respect, and admiration of clients who tolerated pain and hardships without complaining, especially if the clients managed to remain cheerful. They showed admiration for clients who attempted to be self-sufficient by paying their own way in life, for those who cooperated with them and followed their instructions, and for those who tried to improve their health attitudes and practices. As one nurse stated, "They don't have to stick to it, but they should give it a try. If they are not willing to do that I don't bother with them. I have more important things to do." The majority of their visits were made, then, to clients with whom they anticipated change, and withdrawal of services was made to those who were uncooperative or unappreciative.

The behavior of public health nurses was conditioned and determined by a combination of rules set by society, by their profession, and by the agency. But inevitably the rules did not fit many specific situations. Public health nurses, in the setting of the home, experienced conflict between what was expected of them socially and professionally. Their appearance, which was similar in many respects to that of any visitor since they did not wear a uniform, and the social surroundings of the home where the nurses enacted their professional roles symbolized the problem.

Agency policies and procedures prescribed the behavior and activities of public health nurses for certain types of visits, for example, concerning tuberculosis, but not for others such as mental health, partly because of the difficulty of anticipating the type of questions and problems that might arise in the latter instance. Many of the visits made by nurses lacked clearly defined purposes. One of the most difficult problems of the nurses in the study was to make much of their work seem purposeful to themselves as well as to the clients. Also, the vast number of health problems and issues that were presented in some home visits made it difficult for even the most competent and experienced nurses. For example, in one home alone 29 health problems were presented to one of the nurses in the sample. How many of these the nurse was expected to deal with was not clearly defined.

Therefore, as a coping mechanism, the nurses structured their environment by developing their case load in terms of visits that were prescribed by policies and priority for clients for whom they anticipated change in behavior. They further defined their boundaries by focusing on the specific problem for which the visit was initiated.

Public health nurses in the study, reflecting the agency, tended to approach family health problems from the program–disease–client orientation rather than from the standpoint of the family's existing problems. They focused on clients with specific diseases rather than on all the needs of the client or the family. Therefore, when a nurse visited a family in which the husband had tuberculosis, she was inclined to treat the spouse who had multichronic diseases (about which she may have had very little information) as a "side issue." The agency policy called for a thorough follow-up of tuberculosis for the particular client, but it did not extend to the same degree to others in the family. It appeared at times that when the nurses had not anticipated the problems of the spouses or clients and not allotted the time for recording, it was easier to ignore the problems and in that way not deal with them at all. If they acknowledged additional problems it seemed necessary to put them on family records that frequently involved more time than they had designated for the visit.

At times the nurses in the sample ignored the problems presented by the clients and emphasized the agency problem for which the visit was initiated. For example, one client talked about a pain in her back to the physician in the Child Health Conference in the morning. The problem was not discussed there because the clinic was organized to supervise the health of well babies. This did not include the problems of mothers. In the afternoon, at the request of the observer, the nurse visited the same mother in her home. The mother complained about a pain in her back. This was expressed with tears in her eyes. Since the nurse had not gone to the home to discuss that problem she ignored the pain. Later the observer asked the nurse what she thought was the problem of this young mother. The nurse replied, "I guess she had a pain in her back."

Focusing on one problem to the exclusion of many others might have more feelings of guilt for the nurses than it appeared to, except that there exists a vast number of health problems in the community that remain beyond their supervision. By dealing with the diseases and problems that were identified by the agency prior to the home visit, and thus presumably a reflection of the value system of society, nurses met the expectations of the agency, structured their environment to some extent, and coped with the situation. Also, since society places high value on responsibility and achievement, and since the nurses with their middle-class orientation place high value on the future (i.e., improvement), it is possible that the nurses justified the fact that they ignored problems presented on the spot by the amount of responsibility that the client herself "ought" to take for her health.

DISCREPANCIES BETWEEN PRESCIBED PROFESSIONAL BEHAVIOR AND REALITY

There appeared to be many discrepancies between the prescribed behavior and the reality. There were outstanding gaps between the theory that the nurses were taught and their application of the theory to the practical situation. There were lags in the information that the nurses required regarding recent medical knowledge, equipment, and techniques and the information that they possessed. Discrepancies existed between the nurses' knowledge of certain techniques and the nurses' application of these techniques in the home setting. There were gaps between the demands of the agency and the needs of the clients, and the nurses were caught in the middle. There were gaps between the understanding of the agency and the understanding of the nurses regarding the purpose of many of the visits. Finally, there were gaps between the health standards of the clients and those of the nurses.

The nurses attempted to bridge these gaps. For example, they attempted to apply the theory, techniques, and knowledge to the practical situation in the homes although they experienced great difficulties. It appeared that what they were taught as theory inevitably did not apply to the reality of practice (e.g., in interviewing techniques). They tried to make many of the visits appear purposeful to themselves and the clients by expressing a belief in what they thought was practical in the work situation. For example, they believed that reduction of the social distance that was present in the nurse–client relationship could be achieved by such means as addressing the clients by their first names. However, the social distance maintained by the nurses when they interacted with the clients appeared to vary with the type of visits rather than by the manner of address, contrary to their beliefs. It appeared that when public health nurses were required to enforce certain regulations and had the authority to do so they did this by remaining at a professional distance from the clients regardless of the manner of address used.

Agency Control Affecting Nurses' Behavior

Like many organizations today, public health agencies are bureaucratically organized. They emphasize efficiency, organizational ability, record-keeping, and hierarchy of authority. Formally established rules and regulations insure the uniformity of operations of the agency and provide for continuity of services regardless of changes in personnel and thus promote the stability that seems necessary for the existence of the agency. Recommendations were made by the nursing administrator regarding such activities as the minimum number of visits to be made by each nurse per month, the specific hours of work, and the method of recording data. Control mechanisms were set up by the agency to assure consistency and predictability of behavior and performance of the nurses. Rewards, such as promotions, were given for behavior that related to conformity, punctuality, dependability, and efficiency rather than originality and good interpersonal relationships. Sanctions were administered for failure to comply with the rules of the agency. Although the professional nurse continued to render direct service to her clients, the employer established the limits of the service to be rendered, as well as influenced the kind and quality of her services.

By regulating the working hours of employees the public health nursing administrator made an effort to maximize the contributions of each employee and to maintain a certain degree of consistency and dependability of services to the community. Therefore, nurses in the study worked from 8 AM to 5 PM with no variations that were obvious to the researcher. However, major health problems were missed by some of the nurses because of the rigidity of agency policies regarding working hours. These policies appeared to discourage the exercise of professional judgment by the nurses.

Because of the "system," according to one inexperienced nurse, she was unable to reach the young teenaged girls with illegitimate pregnancies, which was the major health problem of her clients. When the researcher attempted to get an explanation for this, the nurse replied, "They don't get home from school until 4 or 4:30 PM. We go off at 5, and report to the office before that." When the observer questioned her about arriving on duty later some mornings and staying later some evenings in order to reach her target group, she said, "Oh, no. This is never done."

This suggests that the demands of the agency frequently interfered with the nurse's professional judgment and discouraged her from looking at some of the major problems in her district. One nurse mentioned that she was unable to gain rapport with one of her clients and thought she was wasting her time and that of her client by repeated visits. She stated, "I wouldn't be bothered going at all except that Crippled Children's Service expects a report." Another nurse (an inexperienced one) did not use her professional judgment on the spot but followed the prior instructions of her supervisor to the letter of the law. This involved a visit to the home of two elderly women who were contacts of a tuberculosis patient. The name of one of them had been submitted to the health department. It was not until the nurse visited that she realized there were two contacts. However, since the nurse was expected to fill out numerous records on one individual and her superior had briefed her on making the visit to one client, she focused on her and ignored the second individual. Thus, one means of coping with the conflict between the agency's demands and the professional ideal is to take a bureaucratic response and follow the rules laid down by the agency.

The agency studied had recommended policies not only in terms of the number of home visits to be made by each nurse per month but in terms of the number of visits to particular clients each year—for example, those with tuberculosis or orthopedic defects. A few of the nurses in the sample stated that the amount of time and effort spent on follow-up of each client with such community health workers as family physicians, social workers, etc., was not accepted by the supervisors as justification for failure to meet the required number of visits. Therefore, the nurses were in a dilemma as to whether they should contact many clients by telephone or increase their visits to particular homes in order to meet the requirements of the agency regarding number of visits. They were also faced with the conflict of whether to attempt to meet the needs of the clients on the particular day they were in the home or to meet the demands of the agency and return another time if necessary to meet the needs of the clients. A gap existed between the demands of the agency and the needs of the clients; however, because of the system of rewards, the demands of the agency took precedence.

System of Rewards Affecting Nurses' Behavior

Shared values provide the fundamental standard by which the behavior of a person in society is judged and regulated with rewards and sanctions. Rewards may be administered for performance that does not require her to enact her professional role or to exercise her professional judgment. Public health nurses were rewarded by the agency, the physicians, and the clients for their ability to organize efficiently (for example, a child health conference), to record concisely and adequately, and to conform. Frequently the comment was made by physicians at child health conferences to the effect that the nurses were "good organizers." In addition the clients were appreciative of their efficiency and expressed their gratitude. Supervisors also rated them on these characteristics.

This emphasis caused nurses to become overinvolved with records, to ask direct questions, to focus on one person instead of the family, or to interact in the home with the person who gave most information for their records about the particular client. For example, one "patient" who had been discharged from the hospital following surgery was visited by a nurse. He was elderly and hard of hearing, but in spite of this he wanted to talk about his operation. The nurse wanted information for her records and for the family physician. Therefore, it was much more expedient to talk to an informative landlady than to the "patient." The frustrated man found it necessary to tell somebody his problems, so he told them to the observer.

The usual distribution of work load for the staff nurses was on the basis of service to the clients in particular geographical areas or districts. The public health nurses in the agency studied were presumably placed in their particular offices and districts on the basis of existing vacancies and the proximity of the vacant district to their living quarters rather than on experience or education, according to the administrative staff. According to the staff nurses, however, the assignment of districts related to a definite reward system. They expressed the belief that when the nurses were first employed they were assigned to the "undesirable" districts (those districts with "hard-core" problem families), and as the nurses earned rewards they were moved to more "desirable" districts. They also felt that nurses were penalized for misconduct by being sent from a "good" to a "poor" district.

If this system of rewards did operate within the agency, and at least 50% of the inexperienced staff in the study were placed in districts with the greatest number of multiproblem families, one wonders at the logic. From the professional point of view, one would expect the clients' interests to be served more adequately by the more experienced nurse: one who had handled similar problems before and who was more familiar with the resources that could be made available to the client. However, if it is felt that the nurse with more experience has little or no effect on the health status of the client, and therefore it does not matter who is assigned, one might wonder whether the public health nurse is the appropriate person for this group of "hard-core" families, particularly when the visit is not initiated by the client.

"Poor" districts often have a discouraging effect on young nurses. They are less able to see results; they are exposed to many problems and subgroups of clients with whom they have had no prior experience; their peers often make disparaging remarks about such clients; and the clients themselves constantly test the young nurses. This kind of situation can lead to a high turnover among staff as they get discouraged and leave their jobs, or it can reinforce bureaucrative behavior over professional behavior.

EFFECTS OF THE SETTING ON NURSES' BEHAVIOR

Widely accepted theory indicates that the setting influences the behavior of participants in interaction. Society has rather elaborate conventions about the appropriateness of topics in the interaction, depending upon the setting and the relationship of the participants.

Administrators of public health nursing programs as well as staff nurses believe that they should be able to discuss almost any subject that may have an influence on clients' health without showing or causing undue embarrassment. Yet guests in a home are not accustomed to discussing such topics as bowel movements or childbirth. Thus the nurses in the public health agency were expected to ask personal questions for the records of the agency in settings in which it was most difficult to enact professional roles. In attempting to obtain certain information for the agency, the nurses often cut across the boundaries of individual rights and ignored the appropriateness of topics for the setting and for maintaining good relationships with clients.

Many factors contributed to making the setting of the home difficult for the nurses. There was usually lack of privacy; they were sometimes treated rudely by the clients or ignored. Effective communication was difficult at times, and frequently it was hard for the nurses to establish an atmosphere in which the clients felt comfortable and relaxed. Most of the usual mechanisms used by professionals to reduce tension and maintain control were not appropriate for the nurses in someone's home.

There were many distractions and interruptions that frequently increased the length of time of the home visits over the time that might have been needed in an office visit. Sometimes it was difficult for the nurse to identify the client from among other members of the family who may or may not have needed, or thought they needed, help. Some of the activities the nurses participated in caused conflict and embarrassment for the nurses as well as difficulties in maintaining good professional–client relationships. For example, it was not too unusual to observe a nurse demonstrate the use of contraceptives amidst confusion and in front of many people.

One might question the persistance of discussing sensitive topics in the home setting. But information was required by the agency, and the nurses were responsible for obtaining it. One alternative action might have been to encourage meeting with the client in an office setting. However, there was not one incident where a public health nurse interviewed clients in a private office. None of the nurses had a private office, nor was one made available for interviewing. The question might be raised as to why there was not a greater effort made by the agency to provide office accommodations for the staff nurses. It has been suggested that many clients would not have kept office appointments for various reasons and home visits may be the most effective way of achieving the results desired by the agency. Also, there was no attempt made at any time by the nurses to discuss health problems with clients in the nurse's car or at a nearby restaurant. Such a setting did not seem to fit the professional image held by the nurses, the administrator, or the clients. This may also be related to the difficulty public health nurses have in defining their role in terms of "talking" instead of "doing," since the customary symbols, such as uniforms, used by professionals to define the legitimacy of the professional–client relationship were absent.

EFFECTS OF INTERAGENCY AND INTERPROFESSIONAL DEMANDS ON NURSES

In addition to the health department, other health and social agencies operate as part of the network of systems responsible for some aspects of "well-being" in the community. Each agency makes certain claims to legitimacy, formal or informal, and may negotiate with one another regarding boundaries and management of health problems.

Health services to the community were fragmented, resulting in gaps and overlaps of services, as well as friction and conflict among the health workers who may have differed from one another even regarding the philosophy of public health. The community may tolerate such conditions of inefficiency partly because these problems are not consciously made explicit and partly because many individuals benefited from the overlap of programs. The client can maintain some control by playing one agency against another. For example, the frequency with which clients in the study informed the nurses of contradictory instructions by social workers and family physicians may have been an indication of attempts made by the client to manipulate the situation rather than attempt to resolve actual discrepancies among the expectations of the professionals.

Occasionally the nurses encountered other health workers (social workers, probation officers, etc.) at the time of their home visits. Many families had several health workers visiting regularly, and there seemed to be little evidence of cross communication. At times the nurses found that other professional workers had contradicted their recommendations regarding health procedures outlined by the family physicians. This made it difficult for the nurses to meet the needs of the clients and maintain their customary professional–client relationships without showing negative differential behavior toward other professionals. The nurses tended to resolve these problems by avoiding open conflict with other professional workers, by showing differential behavior toward them in front of the clients, and by taking a more forceful position in relation to instructions to the client.

On one occasion the public health nurse and the social worker disagreed as to whether the mother was a "fit" mother to have her infant with her. The physician, whom both of them had contacted, would not make the decision. Therefore, both professionals visited this young single woman, but for different reasons. The social worker visited to prepare the woman for the likelihood of her not keeping her child, while the nurse visited to prepare her in some way for motherhood—baby-bathing, formula-making, etc. On one of the two visits the nurse made to this client with the researcher, she found the social worker present. Neither of the professionals communicated to the other beyond a greeting. When the nurse communicated with the client, the social worker rephrased her statements, thus acting as an interpreter. Frequently there appeared to be lack of communication between professional workers over clients, even between divisions within the same health agency. For example, one nurse visited a client regarding the report of an X ray. She discovered that the client had been back to the health department for further follow-up and X rays and that the family physician had been notified. However, as a representative of the agency, she had not been notified.

With advances in technological and scientific knowledge resulting in increased specialization and professionalization, there is evidence of a greater variety of health workers in the community. This suggests problems for public health personnel of providing specialized and high quality services for an entire population while at the same time giving personalized care to each client. This also poses a problem of redistribution of functions among health workers, as well as among health agencies, adding to the problem of communication and interpersonal relationships.

Projection for the Future

Two aspects of the management of the professional role within the administrative organization are how the organization copes with influencing the ideally autonomous judgment of the professional in order to relate effectively with its environment and serve its mission, and how the professional as an individual copes with conflicting demands and expectations when acting as the agent of his organization in interactions with the client.

There are subtle ways in which the application of administrative controls can affect the behavior of the members of the organization by the management of time and place of operations and through both explicit and implicit reward systems. Professional groups control their membership through the development of a professional ethos, a feeling of belonging, and by calling on normative ideals of behavior that come to be represented by a mythology and belief system. In the administrative organization, with a diffuse and general mission, this mythology and belief system of the professional may be incorporated as part of the mythology of the organization. However, actual behavior, as compared with ideal normative behavior, may range widely from the desirable.

We seem to be in a period of transition in relation to formal health organizations and patterns of health practice. With recent legislation requiring a focus on planning in the health field, with regionalization now gaining substantial backing; with emphasis on the "whole patient" and on the role of the consumer in establishing priorities of health, it appears that the professional will be faced with greater uncertainty in his roles that require face-to-face relationships with his agency's clients. If the more formal departmental structures give way to a more flexible arrangement whereby facilities and specialized skills of individuals will be made available where and when needed, without much regard for the jurisdictional assignments that have usually characterized governmental health services, it may well provide the opportunity for the professional worker to exhibit greater individuality and creativity in meeting the needs of clients.

Planning, however, emphasizes the rationalization of activities and the efficient allocation of scarce resources, including the time of professional personnel. As a move toward a more rational health system, health care activities, especially those now carried out by the private physician, will likely be brought into some kind of administrative organization. This study of nurse–client interactions has indicated some of the effects of bureaucratic needs of the organization on the performance and judgment of the health worker at the operational level. As new organizational forms and structures develop for the provision of health care services, it becomes important to study the effects of organizational demands on the role of the professional in the administrative organization. It may be of interest to note that one nurse in the study had a unique role as liaison between a group of private physicians and the agency. She was employed by the agency, but her referrals to clients came from the physicians. (This was a research project in the agency.) There were distinct differences in her behavior compared to the other nurses in the sample. She did not exhibit the same agency authority as did the other nurses; she did not emphasize agency priorities and was free to deal with whatever topic or problems the client presented.

It is essential to recognize that in the design of health service systems efficiency control must be related to effectiveness criteria, especially when integrating the professional into the administrative organization. The behavior of the people within an organizational system is a vital component of the system design.

7

The Professional Association and Collective Bargaining: The Case of the American Nurses Association

Joseph A. Alutto

PROFESSIONALISM AND COLLECTIVE BARGAINING

The terms "professional" and "collective bargaining" traditionally have been considered mutually exclusive. That is, it has been assumed that the very essence of professionalism precluded the utilization of collective bargaining techniques by members of any professional group. Under these conditions participation by professionals in activities such as contract negotiations and strikes were considered particularly inappropriate.

With the passage of time, however, many individuals, both professional and nonprofessional, have altered their conceptions of the relationship between professionalism and traditional collective bargaining activities. That the exclusion of bargaining activities from the realm of appropriate professional action is presently repudiated by many professional groups may be found daily in almost any newspaper. One quickly discovers that across the United States—in areas as diverse as New York, Illinois, Montana, and California—groups of professionals such as teachers and nurses are either threatening to strike or actually are striking their employers.[1] Despite these instances of overt economic warfare, peaceful negotiations between employers and various professional groups are becoming increasingly the rule rather than the exception.

Since over the years designations of "legitimate" professional behavior apparently have changed, there exists a temptation to engage automatically in lengthy discussions of the "elements of professionalism" whenever the work activity of an occupational group is labeled professional in nature. Such explorations have been both numerous and in substantial agreement concerning the characteristics of professionalism.[2] For our purposes it is important to take note of three frequently identified characteristics of most professions. First, professional groups are typified by some form of collective behavior. This collective action is usually taken in regard to the establishment of minimum standards of employment or practice. A second characteristic of professionalism is the existence of one (or more) professional association authorized to act as the representative of individuals practicing within a given occupation. A final recurring theme concerns the nature of professional employment. The very fact of employment by an institution, as opposed to the alleged private entrepreneurial practice of the physician (who may merely work in an organization), is often identified as a major source of dissatisfaction for members of professions as diverse as engineering, teaching, and nursing. At least in an ideal sense it appears that professionalism assumes complete control by professionals over all conditions of their employment (e.g., entry requirements, work loads, and the evaluation of work performance).

Turning to general industrial relations literature,[3] one finds numerous indications that in the past collective bargaining techniques have proven most effective when backed by the unified efforts of some occupational group. These activities also have been most fruitful when employed in attempts to improve working conditions (including wages, working hours, and work loads) deemed undesirable by employees. Finally, viable collective bargaining strategies traditionally presuppose the existence of a formally designated representative for participating employees. Thus it can be seen that the prerequisites for effective utilization of collective bargaining techniques are quite similar to the factors identified as most typical of professional groups. It should therefore not be surprising that efforts by professionals to control their own conditions of employment have resulted in the adoption of collective bargaining activities.

Nevertheless, there appear to be two major difficulties that must be overcome by professionals who attempt to engage in collective bargaining activities. The first problem concerns the very limited conception of professionalism maintained by many individuals. There are those who still believe that professionalism and collective bargaining are incompatible in both concept and practice. It is for this reason that many professional associations advocate the employment of bargaining techniques under the guise of euphemisms such as "professional negotiations" or "informal discussions" (i.e., contract negotiations) and "mass resignations" or "concerted sick calls" (i.e., strikes). To at least a limited extent it appears possible to maintain a conservative image of professionalism by avoiding the use of "nonprofessional terms" while simultaneously exhibiting behavior quite similar to that of traditional blue-collar unionism.

The second major dilemma facing professionals who desire to bargain collectively involves the determination of how one develops, establishes, and maintains control over the organizations required in order to achieve an effective implementation of collective bargaining policies. While this may be considered primarily a question of organizational design, decisions concerning design are crucial since it has been discovered that any structure formed by a voluntary organization for the purpose of negotiating employment contracts tends to increase in power until it dominates the remaining structure—one originally established for the purpose of nursing "democracy" and effective day-to-day operation.[4]

As a species, professionals have not arrived at any consistent response to this question of organizational design. Some engineers have chosen to form unions that operate independently of any professional associations and fulfill the sole function of serving as a vehicle for bargaining over conditions of employment.[5] Teachers have evolved at least two separate and distinct institutions: a militant union-affiliated group envisioned as concerned primarily with issues of "wages and hours" and conservative professional associations viewed as devoted to purely "professional issues." In practice these organizations compete for the membership of teachers since, as indicated during interviews with various officials of these groups, the "union" is increasingly concerned with "professional" issues and the "professional associations" are adopting many activities and policies traditionally labeled issues of "wages and hours." As discussed in a later section of this paper, nurses have chosen somewhat of a middle ground.[6] They have evolved a structure for handling collective bargaining issues that is separate and distinct from the structure devoted to typical "professional concerns," although these structural arrangements exist within the same over-all institution—the American Nurses Association.

While the remainder of this paper discusses the nursing profession in general, the personal and professional attributes of nurses and the characteristics of their professional association are of primary concern. Major emphasis therefore is placed upon an examination of the structure of the American Nurses Association, with respect to both its over-all organization and the structure it has evolved for purposes of collective bargaining. Finally, based upon the preceding analyses, suggestions for future changes in the American Nurses Association structure is developed and presented.

CHARACTERISTICS OF PROFESSIONAL NURSING

Prior to an understanding and evaluation of any professional association a review of the general characteristics of its professional clientele is necessary. As a means of achieving this initial goal we will briefly develop and examine a profile of the "average" nurse:

In term of personal characteristics such an individual would be female (less than 1% of all employed nurses are males).[7] She would be married (approximately 72% of all registered nurses share this status) and somewhere between thirty and fifty years of age.[8] In addition, this hypothetical nurse would probably end her professional career, either permanently or temporarily, soon after reaching the age of thirty.[9] Thus our typical nurse is really not a full-time, career-oriented professional seeking fulfillment primarily through nursing activities. Furthermore, the well-known demands to which she is exposed by virtue of her American motherhood would curtail any nursing employment during her potentially most productive professional years. Finally, as a wife and mother our nurse's income would probably be utilized to supplement that of her husband.

Employment characteristics for our typical nurse would be as follows: She would probably be employed by a hospital (as are 65% of all employed nurses) to work the lowest nursing staff position, that of a general duty nurse.[10] Her pay would be below that of almost all other professional and technical personnel, either within or outside the health industry.[11] Although the current and projected total demand for nurses would be greater than any available supply of personnel, our nurse may or may not find her services highly valued. This will be a direct result of the localized nature of labor markets for nursing personnel.[12] As a wife and mother this typical nurse probably would be loath to travel great distances to reach her place of work and even less likely to move her family in order to capitalize upon wages offered in various sections of the country. She would also find little spare time for participating in after-work activities, such as nursing association meetings, which might result in concerted efforts to achieve higher pay. Finally, since the net amount of her take-home pay may be of primary concern, our typical nurse would probably consider leaving her profession if a better paying, nonnursing position became available.

The professional characteristics of this "ideal" nurse are such that she would have completed a 3-year training program in a diploma-granting institution (as will 86% of all other nurses).[13] In addition, she would not be a member of her professional association (only 27% of all employed nurses are members of the American Nurses Association).[14] This nurse also would be faced with great uncertainty and conflict concerning her nursing duties. She would find herself the recipient of conflicting demands emanating from fellow nurses as well as from her employer and other related medical personnel.[15] Thus our typical nurse would not have the bachelor's degree now regarded as the minimum symbol of "professionalism."[16] She would also have little contact with and receive little direct help from her weakened professional association. Finally, upon entering or remaining in her profession she would be exposed to a degree of role conflict that would increase the attraction of withdrawal from nursing.

Given the above "profile" one is forced to agree with Surgeon General Stewart who recently characterized nursing as a vastly troubled profession.[17] It is a profession weakened by (1) the personal characteristics of its members, (2) the highly segmented and localized nature of its employing institutions, (3) the increased demands for nursing services that have not been accompanied by adequate increases in the supply of nurses, and (4) confusion as to the role nurses should play in medical organizations.

THE AMERICAN NURSES ASSOCIATION

As with all organizations, the present structure and functions of the American Nurses Association have evolved over a long period of time.[18] In 1893, as a step toward standardizing the quality of nursing, the American Society of Superintendents of Training Schools for Nurses of the United States and Canada was formed. This organization was not open to all nurses and, in response to requests for a general membership organization, in 1896 the Nurses Associated Alumnae of the United States and Canada was created. These two organizations, under different names, eventually represented the major interest groups within professional nursing. In 1912 the American Nurses Association (the renamed Nurses Associated Alumnae as of 1911) and the National League for Nursing Education (the new name of the Society of Superintendents) joined in the publication of the *American Journal of Nursing,* thereby making the journal the official organ of the nursing profession.

By 1912 the ANA had evolved as the largest and most representative nursing body. The Association reorganized and became a federation of state nurses associations in 1922, with voting power vested in a House of Delegates.

Professional nurses, however, apparently did not feel adequately represented by the two most prominent nursing organizations (the ANA and the NLNE). Consequently, over the years various special interest groups formed separate organizations which, as a result of competing for members, power, and prestige, threatened to disrupt whatever unity existed within professional nursing. As a result of this danger, a general reorganization of nursing associations was undertaken in 1952. The American Nurses Association was broadened in purpose to become "a professional association of nurses, in which nurses work for the continuing improvement of professional practice, the economic and general welfare of nurses, and the health needs of the American public."[19] Six nursing groups were merged into the National League for Nursing, an association complementary to the American Nurses Association and concerned with general problems of nursing service. Unlike the ANA, this organization was not meant to be a professional association and, therefore, admitted interested nonprofessionals. The purpose of this association was to organize "all members of the health team, agencies supplying nursing service and education, and lay members of the community, representing all races, creeds and national origins, to act together to provide the best possible nursing services and to assure good nursing education."[20]

It was thought that these two organizations would adequately and efficiently represent nursing. However, dissatisfaction with this solution may be found throughout nursing literature.

It is important to note that the American Nurses Association is a multipurpose professional association. The Association is devoted to (1) improving the quality of nursing practice, (2) enhancing the economic rewards received by nurses, and (3) securing an adequate supply of trained nurses. Many of the difficulties experienced by the ANA may be traced to attempts to pursue all three goals simultaneously. It would appear that while greater numbers of nursing personnel may be secured by political action at the national level the first two goals require action at the state (e.g., licensing procedures) and local (e.g., collective bargaining) levels. Most changes in ANA structure, including the most recent alteration discussed below, have had greatest impact at the national level.

GENERAL ANA STRUCTURE

At present the American Nurses Association membership consists solely of registered professional nurses employed in all occupational subdivisions within the nursing profession. Individual membership is categorized as active or associate (referring to nurses who are retired or inactive).

Structurally, the ANA is a federation of 54 constituent associations: the 50 United States, the District of Columbia, the Panama Canal Zone, Puerto Rico, and the Virgin Islands. State associations are in turn composed of constituent district associations and sections. Until 1966 total ANA membership had been divided into district, state, and national sections according to occupational specialties within the nursing profession. While this is presently continued at state and district levels, as of 1967 occupational grouping is achieved through five "divisions" at the national level.[21]

Programs and policies of the ANA are determined by its House of Delegates. Members of state occupational groupings elect representatives to the Association House of Delegates, who in turn vote for the Board of Directors. Between conventions Association activities are conducted by standing and special committees and the Board of Directors. A national headquarters and administrative staff is maintained.

Representation in the House of Delegates is shared by the state associations and existing sections in a state. Through proportionate representation by sections it is hoped there will be assurance that association policies are determined by representatives from all occupational groups. Thus, in effect, nurses have double representation, first through general membership in a state association and second as a result of participating through representatives from occupational specialty groupings.

It is important to recall at this point that the state and district associations all have the same general form of government as does the national association. In each state association's house of delegates there are representatives from the district associations, as well as representatives from occupational groupings within the state. These representatives then elect a board of directors. On the district level a board of directors is elected that consists of some members elected by the total membership and, if possible, the elected representatives of district sections. These associations, national, state, and district, cut across the membership on a horizontal basis rather than on a vertical basis as do the occupational specialty units. This overlapping membership may be viewed as an attempt to combine the virtue of organization in terms of skill levels (as in the case of trade unions) and the advantages of organization on the basis of general participation in an occupation (as in the instance of industrial unions).[22]

As has been stated, in the general structure of the American Nurses Association the sections have occupied a representative role of importance. The ANA recognizes 8 occupational sections: counselors, executive secretaries, and registrars; educational administrators, consultants, and teachers; general duty nurses; nursing service administrators; occupational health nurses; office nurses; private duty nurses; and public health nurses. Upon joining the ANA a nurse becomes a member of the established section representing her occupational specialty.

Of important consequence has been the relationship of occupational specialty units to parent organizations. The Board of Directors of respective nurses associations (district or state) establish sections, approve rules and procedures, allocate funds from the general treasury, and also possess the authority to dissolve a section. While the national association recognizes 8 occupational sections, it is up to the particular state board of directors to determine when a section will be established within that state.

The primary function of any section is the representation of specialty group interests in the development of relevant programs and general policies. All implementation of programs is left to the national, state, and district associations. This also appears to be the purpose of the 5 newly created national level divisions: community health; geriatric; medical–surgical; psychiatric and mental health nursing practice; and maternal and child health. These divisions, however, are designed to serve the somewhat more general purpose of establishing relationships between nursing specialties and related, though nonnursing, medical groups.[23]

Figure 1 may prove helpful in visualizing the previously discussed organizational structure presently in existence.[24] With this idea of the general organizational structure of the ANA in mind, it now is

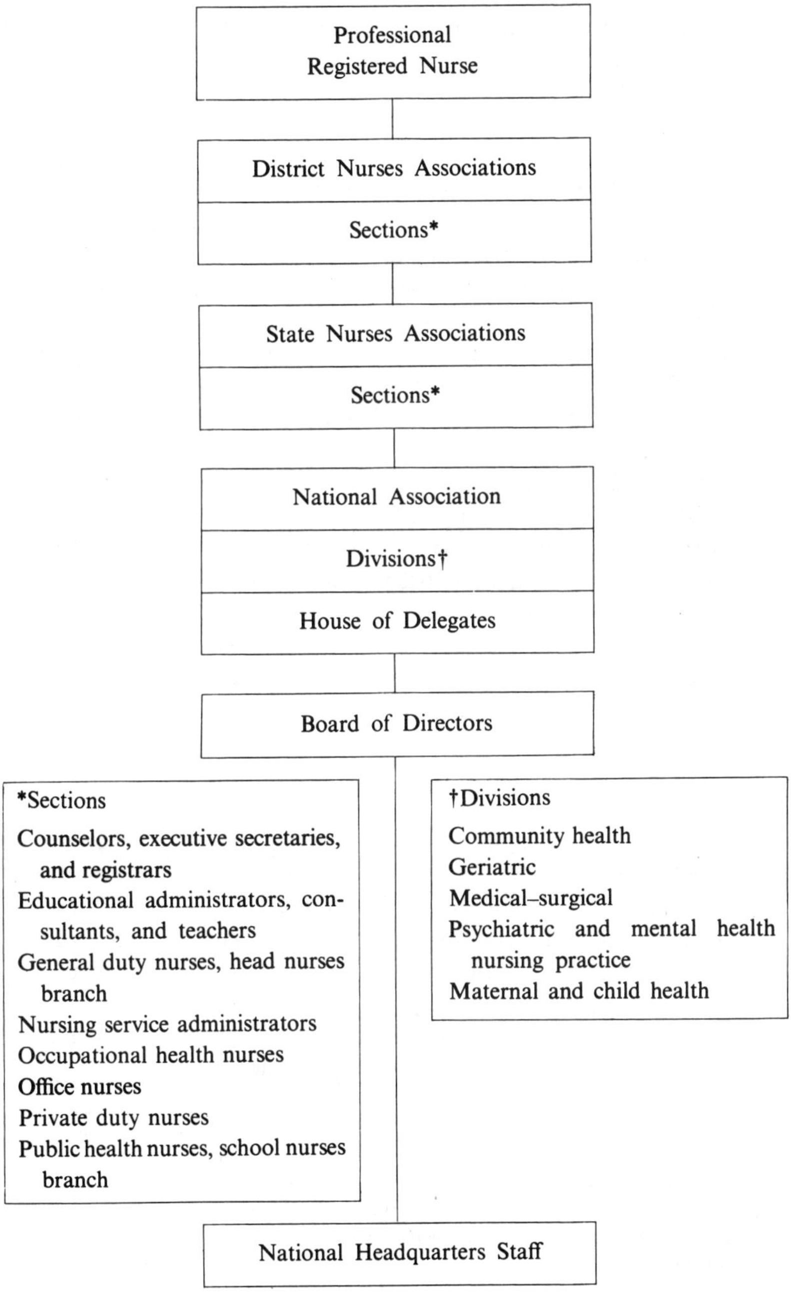

FIGURE 1. *Membership Organization Chart, American Nurses Association*

possible to focus upon the specific structure utilized for purposes of collective bargaining.

NURSES AND COLLECTIVE BARGAINING*

The economic status of the nursing profession traditionally has been considered rather low.[25] This appears to have resulted in great dissatisfaction within nursing and a decrease in the popularity of nursing as a potential career. These two reactions, in addition to a greater number of hospitals in the United States and an increase in the quality of health care (each of which results in a greater demand for nurses), have led to a shortage of nurses.

As early as 1928 some nurses joined trade unions in attempts to increase their economic well-being.[26] It is believed that this movement failed to gain momentum because nurses generally felt that collective bargaining, and the industrial strike with which it became associated, was not appropriate for professional practitioners.[27] Nevertheless, the experience of having nurses leave their professional organization in an attempt to improve conditions of employment served to heighten ANA concern over economic matters.

The depression and consequent unemployment of the 1930s had, as one result, a realization by professional associations that professional idealism did not render practitioners immune from the economics of the labor market. These organizations sought to alleviate the economic hardships of their members by participating in job placement programs and establishing economic standards for the employment of professionals. Thus professionals in general became accustomed to utilizing their associations as vehicles for achieving economic improvement. When the depression ended and the inflation brought on by World War II had its impact, professionals, including nurses, demanded stronger economic action by their organizations.

* "Collective bargaining" is employed in referring to the establishment and utilization of formal procedures whereby representatives of an employing institution meet with representatives of nurses employed by that organization in order to determine the economic conditions under which professional nurses will perform their nursing duties. The term "economic conditions" may include pay, sick days, job assignments, vacations, work schedules, and the host of other activities directly bearing upon whether a nurse will work in any *given* organization. The establishment of licensing regulations, pay procedures, general rules, and guidelines by state or federal law is not considered an indication of the existence of collective bargaining, even though such events may result from ANA activities of a political nature.

In 1946 the ANA officially initiated its Economic Security Program. This program was founded on the principle that while a nurse has an obligation to give conscientious service she is entitled to "just" remuneration in return. Initially stated program objectives offer an indication of what the ANA sought to accomplish through its implementation. Goals of the Economic Security Program were:

> wider acceptance of the forty hour week and establishment of minimum salaries, increased participation of nurses in the actual planning and administration of nursing service through the nurses association, development of collective bargaining techniques by state nurses associations, restriction of nurses to one organization which can act as a bargaining agent, and elimination of barriers to the employment of minority racial groups.[28]

Early in 1950 the ANA adopted a policy whereby professional nurses voluntarily relinquished the right to strike. Therefore, in order to achieve recognition as bargaining agent for any nurses employed in a particular hospital, nursing organizations were forced to rely upon informal influence over the administrator, public pressure, or legislation that compelled recognition by the administrator. This last means is definitely the most effective. Other than in a few cases of special legislation, however, voluntary hospitals, which constitute the majority of hospitals, do not come under Taft–Hartley Act provisions or many statewide "little Taft–Hartley acts."[29] Thus administrators in such hospitals are not legally "compelled" to bargain with or recognize nursing representatives. This has proven to be a serious stumbling block in the utilization of collective bargaining practices by professional nurses.[30]

ANA STRUCTURE FOR COLLECTIVE BARGAINING PURPOSES

The ANA's Economic Security Program was formulated as a means of eliminating employment conditions felt to be inconsistent with the professional responsibilities of nurses. Since the program's inception the ANA has developed guiding principles and policies, a technical staff, and other resources and facilities with which to help state nurses associations implement suggested economic standards. During the development of this program it was believed that the national association could neither function as a bargaining agent nor work closely enough with local groups of nurses to perform the frequently recurring activities required in order to achieve continuous economic improvement. Consequently, the national association's role has always been to act as a *guide, interpreter*, and *clearing house* for the state associations, in addition to being a general sponsor and supporter of favorable legislation on a national level. State associations are responsible for implementing aspects of the economic security program. Therefore, the adoption and implementation of various collective bargaining functions depends upon individual state associations.

Unlike the implementation of other policies, however, the economic security program places great stress upon local units. A local unit is an organization of professional nurses regularly employed at the same level in one institution, plant, or agency.* The primary purpose of such a unit is to bring about specific improvements in employment conditions for a limited number of nurses.[31] State associations usually provide assistance in the form of services from industrial relations, public relations, and legal experts. District or state associations also act as designated bargaining representatives for groups of nurses if, as is common, a local unit requests such behavior.

Local units may be considered the most important structural divisions for evolving successful implementation of professionally recommended employment standards. The ANA's collective bargaining structure *presupposes* strong and active local units. If it is remembered that, unlike instances of general policy implementation by the ANA, in the generation of collective bargaining relationships the local unit is of central importance, it becomes readily apparent that the relative importance and effectiveness of district or state associations is contingent upon developing stable local units.

It is interesting to note that the ANA existed as a national organization prior to the creation of any local units. In this respect the Association's growth differs markedly from that experienced by national trade unions. National trade unions appear to have been created by uniting many pre-existing, though isolated, local unions.[32] Therefore, unlike the ANA, national unions were able to rely upon the resources of ongoing organizations concerned with the everyday, work-related problems of members. The ANA has been forced to encourage and support the initial growth of such basic organizational building blocks.

Figure 2 presents the major structural units involved in implementing collective bargaining and other economic security program policies.

* In most instances this would mean nurses employed in one hospital. However, as in the instance of negotiations with state or governmental agencies the unit may encompass nurses employed in the many hospitals controlled by that agency—e.g., the New York City Department of Hospitals.

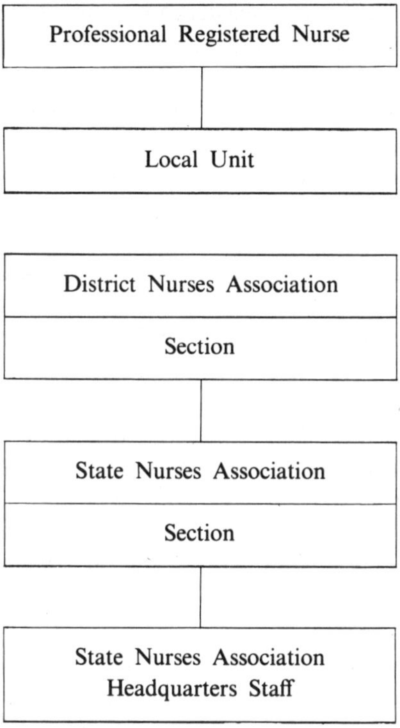

FIGURE 2.

It should be noted that for purposes of negotiating conditions of employment the local unit intervenes between the individual nurse and her district and state associations, as well as between the nurse and her section representatives. This is a significant departure from the general membership structure of the ANA.

PRESENT CONDITIONS

The American Nurses Association has undergone major changes in philosophy and operation in 1958, 1962, 1964, and most recently in 1966. The major purpose for each structural alteration has been the desire to design a voluntary organization that is both effective and truly responsive to its members' wishes, i.e., a democratic and voluntary association capable of efficiently achieving the professional goals of all nurses. As has been noted by Merton and others, this is an ambitious and difficult task because the existence of democratic procedures often leads to the inefficient utilization of time and other resources in the course of decision-making.[33]

While the ANA has certainly evidenced a willingness and ability to change, this dynamism has not been without reason. Latest statistical information published by the ANA indicated that although an estimated 640,000 nurses are employed on either a part-time or full-time basis only 173,000 nurses were classified as ANA members; thus approximately 27% of all employed nurses are ANA members.[34] This compares with a 1960 membership that included 32% of all employed nurses.[35] The problem assumes greater relevance when it is realized that during both periods (1960 and 1967) employed nurses accounted for only about two-thirds of all nurses licensed to practice in the United States, i.e., total ANA clientele. When these additional nurses are included in membership calculations, it appears that in 1960 24% of all nurses licensed to practice were ANA members while in 1967 this figure reached only 20%. Thus the ANA is forced to rely upon only a small portion of the total nursing population in order to both generate resources and determine policies that represent the desires of a majority of nurses.

Given the previously stated aspects of (1) ANA history and structure, (2) its failure to formally attract large numbers of potential members, and (3) its desire to remain an effective democratic organization, what structural change might lead to increased organizational effectiveness—an effectiveness measured in terms of increased membership and the promulgation of policies that reflect the feelings of nurses across the United States? One approach to answering this question is to examine a few of the factors that determine how and why individuals voluntarily participate in organizations.

CORRELATES OF PARTICIPATION

A great deal of theoretical and empirical research has been conducted by behavioral scientists and organizational analysts that focuses upon participation by members of an organization in institutional affairs. The following three propositions are particularly pertinent to our discussion:

1. "Clientele attraction and participation in an organization will tend to be greatest when there exists perceived personal agreement with group goals or policies."[36]

Basically, what is being said is that individuals will be most attracted to, and participate most extensively in, organizations whose policies are most consistent with their own feelings or attitudes. When the obverse is true, and formal organizations advocate policies dissonant with personal predispositions, individuals will be motivated to avoid commitment to and participation in such systems.

This leads one to believe that a crucial issue facing the ANA concerns positions taken on general policies. If the Association advocates controversial policies it can count upon alienating clientele, i.e., both present and potential ANA members. Thus arises the question: Does the ANA wish to be "all things to all people or only some things to some people"? The ultimate decision will be vital in determining the representativeness of the ANA.[37] Will it become an organization representing "fringe" views or, instead, the views of some majority? If individual nurses are professionals they are theoretically capable of censoring and rewarding each other through their professional association. No individual segment of a population of professionals should be able to determine the nature of professional activities, especially when this overrides the wishes of a majority. In fact, due to its "professional" nature it would appear that the ANA must strive to represent the policies of at least a majority of nurses if it is to remain a professional association of nurses and not simply a special interest group.

2. "The greater the degree of participation by individual members in organizational affairs the more similar will become their views and the policies advocated by the organization."[38]

By and large an individual does not agree with all the policies of an organization upon becoming a member. Rather, he usually agrees with policies particularly important and salient to him. A newcomer will tolerate dissonant policies as long as they do not concern his main reason for becoming a group member. In such a situation he will still join and participate in group affairs.

After initial membership is secured, however, this increase in participation leads to an interactive or feedback effect between the member and the organization. The individual affects group policies through participation, and group policies affect an individual's attitudes. Therefore, the greater the member's participation in organizational affairs the greater the degree to which the organization "represents" his views (regardless of whether organizational policies or individual attitudes have undergone the greatest degree of modification).

The dynamics underlying this increased correspondence between personal attitudes and organizational policies are complex. But important factors include (1) the increased exposure of the individual and group to communications reinforcing both individual member and group positions and (2) the importance of quieting any doubt concerning the symbolic meaning of an act of commitment to an organization. The result of these two factors would be an increase in the *perceived* agreement between the attitudes of individual nurses and the policies advocated by the ANA.

In any event, while the Association might be forced to temper or moderate some of its more progressive policies in order to secure greater initial membership and membership participation, all is not lost for the "progressives." As a matter of fact, the chances are very good that over time progressive programs will be more successfully implemented as a result of an initial "go-slow" policy. With greater participation should come greater acceptance and effectiveness of policy execution.*

3. "The greater the visibility of benefits derived from organizational membership to the total clientele the larger the number of individuals who will join and/or participate in organizational activities."[39]

It is not enough for an organization such as the ANA simply to secure benefits for members and any residual clientele. If the Association is to make itself attractive to potential and present members it must make the benefits of joining "visible." As a thinking animal whose time is a precious and scarce resource, a nurse does not wish to know that "it's nice" to join the ANA. Rather, she must find readily apparent the benefits to be received in return for her participation investment.

One solution for this difficulty would involve the utilization of mass communications techniques. Public messages sponsored by the ANA and its constituents would result in general public and nursing clientele acquaintance with at least fringe activities of the ANA. Unfortunately, due to problems generated by the selectivity of perception, many such announcements are "tuned out" and, therefore, of limited effectiveness.

A few studies indicate that a viable approach would be to increase the visibility of ANA benefits right at the work place.[40] For the vast majority of nurses their only contact with other professionals is that which occurs while exhibiting nursing skills. What better vehicle for clarifying the benefits to be derived from joining a professional association than the ever present and important work group? Unfortunately,

* For example, it has been reported that in New York State the state nurses association has increased its membership totals by allowing nonmember nurses to participate in organizational affairs concerning collective bargaining. It appears that many of these individuals eventually join their professional nurses association.

present general ANA structure is such that attendance at nonwork functions is necessary before the advantages of ANA membership become apparent.

ONE STRUCTURAL SOLUTION

On the basis of past performance one may question the appropriateness of present ANA structure for generating an organization in which a majority of nurses participates.* Nevertheless, existing over-all structural arrangements may contain the seed for future survival and growth. This potentially potent mechanism is the "local unit"—an organizational subdivision whose membership is composed of nurses, working for the same employing institution, who wish to engage in collective bargaining activities.

At present a local unit is utilized almost exclusively for purposes of collective bargaining. Since it appears that collective bargaining activities are not currently acceptable to a majority of the nursing population, local units are found only infrequently. The current arrangement requires that nurses approve of collective bargaining techniques *prior* to formation of a unit. It is proposed here that local units become basic general membership units. In so doing the initial formation of these groupings would not be retarded as in previous experience since it would require *no prior* commitment to collective bargaining activities. In practice, ANA members automatically would become members of the local unit attached to their employing institution.

Establishing local units as the basic membership unit would have the following advantages: First, it would allow local nurses to proceed as "progressively" as desired. Nurses might be attracted to the unit and the ANA due to their concern with general nursing problems or, on the other hand, attraction may be the result of their concern over local nursing problems. In any event, local units as general membership organizations would encourage nurses with both orientations to become active in ANA programs.

Second, creation of local units would facilitate the discussion of general professional and specific organizational issues. In the area of labor union administration it long has been acknowledged that the

* This participation need not be in any "physical" sense. As is discussed later, it is possible to participate in organizational affairs through the efforts of others.

interests of organizational members often can be more readily ascertained through informal discussion at the work place than through formal large-scale general membership meetings.[41] Interpersonal communications between organizational members are usually more effective and satisfying than any mass, impersonal dissemination of information. In addition, such informal interaction would result in maximum participation and minimal inconvenience for nurses with nonprofessional obligations, e.g., a family. Even these traditionally inactive, nonjoining, family-oriented members could participate while "on the job" and would be encouraged to do so *within* the unit structure.

Third, officials of these local units could act as quasi-shop stewards and represent all nurses in a hospital at section, district, state, or national activities. Development of these proposed general membership units would not obviate the need for present structural subdivisions. Rather, it would merely provide an opportunity for all unit nurses to benefit from, and be represented by, the work of the few "nursing activists" found on all hospital staffs. In addition, nurses unattached to units might continue to affiliate directly with district, state, national, and occupational specialty organizations.

Fourth, utilization of these local units would increase the visibility of professional association benefits to a greater percentage of the nursing clientele, both present and potential members. As has been indicated, one effective means of securing and maintaining clientele participation is through the maintenance of highly salient, visible membership benefits.

Fifth, these units could take advantage of nursing "work place identifications." Nurses often think in terms of their employing institutions.[42] They identify with a particular employing hospital and focus upon the difficulties encountered there. Local units, however, would certainly not preclude "skill level identifications" as well.[43] Indeed they might even foster such identifications by informing members of the existence and advantages of participating in occupational specialty groups within the over-all ANA structure.

Finally, if unit members ever desired to employ collective bargaining techniques the local unit would provide a ready-made vehicle for initiating and organizing such activity. It would not be necessary for nurses to design and organize a separate organizational structure in order to advance their economic interests. Professional and economic activities would be generated from one structural base, which should lead to more consistent policy implementation.

Of course there are problems inherent in this approach. For example, such a change would result in increased decentralization of decision-making. If for no other reason, this would occur because of the existence of large numbers of units attached to isolated hospitals. In turn this would cause greater emphasis to be placed upon problems of coordination between local, state, and national professional nursing association units. Nevertheless, this very well may be an essential characteristic of any effective professional association. It appears that extensive representation of divergent opinion is a better measure of effectiveness for professional organizations than the development of a highly centralized and efficient decision-making unit of limited representativeness.

SUMMARY

The following ideas have been developed, presented, and discussed in this chapter:

1. Collective bargaining on the part of professionals, including nurses, has become increasingly common. However, two major problems face all professionals who seek to bargain collectively: First, how is it possible to alter the attitudes of the many professionals who believe that such behavior is illegitimate or at best inappropriate? Second, how can the organizations required for collective bargaining purposes be designed in such a manner as to neither accumulate inordinate organizational power nor deter professional associations from achieving more general and traditional client-centered goals?

2. In part due to the characteristics of nursing personnel and their profession, the American Nurses Association has been unable to attract a majority of the clientele it seeks to represent. While the Association has developed a separate, though internal, structure for the purpose of collective bargaining, it has failed to take full advantage of the local unit concept.

3. The ANA is a multigoal organization. Activities of the ANA at the national level appear to be most effective in terms of securing favorable educational legislation supporting basic and advanced training as well as the retraining of those returning to nursing (e.g., the Nurse Training Act of 1964). State associations and sections (or divisions) must achieve goals such as upgrading nursing practices and improving state licensing regulations. In general, state and district associations, operating in conjuction with local units, will be most effective in achieving greater economic rewards for nurses. This proposed emphasis upon local autonomy for nursing organizations

resulted from an examination of (1) the general characteristics of nursing personnel, (2) the extremely localized nature of most institutions employing nurses, and (3) organizational and general behavioral science research concerning factors that lead to individual participation in organizations. In this manner one is led to conclude that in order to generate a broader base of support among nursing clientele the ANA should allocate major resources to the development of strong state and district associations as well as the establishment, operation, and maintenance of local units.

4. Local units would be utilized to full potential if considered to be the basic general membership grouping for ANA members. When nurses desire to employ these organizations for collective bargaining purposes they may, of course, do so. However, the establishment of units should not be predicated upon the prior participation of nurses in collective bargaining activities.

References

1. General reviews of collective bargaining activities among professional employees may be found in A. Sturmthal (ed.), *White Collar Unionism*, Urbana, Illinois: University of Illinois Press, 1966; J. Shister, "The Direction of Unionism 1947–1967: Thrust or Drift?" *Industrial and Labor Relations Review*, 20 (1967), 578–601; B. Goldstein, "Unions and the Professional Employee," *Journal of Business*, 27 (1954), 276–284; and "Nurses Are Making It Happen," *American Journal of Nursing* (February 1967), 285–289.
2. Discussions of characteristics associated with professionalism, in both health and nonhealth related occupational groups, may be found in A. Carr-Saunders and P. Wilson, *The Professions*, Oxford: Clarendon Press, 1933; E. Gross, *Work and Society*, New York: Thomas Y. Crowell, 1958; T. Parsons, "The Professions and Social Structure," *Social Forces*, 17 (1939), 457–467; R. Lewis and A. Maude. *Professional People*. London: Phoenix House Ltd., 1952; F. Kempf, *The Person as a Nurse*, New York: Macmillan, 1951; H. Finer, *Administration and the Nursing Service*, New York: Macmillan, 1952; N. Foote, "The Professionalization of Labor in Detroit," *American Journal of Sociology*, 53 (1953), 371–380; H. Vollmer and D. Mills (eds.), *Professionalization*, Englewood Cliffs, N.J.: Prentice-Hall, 1966; R. Kurtz and K. Fleming, "Professionalism: The Case of Nurses," *American Journal of Nursing* (1963), 75–79; and F. Davis (ed.), *The Nursing Profession*, New York: Wiley, 1966.

3. See N. Chamberlain, *Labor*, New York: McGraw-Hill, 1958; N. Chamberlain, *Collective Bargaining*, New York: McGraw-Hill, 1951; S. Slichter, J. Healy, and E. Liverrash, *The Impact of Collective Bargaining on Management*, Washington, D.C.: The Brookings Institution, 1960; and P. Taft, *Organized Labor In American History*, New York: Harper & Row, 1964.
4. Discussions of differences between collective bargaining arrangements found in voluntary organizations and the structures employed in day-to-day operation may be found in A. Cook, "Dual Governments in Unions: A Tool for Analysis," *Industrial and Labor Relations Review*, 15 (1962), 323–349; B. Karsh, "Union Traditions and Membership Apathy," *Proceedings of the Industrial Relations Research Association*, May 2–3, 1958, pp. 634–647; W. Leiserson, *American Trade Union Democracy*, New York: Columbia University Press, 1959; J. Seidman *et al., The Worker Views His Union*, Chicago: The University of Chicago Press, 1958; J. Barbash, *Labor's Grass Roots*, New York: Harper & Row, 1961; and L. Sayles and G. Strauss, *The Local Union*, New York: Harper & Row, 1953.
5. Discussions of organizational designs adopted by groups of engineers and teachers may be found in E. Dvorak, "Will Engineers Unionize?," *Industrial Relations* (May 1963), 45–65; C. Schock, "The Professional Union—A Contradiction," *The Journal of Engineering Education* (December 1964), 345–357; B. Goldstein, "Some Aspects of the Nature of Unionism Among Salaried Professionals in Industry," *American Sociological Review* (April 1955), 199–205; G. Strauss, "Professionalism and Occupational Associations," *Industrial Relations* (May 1963), 7–31; American Federation of Teachers, *Organizing the Teaching Profession*, New York: The Free Press, 1955; C. Perry and W. Wildman, "A Survey of Collective Activity Among Public School Teachers," *Educational Administration Quarterly*, 2:2 (Spring 1966), 133–151; G. Brooks, "A Case for Teachers Unions," *Monthly Labor Review*, 87 (March 1954), 292; C. Cogen, "Teachers on the March," *IUD Digest*, 7 (Winter 1962), 15–17; and M. Herrick, "Research in the Problems of Organized Teachers," *Proceedings of the Industrial Relations Research Association*, 1957, pp. 249–253. Individuals interested in a general, thorough, current bibliography of major readings in this area should see R. Duino, "Readings on Unionization of White Collar and Professional Employees," *ILR Research*, IX (1964), 15–17.
6. Some research indicates that university professors have evolved a similar though less differentiated associational structure. See J. Belasco, "American Association of University Professors: A Private Dispute Settlement Agency," *Industrial and Labor Relations Review*, 18 (1965), 535–553.
7. *Facts About Nursing*, New York: American Nurses Associations, 1967, p. 12, Table 4.
8. *Ibid*., p. 16, Tables 8 and 9.
9. *Ibid*., p. 16, Tables 8 and 9.

10. *Ibid.*, p. 10, Table 1, and p. 15, Table 15.
11. E. Moses, "Nurses Economic Plight," *American Journal of Nursing* (January 1965), 68–71.
12. See D. Yett, "Demand and Supply of Nurses—An Economist's View," *Hospital Progress* (February 1965), 69–101; T. Hale, "Why the Nursing Supply Is Failing to Meet the Demand," *The Modern Hospital* (September 1960), 101–104, 130–131; and D. Yett, "The Nursing Shortage and the Nurse Training Act of 1964," *Industrial and Labor Relations Review*, 19 (1966), 190–200.
13. *Facts About Nursing*, New York: American Nurses Association, p. 11, Table 2.
14. *Ibid.*, pp. 9, 72.
15. For example, see C. Argyris, *Diagnosing Human Relations in Organizations: A Case Study of a Hospital*, New Haven: Yale University, Labor–Management Center, 1956; K. Benne and W. Bennis, "Role Confusion and Conflict Within the Nursing Profession—What is Real Nursing," *American Journal of Nursing* (March 1959), 380–383; B. Johnson and E. Campbell, "It's Time to be Realistic About the Workload," *American Journal of Nursing* (June 1966), 1282–1285; E. Haas, "Role Conception and Group Consensus: A Study of Disharmony in Hospital Work Groups," Ohio State University Research Monograph No. 117, Bureau of Business Research, 1964; and L. Saunders, "The Changing Role of Nurses," *American Journal of Nursing* (1954), 1094–1098.
16. The American Nurses Association Position Paper on Education [*American Journal of Nursing* (December 1965), 106] contends, in part, that nurses possessing a baccalaureate degree are the only true professionals. This is certainly an interesting position in light of the small percentage of nurses receiving any degree beyond that of the 3-year diploma.
17. W. Stewart, "The Surgeon General Looks At Nursing," *American Journal of Nursing* (January 1967), 65–68.
18. Extensive discussions of general nursing history and the development of nursing organizations may be found in R. Skyrock, *The History of Nursing*, Philadelphia: W. B. Saunders, 1959; M. Roberts, *American Nursing*, New York: Macmillan, 1955; M. Burges, *Nurses, Patients and Pocketbooks*, New York: Committee on Grading of Nursing Schools, 1928; T. L. Ford and D. Stephensen, *Institutional Nurses*, Alabama: The University of Alabama Press, 1954; and F. Davis (ed.), *The Nursing Profession*, New York: Wiley, 1966.
19. "The ANA–NLN, A Joint Statement of Functions and Activities," *American Journal of Nursing* (April 1956), 69.
20. *Ibid.*, p. 69.
21. For discussions of this recent change see F. Powell, "Changing ANA to Meet Changing Needs," *American Journal of Nursing*, Parts I, II, and III (March, April, and May 1964); "The Profession Prepares for Its Future,"

American Journal of Nursing (July 1966), 1548–1557; and "ANA Bylaw Changes Proposed," *American Journal of Nursing* (February 1966), 319–320.

22. W. Galenson, *The CIO Challenge to the AFL*, Cambridge: Harvard University Press, 1960.
23. F. Powell, "Changing ANA to Meet Changing Needs, *American Journal of Nursing*, Part II (April 1964), 111–113.
24. This chart is a modification of the ANA organizational chart appearing in the *1966 Edition of Facts About Nursing*, New York: American Nurses Association, section on National Nursing Associations. No organizational chart appeared in the 1967 edition and, therefore, the author modified the previously traditional graphic display in order to incorporate the establishment of "divisions" at the national level.
25. For extensive discussions of economic conditions associated with the employment of nurses see D. Kruger, "Professional Standards and the Economic Status of Nurses in the United States," *International Nursing Review* (December 1960), 43–48; W. Stewart, "The Surgeon General Looks At Nursing," *American Journal of Nursing* (January 1967), 64–67; E. Moses, "Nursing's Economic Plight," *American Journal of Nursing* (January 1965), 68–71; and D. Kelley, "Equating Nurse's Economic Rewards with the Service Given," *American Journal of Nursing* (August 1967), 1642–1645.
26. H. Northrup, "Collective Bargaining and the Professions," *American Journal of Nursing* (March 1948), 140.
27. M. Roberts, *American Nursing*, New York: Macmillan, 1955, pp. 569–570.
28. *Ibid.*, pp. 565–566.
29. Discussions of the impact of labor laws upon the collective bargaining activities of professionals, including nurses, may be found in H. Northrup and G. Bloom, *Government and Labor*, Homewood, Ill.: Richard D. Irwin, 1963; C. Gregory, *Labor and the Law*, New York: Norton, 1961; G. Taylor, "Public Employment: Strides or Procedures?," *Industrial and Labor Relations Review*, 20 (1967), 617–636; H. Northrup, "Collective Bargaining and the Professions, *American Jnurnal of Nursing* (March 1948), 140–144; W. Scott, E. Porter, and D. Smith, "The Long Shadow," *American Journal of Nursing*, (March 1966), 46–48; A. Mahoney, "Bargaining Rights for Nurses—Convincing the Membership," *American Journal of Nursing* (March 1966), 544–548; and H. Parker, "The Laws Governing Labor–Management Relations in Michigan Hospitals," *Labor Law Journal* (October 1961), 972–990.
30. For an account of the impact of legislation requiring recognition of bargaining representatives for employed nurses see "One Request—One Unique Experience—One Momentous Decision," *New York State Nurse*, XXXV (January 1963), 3–5; and J. Alutto, "Correlates of Nursing Attitudes: A Collective Bargaining Situation," unpublished master's thesis, Urbana, Illinois: University of Illinois, Institute of Labor and Industrial Relations, 1965.

31. *Economic Security Manual*, New York State Nurses Association, March 1958, pp. 4–5.
32. L. Ulman, *The Rise of the National Trade Union*, Cambridge, Mass.: Harvard University Press, 1955.
33. R. Merton, "Dilemmas of Democracy in the Voluntary Association," *American Journal of Nursing* (May 1966), 1055–1061; R. Michels, *Political Parties*, New York, Dover, 1959; B. Karsh, "Union Traditions and Membership Apathy"; A. Cook, "Dual Governments in Unions: A Tool for Analysis"; P. Magrath, "Democracy in Overalls," *Industrial and Labor Relations Review* (July 1949), 501–515.
34. *1966 Facts About Nursing*, pp. 9, 72.
35. *Facts About Nursing*, New York: American Nurses Association, 1964, pp. 9, 77.
36. T. Newcomb, *The Acquaintance Process*, New York: Holt, Rinehart & Winston, 1961.
37. This danger of "take-over" by special interest groups has been recognized in the following: H. Smith, "Contingencies of Professional Differentiation," *American Journal of Sociology* (January 1958), 410–414, and The Editors, "The American Medical Association: Power, Purpose, and Politics in Organized Medicine," *The Yale Law Journal* (May 1954), 938–947.
38. P. Secord and C. Backman, *Social Psychology*, New York: McGraw-Hill, 1964.
39. J. March and H. Simon, *Organizations*, New York: Wiley, 1958.
40. J. Alutto, "Collective Bargaining, Nursing Attitudes and the Local Unit Concept," *New York State Nurse*, XXXIX (August 1967), 13–16; "Nurses Are Making it Happen," *American Journal of Nursing* (February 1967), 285–289; F. Hanes, "Nurses and Economic Benefits," *New York State Nurse* (March 1961), 13–15.
41. P. Magrath, "Democracy in Overalls," *Industrial and Labor Relations Review* (July 1941), 501–515; V. Allen, *Trade Union Leadership: A Study of Arthur Deakin*, Cambridge: Harvard University Press, 1957; and H. Lahne and J. Kovner, "Local Union Structure: Formality and Reality," *Industrial and Labor Relations Review*, 9 (October 1955), 24–31.
42. R. Corwin, "The Professional Employee: The Study of Conflict in Nursing Roles," *American Journal of Sociology* (May 1961), 604–609, and R. Bullock, "Position, Function and Job Satisfaction of Nurses in the Social System of a Modern Hospital," *Nursing Research*, 2 (1953), 4–14.
43. Such identifications have long been recognized as important for the development of professionalism: D. Moore and R. Renck, *The Professional Employee in Industry*, Chicago: The University of Chicago, Industrial Relations Center, Bulletin No. 58, 1955; W. Kornhauser, *Scientists in Industry*, Berkeley: The University of California Press, 1962; and H. Smith, "Contingencies of Professional Differentiation," *American Journal of Sociology* (January 1958), 410–414.

III

THE POLITICAL CONTEXT OF HEALTH ADMINISTRATION

THROUGH THE PROCESS OF POLITICS MANY INTERESTS OF A society are articulated; conflicts in the different values represented by interest groups are, at least temporarily, resolved or ameliorated; decisions are made about the allocation of resources; and the rules by which we are governed are shaped. The political process provides the means by which our social institutions change, adapt, or remain constant. Thus politics is an essential part of any system of action in our society, and the health system is not excepted.

Although politics in this broad sense has been acknowledged by the health professional to be important, there is a strong ideology in the field that rejects politics in the specific sense. Over the past 50 years the professional practice of medicine generally has followed the model of the single, private business entrepreneur, tempered by the ethics of professionalism. Individual political activity by a physician tended to suggest advertising to some of his colleagues, an anathema to the profession's ethics, or it hinted at a possible disturbing influence in the patient–physician relationship. Thus the special interests of the physician as a professional came to be represented by his professional association, and it became his political arm.

Governmental activities, however, could not be so easily divorced from the political process. The physician who worked for government was often perceived by the private citizen as one who could not survive the rigors of private practice. This image stemmed in part from the distrust of governmental employees engendered by Jacksonian democracy; from the conservative's value that government should exert minimal influence; and in part from the dislike of political machine politics that grew in response to the massing of large numbers of immigrants in the cities.

The term public health has generally been equated with governmental activity and as such has been perceived by a large segment of the middle class, economically oriented interest groups as an undesirable (although perhaps necessary in a minimal sense) activity. For example, in 1950, when one of the editors of this book began work for a governmental agency, a friend of the family rationalized this behavior as, "I guess it must be like missionary work."

However, government itself over the past 30 to 40 years has been professionalizing. The broadened extensions of the Civil Service Act in the "progressive era," the passage of the Hatch Act in 1939, and the stipulation in the administration of the Social Security Act that personnel paid by federal funds to state and local govenmental jurisdictions must be employed through merit or civil service systems were reactions against the use of personal influence for personal gain in government. The new occupations of city and county managers and the development of training programs for governmental employees in academic institutions began to reinforce the movement toward a professional ethic of government.

Thus the need for the health professional working in government to improve his status vis-à-vis the medical world and the movement toward professional government converged, giving strong force to the development of an apolitical ideology among public health workers. In some states, for example, the term of appointment of the health officer of the state has been legally made nonterminous with the term of the governor to reduce the "influence of politics." This apolitical ideology, coupled with the ideology of the ethics of medicine, was accepted as part of the normative behavior of the health professional and has been particularly strong in the field of public health.

Although the professionalization of public health has led to a more uniform quality of activity, it has had the dysfunctional effect of developing a cadre of persons ideologically committed to a negative view of the political process. Furthermore, because of this negative view health administrators are often politically naive and unaware of strategies that might more effectively achieve their goals.

The chapters in this part provide an overview of some of the political processes with which health administrators are intimately concerned. They are presented as illustrative cases in point, rather than as one particular model for viewing the political context of public health.

8

Emerging Patterns of Federalism: The Case of Public Health

David G. Smith

It is generally accepted that federal institutions affect health, education, and welfare policies, although the effects are difficult to trace. Variety, or disparity, in program levels seems to be the main effect, although federalism may be equally affected in its institutions and ideas by the development of programs and their political institutions and administrative momentum.

The "new federalism" created by the Social Security Act was characterized by the redistribution of responsibility for programs to the federal and state governments from what was formerly a state–local responsibility; by the shift of fiscal balance whereby federal grants became more a necessity than a supplement in some programs; and by the alteration of practice in a few professionalized programs through the stipulation of federal standards attached to grants.

Today, however, there is evidence of a "new, new" and a "new, new, new" federalism in the "direct federalism" of federal grants to local governments and the "private federalism" of federal grants to individuals and institutions: e.g., universities, clinics, and community action programs.[1] The following outline of policy and administrative changes in public health is illustrative of changes in federal administration in response to substantive policy.

Historically, Public Health Service relations with the states were a good example of the traditional "layer-cake" federalism. The PHS collected vital statistics, enforced interstate sanitation and quarantine, and provided technical assistance to state departments of public health. As a field of administrative endeavor, public health prior to 1936 was understood to be almost exclusively "preventive medicine" with a sharp line of demarcation between public health and "medical practice" or fee-for-service medicine. This traditional "Haven Emerson" public health fit with layer-cake federalism: state aid to local units and federal aid to the states, each superior layer of government providing subsidies or grants and technical assistance to complete the spread of local services and improve them, but not to transform practice or public–private relations in medicine.

As a matter strictly of legislative history, the modern era in federal–state relations for public health began in 1935 with Title VI of the Social Security Act, which authorized $8 million annually for training and technical assistance to state and local health work.[2] More important, however, for the administrative history of the contemporary PHS was a ferment engendered by World War II, especially in the period right after the end of the war. In 1943 and 1944 the PHS leadership began taking the measure of trends anticipated for the future in patient need, medical treatment, and professional training. After the war supervening political influences combined with administrative planning to urge the PHS toward a new pattern in federalism.

Technical trends were probably more important in postwar policy development than was politics. One of these trends—thanks largely to the PHS itself and to the discovery of wonder drugs—was the precipitous and continuing decline of communicable disease. Scientific and medical interest turned increasingly toward the chronic, killing, and crippling diseases such as heart disease, cancer, and arthritis. Professional sophistication also increased rapidly after the war, marked especially by more specialization and by interest in clinical and basic research in medicine. By and large the PHS and other professional leaders in health foresaw the first of these developments and its importance, but not the rapid shift toward specialities or the impact of the postwar "information explosion" upon medicine.

The postwar program put forward by the PHS was a mixture of old and new philosophies of federalism, intended to be responsive to future needs as the Service assessed them. On the one hand, New Deal "cooperative" federalism was represented in the famous Joseph Mountin–Thomas Parran "integrated hospital system."[3] This scheme for regional hospital complexes and service areas was intended to make medical care broadly available, to integrate medical specialties efficiently, and to insure continuing improvement in the health professions. Establishment of the local health units and categorical support for weak program areas would strengthen the "continuum of care" by aid to nonprofitable medicine and help create an equitable "partnership" with private medicine.

How well this postwar plan would have worked in practice is debatable. Hill–Burton, which was the modified version of the hospital part of this plan, has shown how difficult planning or direction is when it relates to an assemblage of health professions, public and private institutions, and multiple constituencies. The scheme for public health units seems, with the perspective of twenty years, curiously anachronistic and parochial. These observations, however, point up the difficulties of public leadership in the health field in attempting to determine in advance the goals that will win the assent of a host of professions and provide a guide in a rapidly evolving field.

As professional developments and trends in demography and mortality and morbidity tended to underline the importance of manpower, training, and physical facilities for the future, so the politics of the period also favored a move to "private" federalism. More specifically, the debacle of the Ewing Plan and its defeat left the PHS politically weak. A new Surgeon General from the National Institutes of Health and the prevalent need of the Eisenhower era also tended to emphasize a program direction away from vigorous and active involvement with state and local governments toward less contentious relations with the professions, the medical schools and hospitals, and the local "community."

There were two important developments in PHS grants administration during the twenty-year period since the war. The relative importance of different grants to the states changed radically: decline of the general health grant, the absolute and relative increase in categorical grants, and finally the growing importance of project and research grants relative to both of the preceding kinds. Second, biomedical research and research training increased vastly relative to other programs and ultimately displaced them as the main elements of PHS program development. The first change related especially to the more traditional branch of the PHS, the Bureau of State Services (BSS); the second, to the National Institutes of Health.

The general health grant fit nicely a traditional conception of public health as largely governmental rather than private and a federalism that emphasized strong national leadership in a hierarchy of governments. The grant was especially important for the states' programs because it could be used to pay administrative costs, support local health units, or fund projects that gave "visibility" and popularity to public health efforts. Under Surgeon General Parran (1936–1948), the grants structure for state aid expressed this philosophy faithfully: Categorical support was not a *deduction from* general support but an *addition to* it, strengthening the program in weak areas. After 1948, for reasons explained below, categorical grants grew both absolutely and relatively at the expense of general health support, making the latter increasingly residual in character.

One reason for the relative increase in categorical grants was change in the sources of program support and innovation. Locally, efforts to organize a heart disease control program or build a hospital brought together little clusters of doctors, fund-raisers, and health and welfare associations—not public agencies or governments. At a higher level, professional interest and associational efforts centered upon mental health and cancer, upon disease categories, and not—except for The Association of State and Territorial Health Officers (ASTHO)—upon the cause of state or local public health departments. Furthermore, the period was one of changing conceptions of medical practice, yet of uncertainty about the point at which new conceptions would converge. Prudent administrative planning dictated that public health personnel both locally and in the PHS itself maintain close contact with the professions and voluntary associations in areas of categorical interest. At the very least, these "clusters" provided alternate routes for program development. At the most, they might well represent the character of things to come.

The trend to categories also had a political rationale, depending partly upon the professional and associational support for these programs and partly as well upon unique aspects of the American political system. Public health programs cover wide fronts—scores of separate programs supporting in turn hundreds of different kinds of services and projects. Categorical efforts—so many kidney machines, heart control surveys, and cases treated—can be made "visible" to the legislator and public alike. Categories give the legislator, especially through annual appropriations, a way of directing programs by giving or withholding funds in return for administrative responsiveness to his wishes. Also, by becoming Mr. Water Pollution Control or Mr. Health in Congress or by associating himself nationally or locally with such causes the legislator can acquire a power base in the Congress or the praise of newspapers and associations locally for his patronage of a beneficial, nonpartisan cause. By contrast, the more traditional public health—resting upon the states and localities—was supported by a fragmented constituency, out of the professional mainstream, and lacked "visibility" for securing appropriations or legislative support.

How powerful or important these political influences may have been by themselves is impossible to determine. In politics, however, what is the case matters less than what is believed to be the case. Specifically, with respect to the categories versus the general health grant, an important fact was simply the belief that aid to the states as such had little support and that categorical programs did or would get support. This was a belief shared overwhelmingly by interest groups—including ASTHO and the APHA—by the PHS leaders, by the Bureau of the Budget,* and by congressional appropriations staff.

The decline of the general health grant and an increase in the relative proportion of categorical aid expressed particularly one aspect of a general trend toward "private federalism"—the importance of professions and health associations for administrative initiative and political support. The rapid increase of project and research grants relative to both of the preceding kinds of grants was responsive especially to the changing substance of public health programs.

Conceptually, although the general health grant fits a program logic of conventional service or regulation, the project grant on the other hand fits most closely the rationale and administrative methods of scientific research and development. In the 1940s these grants were used particularly for individual research and demonstration projects that would lead quickly to usable clinical or laboratory knowledge, demonstrated technique, and sustaining programs. Since the 1950s they have been used especially as a way of lengthening and broadening the research and development "continuum." Research and development has been stretched out to include at one end more basic science and at the other projects that were formerly sustaining formula-supported state programs. It has been supported or "broadened" with projects designed to stimulate services, build facilities, and train professional manpower.

In community health the contrast noted above is important for an understanding of the project grant and its role. In the earlier period the emphasis was upon cooperative research and development—projects undertaken jointly between federal and state or public and private agencies and aimed at closing expeditiously the distance between scientific discovery and public health practice. As the distance between public health program needs and actual or potential state performance grew—because of weak PHS leadership and lack of state responsiveness, because of changing needs for professional services and health facilities, and because of advances in the technology and practice of medicine—the project grant was used with varying success to stimulate public or private activities or to close the distance between the two.

The project grant evolved pragmatically, in response to specific needs or program gaps as they developed. For instance, Hill–Burton and

* The Bureau of the Budget, despite the "staff agency's" dislike of categories, came to support this trend, especially to gain increased political support for the programs.

water pollution construction money were needed by cities and regions. The formula–project grant provided a way of putting the money where it was needed. Clearing out "pockets" of VD and TB required a concentrated, short-term effort in a particular area and the organization of a locally coordinated attack. The terminating project grant lent itself to this job. Outpatient or Chronic Illness and Aging services called especially for expanding the hospital's endeavors and for joint public–private activity; thus, it was used for project grants directed at hospital services and tying them with community efforts.

The important point about the project grant is its appropriateness for utilizing the services of professional groups or private institutions. The project grant could be funded without going through an intervening layer of government and without adhering to civil service regulations. It was awarded, typically, on the basis of a project design originating in some local, professional, or scientific interest and aimed at some "problem"[4] of public health practice or needed research. It was judged by a panel—an administrative panel for a service project, a "study section" of professional "peers" for research. In principle, the project grant allowed a maximum of flexibility in the utilization of personnel, in combining public and private efforts, and in a selective program emphasis. At the same time the combination of initiative from the project proposers and judgment by professional peers or departmental committee provided an administrative technique responsive in differing measure to community developments, to professional progress, and to PHS objectives.

The project grant, so far as community health or the more traditional PHS programs were concerned, was an administrative device sought for by the Service but stoutly resisted by the states, by ASTHO, and by President Eisenhower's staff, who disliked "direct" federalism and especially project grant authorization—appropriately enough, inasmuch as the project grant is especially suited to "frontiersmanship." After 1960, project grants in community health quickly grew to rival categorical aid, completing the reduction of the general health grant to a small, residual slice of the total program.

These trends in community health, toward increasing categorization of aid and the use of project grants, show in particular changes *within* a traditional federal program in aid of the states—changes responsive to evolution in the whole health profession and its objectives. Much more important, however, than these changes within the traditional program was the development of an independent approach toward ultimate delivery of service based upon the program logic of scientific research and development and centering upon the NIH.

Again, in the choice of the NIH route for the major PHS effort, secular trends extraneous to government conspired with contemporary (and fortuitous) political circumstance. The postwar years brought an interest in basic science, including biomedical science. The PHS, wanting a stronger research arm, welcomed this trend and expanded NIH over the years, looking also toward a larger future role for biomedical sciences and research and development generally in the delivery of health services.[5] Had it not been for President Eisenhower, though, the NIH would likely have remained a service agency within a traditional PHS mission. Frustration with the President's weak support for public health or medical progress, Marion Folsom's energy and interest in health, the opening of a route through two appropriations committees, and administrative capability in the NIH combined to encourage a path of least resistance: the route of private federalism and of subsidy to science, the universities, and the professions.

The major "breakthrough" came in 1956, ratified by the President's health message of that year. In the message, research came first, with an emphasis upon "basic research." A second item, support for health research facilities (regional nonfederal centers) provided only "bricks and mortar," although to the extent of $250 million spread over five years. This legislation, by extending the NIH mission along categorical lines of "killing and crippling diseases" to include a primary responsibility for supporting regional facilities, strengthened both the categorical approach and the alliance of the NIH and the universities and research centers. Support for the training of nurses and public health specialities was a weak third to this trinity of science, facilities, and health manpower and had rough going in Congress because of First Amendment traditions; but this program began the intensive study of health resources and manpower needs, with the ubiquitous advisory committees and task forces. The practical effect of the legislation during 1956 was to give approval to an expanded NIH research mission and to assign to the Institutes, in principle, a large and undetermined future responsibility for health resources and operational activities related to medical research and development.

The interplay of congressional appropriation, the visibility of the "big categories" represented by the Institutes, and broadened NIH program responsibilities produced spectacular results. In a period when domestic services were on the whole faring badly, NIH appropriations increased by approximately $100 million a year to reach a ceiling of $1 billion. The budget request for 1965 was $1.1 billion. By way of contrast, the total of *all other* PHS programs, including community health, environmental health, the medical services, and government hospitals, was $600 million.

The creation of the NIH research empire was a response both to political circumstance and to professional trends extraneous to government. The NIH's rapid growth and great popularity invite comment, particularly with respect to some of the special strengths of "private federalism" in biomedical science. For one item, the NIH represented subsidy with few strings attached.[6] A NIH project grant to scientist or university supported what they already *wanted to do*, and did not—at least immediately—deprive anyone else. Furthermore, the grants went especially for research and traineeships in medicine and biomedical sciences, rapidly moving fields of inquiry and professional development, with a traditionally low rate of investment except for the bread and butter of training and service. Finally, effective program organization—through national advisory councils, study sections, and committees of university administrators, scientists, and government bureaucrats—coincided almost perfectly with effective organization for political support and congressional lobbying. The private federalism of the NIH rested—and rests—upon an enormously powerful and politically legitimate constituency of able, energetic people in frequent communication, sharing a common goal and interest, and capable of advancing their cause indirectly through universities and professional associations or directly, with access to the "corridors of power," at the Cabinet level, with congressmen and senators and the President himself.*

NIH programs have continued since 1956, and especially since 1960, to grow not just in authorization and appropriation but in scope and jurisdiction as well. In the latter category of change, four items deserve brief mention.

A decisive step in extending research and development toward eventual delivery of services was the establishment of large-scale project support, especially after 1959–1960, for categorical and general clinical research. In 1957 Congress authorized bricks and mortar. Beginning with 1959, funds were earmarked to train manpower and provide block grants to medical schools and clinical centers for program support. Inasmuch as "research" supported facilities, manpower training, and treatment costs—especially, for instance, in program projects—research and development became in fact a device to provide

* The various Presidential task forces, advisory commissions, and policy committees from Kennedy's Health Policy Committee of 1960 to Johnson's Commission on Heart–Cancer–Stroke have been staffed by the leading lights from the biomedical sciences, the medical schools and clinical research centers, and especially the Lasker Foundation group. Much of the politics of program innovation in health and welfare relates to the planning, initiating, and staffing of such advisory commissions. An important additional item is that "old line" bureaus and divisions within the DHEW suffered because they did not have direct access to the President.

the manpower (educate it) and to deliver services (albeit selectively) to patients.

To compensate for some of the side effects or "externalities" produced by heavy investment in research, the NIH also assumed a responsibility for the general welfare of the research institutes, medical schools, and university departments involved in biomedical research. To fulfill this responsibility the NIH has sought increased payment for indirect costs, funds for instrumentation and special research resources, and block grants for general research and the general medical sciences (as distinguished from the clinical specialities).

A third area of NIH program expansion was manpower development. This responsibility, however, went far beyond more support for scientific training. It included training of health manpower generally, though mainly under the guise of research training. Also, support for training was used for wider purposes. For instance, development and career fellowship—similar to five-year and tenured academic appointments—both developed scientific manpower and provided a source of "hard money" (reliable income) for the institutions. With respect to some of the clinical fellowships, and especially the NIMH traineeships, the responsibility assumed was even larger, transforming the conception of practice while training the manpower to implement the new conception.

In broad, inexact terms, NIH program development from 1956 to 1966 could be viewed as supplementing a scientific research and development mission with clinical (applied) research and support for facilities and manpower development. The ultimate step completing this hugely successful experiment in "private federalism" was to go "operational." The NIH took this step in 1965 with two programs: staffing grants for the community mental health centers, supervised directly by NIMH, and "regional medical programs" (originally, Heart–Cancer–Stroke), designating the path of the region, the medical "multiversity," and the clinical research team toward improved medical services to the patient.

As a comment upon the relative ascendency of "private" over "public" federalism, these same years brought little new responsibility for the traditional branches of the PHS. For instance, few believed that the PHS should administer Medicare, the most important health legislation in a generation. The two other most important health service programs—mental health and the regional centers—were made NIH rather than BSS responsibilities.

Some of the factors that have encouraged "direct" federalism were also at work in the public health field—hard-core needs concentrated in metropolitan centers, antiquated state administrative systems, and parsimonious traditions of public expenditure in health and welfare.

The shift toward "private federalism" both in more traditional BSS programs and independently of these, through NIH extramural grants, depended more basically upon factors extraneous to politics: upon changing patient populations, trends within the health professions, the excitement and challenge of science, and the internal politics of the biomedical constituency itself.

Biomedical politics deserves a separate comment. Public health programs organized along traditional lines have been notoriously weak, tending toward fragmentation, political contention, and program *stasis*. By contrast, the new style "pressure group" of health professions, medical schools, and clinical centers has shown an enormous potential for innovative leadership and mobilization of political resources. Insofar as the issue is more for all—subsidy rather than reallocation or regulation—biomedical statesmen also have shown a unity of purpose and interest greatly enhancing their political effectiveness.[7] A latent Populism moves some, including old-line public health officers, to denounce the NIH, the Lasker Foundation, and the biomedical constituency for their raids upon the public treasury; but the critics are also disarmed because the biomedical politicians are, beyond any question, doing the works that need doing. One PHS official commented in retrospect, "They beat Eisenhower when no one else could." At the present time, the same alliance continues to provide much of the élan and political power to continue the momentum in the health field.

Probably private federalism in public health will lead to some extreme examples of the "dualism" characteristic of contemporary American federalism. Many of the trends we have described are recent ones. Yet there is ample testimony and some evidence that the project grant, scientific research and development, and manpower development in the field of public health tend in the first instance to afford opportunity mainly to the already competent and resourceful and to benefit for the longer run primarily those able to implement new discovery and to attract and hold trained manpower. Strictly speaking, the rich do not necessarily get richer and the poor poorer, since many institutions and public authorities with modest resources can through disproportionate effort do well for themselves. However, the less well-endowed community or institution tends to share less in the total grants package and especially less in the livelier aspects of health and medical developments. In concrete terms, elite universities and well-established medical complexes in California and Michigan and New

York City do extremely well while others do less well. Universities, hospitals, and professional groups have often benefited enormously; public programs have often tended to benefit proportionately less, to be out of the "mainstream"—more so in backward states and cities, but also everywhere.

Some of the rancorous controversy over Medicare, and especially the early stages of implementing the program, indicate other potential tendencies of "private federalism": disputes over the balance of public and private in programs; implicit regulation of one profession by another; and conflicts of interest in the dealings of health personnel with the government and with patients. It is worth adding that the politics of the biomedical constituency and the administrative organization of health programs are especially well suited to obscure just such issues, particularly in the initial stages of program development.

This historical account would be misleading without a recognition that administrative leaders and in this case the PHS are mindful of undesirable aspects of private federalism. With respect to the PHS, for example, the Surgeon General in the recent past took two important steps: One is abolition of most categorical grants to states and an attempt through encouraging "comprehensive planning" to strengthen state public health programs. Another is the assertion of the authority of the Surgeon General's Office over the NIH with the implication—not yet an accomplishment—that the NIH will tend increasingly to become a "health" rather than a "science" agency. Both of these measures would tend to limit "private federalism" and take an important step toward a larger public role. Whether the established trends and the existing categorical and professional interests will prove too powerful remains to be seen. In any event—and this is another important aspect of "private federalism"—the struggle will be largely a secret one understood mainly or only by administrative or professional "insiders," and the decision itself will be ultimately in the keeping of a few men, many of whom will not be in government at all.

References

1. A much more extensive discussion of American federalism is found in Charles E. Gilbert and David G. Smith, "Modernization of American Federalism," in Murray Stedman (ed.), *Modernizing American Government*,

Englewood Cliffs, N.J.: Prentice-Hall (Spectrum Books), 1968, pp. 122–152. Much of the material presented in this chapter also appears in their book in substantially similar form.

2. Edwin E. Witte, *The Development of the Social Security Act*, Madison, Wisconsin: The University of Wisconsin Press, 1962.
3. *Wartime Health and Education*, Part V, Subcommittee of the Committee on Education and Labor, U.S. Senate, 78th Congress, 1944, pp. 1173–1207.
4. Compare T. D. Weldon's distinction between "problems" and "difficulties": *The Vocabulary of Politics*, London: Penguin Books, 1953, pp. 75–83.
5. Donald C. Swain, "The Rise of a Research Empire: NIH, 1930 to 1950," *Science*, 138 (1962), 1233–1237; *Federal Support of Basic Research in Institutions of Higher Learning*, Washington, D.C.: National Academy of Sciences, 1964.
6. Compare Theodore J. Lowi, "American Business, Public Policy, Case-Studies, and Political Theory," *World Politics*, 16 (1964), 677–715, where the distinction is made between "distributive," "regulatory," and "redistributive" policies.
7. Note Robert A. Dahl's concept of the "potential for unity" of an elite: "A Critique of the Ruling Elite Model," *American Political Science Review*, 52 (1958), 463–469.

9

Health Organization: The Public Administrator's View

Morris Schaefer

Health administration in the United States has had a long and honorable concern with the organization and reorganization of health agencies to meet changing needs and conditions. Historically, the central aim in reorganization has been the delivery of better health services.

A landmark in the birth of modern public administration, interestingly, was the first major study conducted in 1906 by the New York City Bureau of Municipal Research on the organization and administration of the New York City Department of Health.[1] In the intervening years public health has seen itself pass through a number of major phases in its continuing concern with organization. Each of these phases has had a particular focus—the establishment of state leadership in public health, the county health department movement, the development of effective hospital administration, the extension of professionalism, and the emerging concepts of community health. While the advocates of these focuses enunciated goals, values, and ideologies, their extension and development in practice was uneven and spotty. In each instance the thrust of organizational reform was limited by the pluralism of power and discretion inherent in a federalized system of government and an open society—a condition that current and future movements for organizational reform in health administration must take into account.[2]

The years of this decade have seen health administration confronted with new challenges—increased urgency attached to old problems, new responsibilities and functions, regionalism, and comprehensiveness.

Moreover, these challenges have presented themselves at an increasingly rapid rate. And each of these challenges has raised anew issues of how organization shall be structured so as to respond to continuing changes and yet maintain the stability necessary for effective service.

New administrative demands upon the health professions have led to consequent questions by health administrators on the fields of administrative theory and, perhaps even more relevantly, political theory. How can the questions be framed? And what answers can be expected?

THE PAST IS STILL PRESENT

As health administration faces a new day, it does so with a hangover. Unsolved long-standing problems of organization must affect solutions in the future.

The contemporary health administrator faces a clamor of demands in unfamiliar areas of service, attempts to respond to these demands despite a shortage of personnel and other resources, tries to plan under conditions of uncertainty, and tries to comprehend the swift changes in his environment. The new day is different, if only in the tempo, scope, and number of demands upon his agency. Official health agencies, only a few months or years removed from the comparatively settled functions and responsibility of "public health," may look nostalgically to the recent past as "the good old days." No longer is the job of organizational analysis limited to designing that agency structure that will maximize effectiveness or permit increased services or new activities within the same budget. The old need to minimize frictions within the agency—always a neat trick in an enterprise so varied in program, goals, and the relevant scientific disciplines—has suddenly become vastly more complicated in its community-wide dimensions.

We can only speak in relative and general terms, of course, but in "the good old days" relations among governments were fairly orderly. Target populations were limited and usually known. The responsibilities of the health agency were comparatively stable and familiar. Expertness in function by and large was achieved. "The public" was usually quiescent, except for an occasional scrap over the budget, and more often than not had to be stirred up over health problems. Relations between the official and nonofficial sectors of the health services industry tended to be polite and comfortably distant, with fairly clear distinctions among roles. What was desirable in a public health system was fairly well known; textbooks were relevant, useful, and changed little between revisions; the American Public Health Association could issue an evaluation schedule to act as a standard for community health services —or so it all seemed.

Not all of the problems of organization were amenable of solution. Indeed, none of them was ever more than partially solved. To be sure, the machine model, generated out of the application of the scientific management movement to public administration, provided a basis of order, a distribution of social and functional territories within the agency, and a mechanism appropriate to the key processes of budgetary and personnel administration (which also have changed). But the organization chart that adorned the office wall of the health officer and his key lieutenants only barely concealed the tensions and contradictions of the typical structure. The struggles between agency headquarters and their field units were (and are) classic examples of the effort to find a balance between the expertness of the specialist and the integrative responsibilities of the generalist. The tensions between state and local governments remained (properly perhaps) a persistent problem. Although administrative theory suggested that agencies could be organized according to program (tuberculosis control), process (personnel administration), clientele (mothers and children), and area; public health administrators found their agencies had to use all these bases plus organizational units based upon particular professional disciplines (nursing, social work). An inevitable augmentation of tensions and struggle for loyalty resulted.

While consolidation and integration continued to be ideals in health administration, various public health functions struggled to become autonomous and self-sufficient. At various times and places, either within the agency or by the organization of special governmental districts, tuberculosis control, public hospitals, mental health, and medical services to the indigent achieved organizational and fiscal identities of their own.

Health needs generated special units, and the special units found and used constituencies to maintain identity and to present claims. Where political power was insufficient to resist the "encroachments" of administrative and budgetary analysts—and the health officer himself—the intricacy and mystery of the specialty itself frequently served as a defense.

Despite publicized definitions of the boundaries of public health, the frontiers were uneasy. It is difficult to say whether aggressions from the outside or a sense of irredentism (e.g., school health) within the agency itself was more powerful in this unease. There were patrols and excursions and skirmishes along the borders in efforts to alter the boundaries that lay between the public health agency and other governmental agencies with health responsibilities, and there was a consistent feeling-out of strength between the official and nonofficial sectors.

In retrospect it is clear that the fundamental dynamism of health administration could not really be denied or rejected by freezing it into a tidy organization chart. The history tells us, further, that the old and well-propagated myth of the nonpolitical character of public health was a delusion—except, sometimes, in the sense of partisan politics. That the "nonpolitics" myth persisted as long as it did (and does) suggests that many opportunities were lost and many conflicts were generated because health professionals too often lacked the clarity of vision or the stomach for the rough and tumble of program and interagency politics.[3]

To the extent that the myth continues and has spawned an antipolitical ideology, and to the degree that organizational problems have not been solved, health administration faces its new challenges with a burden. Because some of these problems are ultimately insoluble —and because some current problems are extensions and intensifications of those of the past—the hand of the past lies upon the future.

EMERGING ISSUES OF HEALTH ORGANIZATION

The above is not the full limit of the issues in the organization of health services. The social clock has moved, perceptibly and significantly. The shape and the expression of American society has altered. These changes make a difference.

Place of the Local Governmental Unit

The rise of suburbia and development of communications and transportation has made the resources of major metropolitan centers accessible to scattered populations, while technological developments have greatly expanded the effective reach of administrative and service mechanisms. It is not difficult to hypothesize articulated systems of health services—such as medical care services—on a regional basis, with elementary and basic services performed at the locality and more complex and specialized activities concentrated at the center.

In most places, there are three barriers to activating these ideas. First, there is the existence of vested interests in practically sovereign local governments. Second, there are the values and emotions that attach to the idea of small government, whose decision-makers are accessible and responsive to relatively small-sized publics. When these values are maintained and are coupled to antipathy toward the metropolis and the prevalent social deterioration there, the development and maintenance of a balanced, rational distribution of responsibilities, tasks, and resources become difficult. Experience in the Hill–Burton programs for the construction of inpatient facilities demonstrates that even financial sanctions may be insufficient to overcome the resistance of smaller communities against becoming dependent upon larger centers for hospital and related services.

The third difficulty is that the regional level of administration is inherently weak. The region has no political or fiscal base of its own. It has no legislature to which it can turn to make its claims for authorization and funding. Its political executive will be the distant chief executive of the state (and his health officer) in an intrastate region; in interstate regional organizations there is no single political executive to whom the regional administration can turn for support. Thus regional administration is caught between the demands imposed from above and the resistance that arises from the local level.

Yet the ideology of regionalism in health administration grows stronger, without necessarily addressing itself to the strong tradition of localism. Even more difficult than establishing regional administration over areas lacking effective organized health services is the establishment of regional administration over effective units already in existence.

Bases of Field Organization

Another dimension of the areal issue centers on the questions of (1) whether field units shall be organized according to how health problems and resources are distributed or (2) whether such units should be organized on a standardized, coterminous administrative basis.

Taking three leading problems for regional administration—water and air pollution and articulated systems of medical care—it is most probable that each will have different distributions of their geographic and economic factors and that political geography is likely to be irrelevant to all three. Drainage basins differ from the combination of industrial locations, population concentrations, and geophysical features that affect air pollution. Medical care programs have to be based upon the distribution of facilities and human resources as well as how people move and communicate. The "natural" conformation of all three programs is likely to have only accidental relationships to the boundaries of cities, counties, or even states.

A number of approaches to this issue promise to maximize cooperation and coordination among political jurisdictions. Each of them, however, involves either sacrificing existing social values (e.g., by absorbing local programs into new supralocal organizations) or increasing the number of organizational fragments by creating inter-jurisdictional confederations based on particular problem or resource distributions. In the latter instance, while coordination of the new fragments may be possible, it can be extremely difficult and expensive for a regional organization to do this, and in some instances the geography of the problem may make interregional coordination necessary as a further complication. These difficulties, then, tend to drive program administration to the state level or even higher—to the further detriment of the values of localism.

In some measure these difficulties can be eased by the development of improved information-gathering and exchange systems, employing automated equipment. But such developments will not by themselves obviate the necessity for more sophisticated patterns of management than now exist. And it will require the highest order of epidemiological planning and political insights to discern how local interest and initiative can be harmonized with broader views of specific problems and how problems and activities can be better related to each other. The achievement of these objectives and new equilibriums will involve a need for imaginative and highly capable executive action, as well as a level of competence in information technology that we are only approaching.

The Definition of Integrity

Quite aside from the problems of political geography and program geography, the established boundaries of official health agencies have been brought into question by the related factors of size and status. Already in the larger public health jurisdictions, the sheer size of certain programs not only puts enormous strain on the coordinative abilities of executives but also generates claims for independence. For example, as official health agencies assume responsibilities and assemble resources for massive programs of water and air pollution abatement or regulating the quality and financing of medical care, program directors find themselves developing relations with and dealing in areas unfamiliar to the executives of the official agency. The rationale for their continued affiliation with the health agency comes into question. They have before them the examples of major programs in mental health, industrial hygiene, and school health, organized outside the public health agency, more often than not. Long-standing tensions among the professional groups involved in public health come to the fore and foster aspirations to greater discretion and status through the separation of these programs from the health agency and the achievement of equal status with that agency.

Looked at objectively, the choice among organization values is cruel. On the one hand there are opportunities for the program: to escape from having to conform the program to the rules of the agency; to augment the political potentials of the program by giving it greater visibility; and to move faster by shortening lines of communications with central control agencies, the legislature, and program constituencies.

On the other hand the independent organization of these and other programs represents a loss of potentially fruitful melding of research and services addressed to the environment and to the person. Administratively there will be costs of duplicating supporting services in several agencies, increasing the span of oversight of the chief executive of the governmental jurisdiction and increasing the competition for personnel and other resources and still further complicating—perhaps to the point of impossibility—the coordination of services.

The Clientele Approach

The emergence of massive programs oriented to specific clienteles, notably the War on Poverty, raises still another issue for health administrators, among others. Such programs represent a protest against existing fragmentation of responsibilities among agencies and against traditional ways in which agencies do business. When the urgencies of the problems affecting a particular group in the population impresses itself on political leadership, the official health agency is faced with the choice of responding to these strong signals either by liaison or by reorganization. Liaison implies the introduction of "clientele specialists" to coordinate and stimulate contributions from various units within the official agency. It may result in the least disruption, but it is also likely to be less responsive to political claims.

Reorganization, by establishing special units to be concerned with the problems of a particular clientele, will involve costs of duplication and tension. But it will tend to be politically responsive by giving the clientele representation in struggles for allocations, authorizations, and visibility.

The Sectoral Boundary

Recent federal legislation has involved health agencies deeply with problems of medical care that until recently were matters of interest but not responsibility. The issue before official health agencies is this: Where is the new boundary of the official sector vis-à-vis the private and voluntary sectors to be set? Realistically, the answer to this question will evolve over some years. So long as it remains an active question, a strong element of uncertainty must continue to exist in the organizational planning and actions of official agencies.

The Title 18 and 19 amendments to the Social Security Act, the regional programs for heart, cancer, and stroke, and the legislation for comprehensive health planning (P.L. 89–749) all involve official health agencies more intimately with the private and voluntary sectors. In certain states and large municipalities additional legislation intensifies involvement in such areas as medical audit, approval of construction for inpatient facilities, financing of those facilities, and major programs of medical research.

In some instances the legislation is partly a hunting license and partly a promissory note. Beyond certain core authorizations the interests concerned are left to negotiate and otherwise develop the extent and character of their respective participation. Uncertainty in structuring and managing organizationally results. Not only do the boundaries, which define the scope of the agency, remain ambiguous but the agency may need to reorganize itself more than once within a relatively short span of years in order to attain and maintain a structure of authority and communications that will respond to a changing situation.

Place of the Planners

Under the impetus of P.L. 89–749 and various governmental efforts in Programming–Planning–Budgeting Systems (PPBS), a quiet revolution has begun to take place in the planning of health programs and activities. Earlier—and not notably well-developed—planning efforts by official public health agencies were concerned mainly with mounting effective programs of limited scope. By contrast, contemporary planning efforts are to be directed toward policy formulation, to use highly sophisticated statistical information and planning technics, to emphasize values of coordination and holism, and to become involved with the private and voluntary sectors in varying ways.

These expectations are substantial enough to require the development of specialists in health planning prepared in a more rigorous and professionalized basis than heretofore: Indeed educational efforts to develop such specialists already are under way. The emergence of such health-planning specialists will challenge the assumptions that previously governed the organization of the planning process. These assumptions were (1) that planning was but one aspect of managerial or executive activity, (2) that the training in planning contained in the typical public or business administration curriculum provided adequate expertness to the health agency, and (3) that through a minimum of training and progressive experience health officers and other executive personnel without professional administrative training could contribute the necessary guidance and direction to planning efforts.

Beside these assumptions stands the conception of planning as a major social process and institution, equal (if not superior) to budgeting in guiding the outcomes and direction of governmental and quasi-public agents. In this view planning is coordinate with health, education, public works, and other public functions. Central planning agencies legitimately would make claims upon planners in health agencies as their counterparts[4] and supporters.

While such an ideology may have an intense and shocking impact upon health agency organization, it appears likely that to view planning as being simply another of the functions of managers will not be a socially or politically viable position in the years to come. The finding of a middle ground—and obtaining acceptance for it among the parties concerned—is becoming an urgent problem for health leaders. Nor will this be the last "new" specialization to emerge.

CONCLUSIONS

It appears that—beyond the continuing problems from the past—health agencies are faced with problems of organization centering upon levels of governmental authority, programmatic versus community bases of organization, the needs of special clienteles, the divisiveness of disciplines, the relationship of governmental efforts to voluntary and private efforts, and the impact of new processes and specializations. What is striking about these problems is that they are not so much administrative in character as they are political. They have to do with the structuring of authority and power.

Search for a Theory of Organization

If the above is true, then health executives cannot go about finding resolutions of these issues by simple reference to the body of administrative theory. It is not that administrative theory is useless—indeed, it has provided the framework for the preceding analysis of organizational issues. But it cannot be expected to provide formulas and clear solutions, mainly because the nature of the emerging issues go beyond the issues with which conventional administrative theory has been concerned.

The two most influential and most complete bodies of administrative theory seem to be inadequate to the task that faces health leaders. Both scientific management theory (also called traditional or O & M) and the human relations variant are probably inapposite to the most crucial of these issues because each uses an equilibrium model, seeking to define a pattern of organization that will operate with a minimum of friction and conflict.[5]

A third body of organization theory—behavioralism—to date has produced only fragmentary findings and may be generically incapable of developing a general body of theory. The fourth body—general systems theory—is as yet insufficiently developed, particularly with respect to nonphysical processes.[6]

This deficiency is more than an academic matter, because the theory that health executives absorb and observe tends to govern their expectations, ideals, and behavior. Theories that assume clear boundaries, stable goals, settled relationships, and lasting divisions of responsibility and function will not be responsive to the needs of community health at the present time. Such theories cannot adequately orient executives for innovation, bargaining, modifying, and planning under conditions of uncertainty. They cannot raise the administrator beyond the level of coping with conflict—to dealing in it.

Certain elements of administrative theory may be applicable and useful, but they will not be completely relevant unless they are joined to certain elements of political theory appropriate to the character of the problem. Consensus-building, constitutionalizing, bargaining, coalition formation, compromise, and trade-offs may sound strange in the lexicon of community health administration but they are the keys to the future.

Yet because these terms and concepts may not only be strange but even abhorrent, the first step of attitude reorientation may be the most difficult to take. So long as the myth of the nonpolitical character of public health prevails, too many health leaders will be frightened off by the label of politics. If this behavior persists, we may be signaling our incapacity to appreciate the character of the problems we face and our inability to select the analytical and predictive instruments appropriate to those problems.

References

1. Fritz Morstein Marx, *Elements of Public Administration*, 2nd ed., Englewood Cliffs, New Jersey: Prentice-Hall, 1959, p. 24.
2. National Commission on Community Health Services, Task Force on Organization of Community Health Services, *Health Administration and Organization in the Decade Ahead*, Washington, D.C.: Public Affairs Press, 1967, pp. 9, 13, 17–21, Chapter V.
3. Morris Schaefer, "Area and Function in the Administration of Public Health in New York State," Chapter VII, unpublished doctoral dissertation, New York: Syracuse University, 1962.
4. H. E. Hilleboe and M. Schaefer, *Papers and Bibliography on Community Health Planning*, Albany, New York: Graduate School of Public Affairs, State University of New York, 1967, Part 1.
5. Sherman Krupp, *Patterns of Organizational Analysis*, New York: Holt, Rinehart & Winston, 1960, Chapters 6 and 9.
6. M. Schaefer and H. E. Hilleboe, "The Health Manpower Crisis: Cause or Symptom," *American Journal of Public Health*, 57 (January 1967), 6–14.

10

Community Politics and Health Planning

Mary F. Arnold & Isabel M. Welsh

The desires and dreams of the future are deeply embedded in any discussion of planning, because the very word implies a rational endeavor to achieve a desired outcome. When the process of planning is institutionalized in a society, as in the implementation of legislation such as Public Law 89–749 in the Federal Partnership for Health program, there is an indication that the society is not satisfied with its image of what the unplanned future will bring.[1] On the other hand, the idea of planning conflicts with some of the strong values of our society—our emphasis on individualism and on freedom of action for the individual, our desires for local autonomy and home rule, our fears of an all-controlling, all-encompassing "big brother," and our desires for protection from invasion of privacy. Thus, in the development of our statewide and local planning organizations we seek to preserve these things we hold dear. The requirement for consumer representation in health planning advisory councils is a manifestation of a concern that the many interests of the community be incorporated into the planning process. Most of the discussions in the other chapters of this book imply an underlying value premise that the achievement of a planning society is to be desired over the development of a planned society. In order to develop the organizational mechanisms for a planning society it become important, therefore, to understand the political decision-making processes of our society. One of the characteristics of a planning society in a democracy is that participation in the planning process should be initiated at the most decentralized level possible. Thus the political decision-making process in the local community is of particular concern to the planner.

There is a crucial question, the answer to which is of fundamental importance to the health planner: "In a political system where nearly every adult may vote, but where knowledge, wealth, social position and access to officials and other resources are unequally distributed, who actually governs?"[2]

Ideally, the answer to this question should aid the health planner in his broad and longer range calculations concerning possible ways of using community resources or gaining access to resources outside the relevant community. The answer should help the planner better understand the issues on which the community might be persuaded to expend these resources and the perception that different groups within the community might have of the political costs and benefits from alternative uses of resources. More specifically, the answer to the question of who governs should help to identify and characterize the participants in political decision-making, determine who gains and loses from decision outcomes, and suggest how successful participation in the community's decision-making can be achieved.

Community Power Structure

Ready acceptance by public health practitioners of the findings of the early studies of community power by Hunter,[3] Mills,[4] and the Lynds[5] has led to a popularization of the term "community power structure." From this has stemmed a kind of folk belief that if one could find a way to influence this power structure, success in achieving community change would be assured. However, a growing number of relevant studies by political scientists and sociologists reveal considerable inconsistencies in the structure of political power in different communities across the United States. Some investigators argue that several elites, usually with a degree of overlap, share local power. Others argue that business dominates the local scene (this was the point of view of the classical study on community power structure by Hunter). Still others claim that power structures are an artifact of a method of study. There is a sizable literature in the sociological and political science journals expanding the theoretical and methodological arguments. However, the issue argued is essentially whether the American community can be characterized as being governed by a monolithic or coalitional power elite or whether it can be characterized as pluralistic where decision-makers may vary depending upon the kind and scope of the issues.

For the planner, Walton's review of the current status of research on community power structure is helpful.[6] Walton analyzed 33 studies that dealt with 55 communities and tested a number of hypotheses that have been suggested about the association of community power with various other characteristics of the community. His most significant contribution to the debate over the nature of community power is the finding that the method of study of community power is associated with the type of structure identified. The reputational method (informants are asked to identify key influentials in the community in a variety of ways) tends to identify pyramidal structures, while studies of decision-making (the study of specific issues and corresponding leadership activity) reflect factional, coalitional, or amorphous types of power structures. Social integration, as well as regional differences that may reflect something of the community's political life, is moderately associated with a less concentrated power structure. Finally, there was some slight evidence in his study that the more industrialized communities were associated with less concentrated power structures.

Thus there is no simple guideline for the planner for discovering a clear-cut power structure in his community. Any or all theoretical positions about the patterns of community power in American communities may be empirically sound, and this inconsistency may reflect the genuine differences in power structures across the United States: "At the national level inconsistent findings of this kind would have to be reconciled; at the local level they may indicate not inconsistency but historical and social diversity."[7]

It is our belief that the planner who makes no a priori assumptions about the distribution of power within the community for which he is planning, but rather sets out to discover the community and its power structure by asking and answering three very important questions, may provide himself with a more accurate guide to the political scene than the planner whose ideological preferences cause him to opt for a more rigid and possibly inaccurate position. The three questions that need to be answered are: Who participates in the community's political decision process? By what rules are decisions made? What kinds of power are needed to influence and implement policy decisions?

WHO ARE THE PARTICIPANTS IN THE COMMUNITY'S DECISION-MAKING PROCESS?

Participants in the decision-making process may be classified as voters, interest groups, or influentials. The first category reflects one classical approach to the nature of the decision-making process in a democracy—the individual citizen's views and preferences will be taken into account by virtue of his power to punish at the polls. Interest groups, as a category, are premised on assumptions that individuals or organizations of a private or public governmental nature will unite and act to defend or press for limited objectives. Interest groups are usually characterized as highly specialized and, especially in the instance of governmental agencies, highly professional. It is generally assumed that they operate from a relatively narrow base, as distinguished from the larger stream of public opinion. The influential is so called because he has access to and controls certain skills of influence.

Voters as Participants

Banfield and Wilson, in their analysis of city politics, argue that there are two fundamentally opposed conceptions of politics. One, with origins in the Protestant ethic, is essentially public-regarding and is generally accepted as a middle-class norm; the other, with origins in our history of immigration, is essentially private-regarding. These authors put forth five hypotheses that should be of interest to planners:

> (1) that in all social classes the proportion of voters who are decidedly public-regarding is higher among Protestants than among other ethnic groups; (2) that in all social classes the proportion who are decidedly private-regarding is higher among those ethnic groups whose conception of politics is, in the relevant respects, most opposed to the Protestant one; (3) that people in the upper-middle and upper classes are more public-regarding than those in the lower-middle class; (4) that people who are decidedly public-regarding or decidedly private-regarding on one matter tend to be so on all matters; and (5) that decidedly public-regarding and decidedly private-regarding voters tend to be further apart on all matters, including those which have no public–private dimension, than are other voters.[8]

Studies showing differential patterns of voting by religion, class, and ethnicity may find an explanation in this public/private regardingness ethos postulated by Banfield and Wilson. These authors suggest that techniques to measure public (or private) regardingness might be interviews or attitude-scaling techniques or one might classify all those as public-regarding who, on some occasion, voted for an expenditure that would yield no private benefit. Thus one might be able to predict tendencies for these groups to vote decidedly one way or another. Suburban communities, according to these authors, are most likely to vote in terms of the predominant ethos of the "kind of people" that gravitate to the particular suburb. As many suburbs become middle class in character, one would expect a voting behavior more toward the public-regarding ethos. Issues such as fluoridation seem to bear out the authors' hypotheses.[9]

Interest Groups as Participants

While the planner must keep in mind the ultimate authority of the voter, he should be well aware that voting is not in itself an adequate measure of political power. Interest groups also serve to articulate demands of individuals and groups. One can classify interest groups in terms of the type of group and the type of access channel through which its message comes. There are *nonassociational* groups such as ethnic, regional, and family who express their interests only occasionally through an individual. An example might be a small group of persons appearing at hearings of a City Council to request a stop sign at a particular corner. These groups are of an intermittent nature and do not have a long-lasting organization for communicating their demands. Almond and Powell argue that this type of interest group is limited in our complex society because of competition from organized interest groups and because their lack of organization makes maintenance of continuity of the group difficult.[10]

Two other types of interest groups are *institutional interest* groups and *associational interest* groups. The former are found within such organizations as political parties, legislatures, and large organizations such as governmental agencies. As either corporate bodies or smaller groups within corporate bodies, they may articulate their own interests or interests of other groups in the society. Employees' associations, special cliques with a bureaucracy such as a church or a governmental agency, special skill groups, and so on, may be quite powerful because of the strength of their organizational base.

The associational interest groups are generally organized for the purpose of expressing their particular interests in the political arena. Their special characteristics are explicit representation of the particular group, usually organized with a full-time professional staff, and orderly procedures for the formulation of interests and demands:

> As the importance of associational interest groups in interest articulation has been recognized, they have been the object of many studies

> in the more developed societies. Where these groups are present and are allowed to flourish, they tend to regulate the development of the other types of interest groups. Their organizational base gives them an advantage over nonassociational groups; and by representing a broad range of groups and interests they may limit the influence of real or potential institutional interest groups and of self-representation.[11]

The organizational structure of these groups is important in enhancing or decreasing their ability to mobilize the support, energy, and resources of members, and this in turn will determine a group's effectiveness. A loose, voluntary group will probably be less effective than a tightly organized group. On the other hand, the tightly organized group may come to represent only the leaders' interests and not those of the rank and file of the organization. The amount of control over the membership is also of importance. In organizations that depend upon membership loyalty and motivation for maintenance of the membership, the interest represented by the group as a whole will likely represent the interest of the majority of the members. But where access to the group is important for other aspects of the members' lives, as in labor unions and membership-controlled professional occupations such as medicine, the interests articulated may be those of the leadership rather than that of the majority of the members. This leadership may be representative of either the most conservative of the members or the most liberal. The ways in which interest groups penetrate the political arena will be discussed later, but it is important here to note that it is seldom that access to the public media is effective. Instead, interest groups must usually find special channels through which to express their demands to the decision-makers. Of interest today is the fact that through the Economic Opportunity Act, in the Federal Partnership for Health program, and in the Housing and Urban Development's Model Cities program, the requirement of consumer representation has been a conscious national effort to develop interest groups among those persons who have been alienated from the political decision-making system regarding the health values or have not had an adequate organizational base from which to articulate their interests.

Interest groups possess or control means or facilities for influencing decision-makers. Such means or facilities may include education or professional skill (for example, legislatures may depend greatly upon highly knowledgeable lobbyists), social standing in the community, liquid resources such as cash or credit, control over jobs, information, or mass media, and control over values (for example, incumbency in certain professions concerned with the interpretation of cultural values). The planner must not only be aware of these various resources but also be apprised himself of the nature of the distribution of these resources. In some communities possession of one resource usually entails possession of most of the other resources (especially those significant for influencing decision-makers). This situation has been characterized by Dahl[12] as one in which there is a "cumulative" possession of resources as distinguished from a situation in which possession of one or more resources does not entail possession of other significant resources—the "noncumulative" possession of resources.

The importance of the investigation of the distribution of these resources should not be underestimated; it is one of the most crucial ingredients for the planner's determination of his tactical moves, because it aids him in outlining possible techniques of intervention. He has two alternatives: to use or bargain with individuals or groups possessing dominantly influential resources or, if the situation requires it, to mobilize individuals or groups possessing resources that hitherto have been relatively unexploited and, hence, have not given these individuals or groups significant access to influencing the decision-making process.

It should be pointed out that in addition to the determination of the nature of the distribution of these resources the planner must add the ingredient of uncertainty that occurs especially in situations of dispersed or noncumulative distribution of power. Interest groups or individuals may possess potential and actual influence independent of a specific issue—they may not choose to expend these resources in all policy areas. Moreover, their influence may vary at different stages of the political decision-making process.

Influentials as Participants

As mentioned earlier, the method of identifying leadership in a community will affect the type of power structure that is identified. One approach is to assume that active participation in decision-making in the community is leadership. Another is to assume that formal authority is an index of leadership, while a third approach is the study of social participation with high participation the index of leadership. A fourth approach to the problem of identifying leaders in the decision-making process is to seek out those who have a reputation for leadership. Freeman et al.,[13] in a study in Syracuse, tested out these various methods and found, for example, that reputation seems to derive more from position than from participation and that participation by organizations seems to be highly associated with which leaders are identified by reputation and by position. In their study the personnel of the largest organizations had the highest participation rates. The individuals who are high participators seem, by virtue of the extent of their participation, to be professional participants, often employees of governmental agencies or executives of voluntary interest groups. These authors identified three kinds of leadership: *institutional leaders*, who are the heads of the most actively participating business, professional, industrial, governmental, political, professional, educational, labor, and religious organizations; *effectors*, who generally were governmental personnel and professional participants and others in the employ of those organizations from which the institutional leadership comes; and the *activists*, people who are active and may hold office in voluntary organizations but who lack the positional stature of the institutional leaders. The authors suggest that communities in different stages of development and diversification will show different patterns among these types of leaders.

Studies of the characteristics of high participators in community affairs indicate that they tend to be of higher education and social class than low participators, and a high proportion are professionals. This reinforces the idea that out of associational interest groups a cadre of professional participators is formed as the community becomes more diverse and complex. Additionally, it should be noted that since the 1940s there has been a trend of economic centralization:

> But what was significantly different then [before the 40s] was that the owner-managers of that earlier age had to sink or swim with their communities. They provided a continuing pool of community political leadership that remained at home in good times and bad. The new centralization of economic control, on the other hand, began immediately to drain communities of their best manpower and to divorce men with local economic power from serious community concerns. The most talented men of the country were rotated from community to community, sinking no roots in any one of them. Even the interests of those who were not transferred were turned away from the local scene.[14]

The type and scope of issues also affect the kind of leadership that emerges in political decision-making. Rossi argues that although companies expect their young executives to become active in community affairs, there is a risk for them in affiliating with issues or programs that have an aura of nonsuccess about them. For example, welfare programs in many ways represent the unsuccessful, and since these young men who are upwardly mobile in their occupations tend to affiliate with issues in which they can be seen as successful, they are not likely to be concerned with welfare-type issues.[15] Miller's study of community health action also indicated that the business leadership tended to affiliate with projects such as hospital construction where economic values were most important. When the organization of local health departments was the issue, welfare values seemed to take precedence and the leadership seemed more to come from the women in the community.[16]

In very recent years new groups of political activists have formed, stemming not only from the dissatisfaction with the war in Vietnam but particularly from the demand of the black community for autonomy, the self-esteem of power, and control over some portion of their lives:

> Today the black ghettos resemble nothing so much as newly emerging nations faced with extraordinary demands and few resources. There is the same ambivalance toward "foreign" aid: you must have it and yet you hate the giver because of your dependence on him. Highly educated and skilled people (black as well as white) are deeply resented because of the well-founded fear that they will "take-over." The greater the disparity between aims and accomplishment, the greater the demagoguery and destructive fantasy life.[17]

Many of these groups are in the process of forming their organizational base but have not yet become integrated into the general political transactions of the community. This in itself is a political problem in our society, and health-planners in the near future may have a major role in its satisfactory (or unsatisfactory) resolution.

BY WHAT RULES ARE POLICY DECISIONS MADE?

The answer to the question of what rules are employed has at least two components. One is that the nature of the transactions among interest groups or individuals attempting to influence the decision-making process involves choices by participants of strategies in either competitive or cooperative action. The other component concerns the image of the role of government held both by governmental officials and members of the various organizations and interest groups within the community. This image of the role of government may greatly influence the definition of what community/government relevant functions are.

Strategies in Political Decision-Making

It is useful for the planner to think of the transactions among protagonists in the political decision-making process as an exchange relationship. Blau's analysis of the process of social exchange transactions and power relations argues that association with others is maintained because the outcomes of such association are mutually rewarding. When the transaction no longer serves to meet the needs of both parties to it, it dissolves. However, when one party has something to offer that is needed by another but has no need that can be immediately served by the other, the association will be differentially attractive. The party in need of help has several alternatives—he can force the other person to provide for his need; he may seek another source of help; he can find ways to get along without the help; or he may obligate himself, giving the supplier of the need power as an inducement for furnishing the needed help. "The power to command compliance is equivalent to credit, which a man can draw on in the future to obtain various benefits at the disposal of those obligated to him. The unilateral supply of important services establishes this kind of credit and thus is a source of power."[18]

Since this kind of relationship seldom exists in isolation, power relationships continually change depending upon the social alternatives available to the subordinates. In the relationship of or in order to maintain the superior position in the power relationship, the association must be satisfactory for both parties. When a group of persons obligate their support to a leader, they have influence over his actions in that he must continue to meet their needs in competition with other social alternatives they may acquire. Power as a credit for future obligations is like money in the bank; once it is drawn upon, it is no longer available. Thus the planner should consider the varying effects of the use of influence on the social transactions involved: What obligations will be disturbed if power is committed to an issue? How will this affect the power relationships among individuals and groups in the future?

One reward in social transaction is to accord the supplier of needs a higher status. But there is a risk attached to the exercising of this power credit because if the power holder is unsuccessful in meeting the needs of those obligated to him, he may lose his ability to maintain the relationships that are the social base for his power. Lack of success in community action, even though it may not directly involve the participants in a particular power relationship, will change the expectations of the subordinates in that power relationship, and the value of maintaining the relationship may be decreased.

From the viewpoint of the particular actor in a transaction, whether he be an individual or a group, there are three basic strategies available to him, depending upon his needs, that can be met by the other actors in the transaction. These strategies can be competitive, cooperative, or exclusive. *Competition* implies rivalry between two or more actors that is mediated by a third party; in other words, two or more parties can fulfill the needs of the third party and are competing to enter into a transactional relationship with him. Levine and White have suggested that health and welfare organizations may compete for clientele, for financial support, for functions to be performed, or even for a particular disease domain.[19]

Cooperative strategies may include bargaining, co-optation, or coalition. In this case the transactions start from a point where both parties have needs to be fulfilled by each other. *Bargaining* implies a negotiation of an exchange between two or more individuals or groups. In order to make the transaction mutually attractive, each has to compromise and adjust to the other. *Co-optation* is the strategy of absorbing new elements into a leadership or policy-making structure of one group to maintain its own position and stability. For example, the practice of placing a representative of organized medicine on a board of health is a co-optation strategy. Finally, *coalition* is the formation of a combined organization to serve a common purpose: "The enterprise that competes is not only influenced in its goal-setting by what the competitor and the third party may do, but also exerts influence over both. Bargaining, likewise, is a form of mutual, two-way influence. Co-optation affects the co-opted as well as the co-opting party, and coalition clearly sets limits on both parties."[20]

Exclusion is a strategy where the transaction is avoided because it is to the advantage of the group to not enter into the transaction. There are two ways in which this can happen—either the actor is so highly rewarded through other social alternatives that the particular transaction has low salience or the transaction would be so costly to the participant that he chooses to seek out other alternatives or do without the needs that could be served by the transaction.

There is a rationale to the use of various cooperative strategies that depend upon two dimensions—the amount of agreement among the parties about preferences for outcomes or objectives and the congruence among the parties' beliefs about the means to achieve the goals. Figure 1 has been adapted from a model by Thompson and Tuden[21] and later expanded by Thompson.[22] When there is agreement (or certainty) about preferences for desired outcomes and there is also agreement about the appropriate means of reaching the outcomes, the strategy is merely computational, because in this case there is no need for one party to influence the other. However, where there may be agreement about outcomes but disagreement about means, a judgmental strategy is operative. If there is disagreement about the preferred ends but common means are available, bargaining is the strategic move. In the case of a judgmental strategy, an adaptive process is used to test different means over time since there is agreement by the parties involved as to the preferred outcome. However, when there is disagreement about the scale of desirability of potential outcomes, the parties must enter into a negotiation to find a compromise solution.

		Preferences About Possible Outcomes (Ends)	
		Agreement	*Disagreement*
Beliefs About Appropriate Means	*Agreement*	Unilateral action based on dominance or shared control — Computation	Bilateral action based on compromise — Bargaining
	Disagreement	Multilateral action based on action and reaction — Judgment	

FIGURE 1. *Cooperative Decision Strategies*

Obviously, where there is no agreement, no strategy between the parties can be effective. In this case either the competitive strategy where a third party is involved or the exclusion strategy is likely to be used. Thompson argues that the strategies of co-optation and coalition are means of reducing the uncertainty or disagreement to the point where a certain amount of agreement is developed either about means or ends so that an appropriate cooperative decision strategy can be used. Thus strategies for influencing the decision process are dynamic and continuously change as the social relationships in the transaction and in the environment change.

A few examples show how this operates in the health field. The mission of school boards, for example, is that of education, while the mission of the health department is the enhancement of health. But health services for school children can serve both goals, and one finds many kinds of negotiated contracts between health departments and schools for health services. If the means no longer are agreed to serve each organization's outcomes satisfactorily, the alliance will be re-negotiated or terminated. This is the bargaining strategy. The judgment strategy is similar to that of Lindblom's "disjointed incrementalism" wherein each party moves in the preferred direction and then adapts as the situation about means becomes more clear. Disagreements—for example, as to who shall serve what aspects of a client's needs, as in rehabilitation—may be solved on a cooperative basis by an agreement by each agency to serve specific types of clients or to provide one part of a series of services to the same client. The use of case conferences among agencies to work out appropriate means of serving clients is an example of a judgmental strategy.

In different communities, depending upon the history and other factors, the above tactical strategies of finding appropriate means of working through disagreements in political decision-making may become stabilized as a preferred way of working in the political arena. The political transactions become locked into a particular set of relationships, and those individuals and groups who do not have access to resources for entering into the political decision-making system are likely to become isolated and impotent. This, in turn, leads to disequilibrium when such groups are exploited or begin to gain enough access to other power resources to disrupt the established patterns of decision-making. In addition to patterns of preferred ways of resolving differences in a community, one finds variations in political ideologies—that is, beliefs about the proper role of government.

Beliefs About the Role of Government

A political ideology may be defined as a body of concepts held by individuals or groups that have the following characteristics:[23] They constitute an argument—that is, they are intended to persuade and to counter opposing views; they integrally touch upon some of the major values of life; they embrace a program for the defense or reform or abolition of important social institutions. They are, in part, a rationalization of group interests but not necessarily the interests of all the groups espousing them. But more than this they are normative, ethical, and moral in tone and content. Essentially they deal with such questions as: Who ought to rule? How will rulers be selected? By what principles will they govern? What is the social nature of the community? What is the image of the proper role and scope of government?

For example, the planner should recognize that there may be quite disparate views in the community as to whether political leadership would come from the affluent and the propertied (those that have a significant economic stake in the community) or whether political leadership should represent the lesser advantaged or come from a combination of social elements of the community.[24] Additionally, the community may be seen as composed of classes or status groups with different interests or needs, as an organic whole with a common interest and a recognized interdependence among its members, or as a collectivity with a single set of interests defined by one section of the community. Government may be seen as the instrument of community growth, the provider of amenities, a caretaker (limited to certain functions), or the arbiter of conflicting interests.

These varied points of view about the role and scope of government that represent different political ideologies are important factors in the political structures which exist and which arise to meet new contingencies. They are particularly important in establishing the bases of conflict and cooperation within the community. For example, in a study of reported community conflicts in a variety of geographic areas, Coleman found that when the normal processes of political give-and-take broke down and issues became public issues, there was a tendency for the issues to become polarized and for ideological leaders to emerge. When the issue became one of ideological differences, it was more difficult to come to a satisfactory resolution of the conflict.[25]

Depending upon the power structure, the political decision-makers, as well as other sectors of the community, may operate within single or among multiple ideological positions with differing measures of divergence or convergence between them. Moreover, the planner must recognize the possibility of a discrepancy between the ideological premises espoused by individuals or groups and the extent to which their operationalization of the premise, when confronted with a particular program or policy, is at variance with these premises.[26] Free and Cantril noted a discrepancy between results on the operational spectrum, which revealed consensus on the liberal side, and those on the ideological spectrum, which leaned toward the conservative side.[27] Many individuals were found to express operational liberalism along with ideological conservatism and failed to note any contradiction or express any cognitive dissonance.

POWER NEEDED TO INFLUENCE AND IMPLEMENT DECISIONS

Although we have not previously defined power in this chapter, it has been assumed that the person who has power has access to resources not available through other alternatives to those needing these resources.

As mentioned earlier, however, there is a subtle difference between power as an ability and willingness to commit resources as compared with power as a potential of resources or credit. There are a variety of assets or resources that are desired in social interaction—liquid resources such as cash or credit, jobs, social standing in the community, special skills, and abilities. There is, in addition, the legitimate authority of encumbency in office, whether in governmental or nongovernmental organization, through which the resources of an organization can become available.

Therefore, for the planner it becomes important to identify the kinds of decisions that are made in the political context and those that will be made outside of the particular political arena in order to ascertain the likelihood of actual use of power resources. Diesing argues that political decisions are those that "have decision structures as their special subject matter"—that is, that are concerned with the organization, the supply or resources, and the value transactions in social organization.[28] Others argue that political decisions concern "publicly authoritative allocations of public values" and that political decisions differ from private transactions in that the formal or informal group rather than the individual consumer or producer is the basic unit, that the budgetary process rather than the price mechanism is the means, and that the public "products" are not for the individual good but are rather for the collective good[29]: "Public policy actions involve far more chains of decision than private."[30]

The way in which political decision-making occurs is central to what powers are needed to influence or implement decisions. Robinson and Majak suggest that there are three kinds of subprocesses in decision-making: the intellectual, the social, and the quasi-mechanical: "Problem-solving, collecting and analyzing information, defining situations, formulating alternatives and similar activities are intellectual processes."[31] These are analytic in nature, although they depend upon the subjective cognitions, insights, intuitions, and perceptions of the participating parties.

The social processes, on the other hand, are the means by which resolution of differences among the parties can be achieved. As described earlier, cooperation, competition, or exclusion strategies may be used. These seem to take significance when consolidation of the various interests is required to actually implement collective decisions. Finally, the quasi-mechanism processes are those that emerge almost automatically because of previous commitments of the various parties, present power relationships, or patterns of organization. For example, the regulation under P.L. 89–749 that the decentralization of state health planning bodies be by geographical configurations sets certain limits to the patterns of planning processes that can occur and, in a sense, limits in a quasi-mechanical way the kinds of intellectual and social decisions that are possible.

The capacity for gathering power in political decision-making and for influencing social decision-making is dependent upon both the informational resources needed for influencing the intellectual decision process and the constraints imposed by the structural context in which the decision-making occurs. For example, within the local community most health and welfare organizations are not free agents but rather have ties to constituencies both within and outside of the relevant community. Local governmental agencies, such as the health department or the welfare department, are closely tied through funding and other regulatory mechanisms to relevant state and federal agencies. Many voluntary agencies are affiliated with or receive charters through national organizations. Additionally, those organizations, whether governmental or nongovernmental, who have a high proportion of professionally oriented personnel find constraints through the articulation of professional values. These are quasi-mechanical limits to the ways in which resources in the local community can be allocated. Additionally, by the very nature of their responsibility, there is a tendency for administrators of agencies to perceive the problems of the community in terms of problems of achieving an agency's immediate mission.[32] This tendency restricts the intellectual decision processes of assessment and problem identification and of finding a diversity of alternatives toward solving community problems. Two prime functions, therefore, of an area-wide planning agency would be to facilitate the intellectual processes in decision-making through expansion of the sources of information available to the planning group and to enhance the opportunities for the development of new social transactions within the limits of the local powers for decision-making. A third function is to bring together the various factions within the community in order to consolidate power for influencing decisions that are outside of the relevant community's domain.

In Chapter 15 there is a discussion of skills of influence as one kind of tool for planning. The skills of expertise and knowledge, of communication, and of prediction of the effects of action (or nonaction) can be brought to bear on the problem delineation process—the intellectual aspect of legitimating action, organizing and arranging people and resources, bargaining and conflict resolution, and the development of trust and enthusiasm are operative in the social process aspect of political decision-making.

There is little empirical data available that can aid the planner in predicting the final outcomes of particular decision processes. There is some evidence—for example, that, taking into account such things as per capita income, the greater the competition between a state's political parties the greater will be its welfare efforts.[33] But this information is not of particular operational value to the planner. The implementation of plans generally requires that some change occur in the existing social transactions that form the social base of political power. However, in any situation the power equilibrium is dynamic and in a continuous change process. Therefore, a major skill of planning for implementation is that of extending the variety of means by which decision will be made by the many kinds of participants in the political decision-making process.

Therefore, when analyzing the resources he has for influencing political decision-making, the planner must consider all of the following:

1. The nature of the power structure. Is it concentrated or diffuse? Does it have an economic base or is the base dependent upon the type and scope of the issue? What prospects are there for change in the power structure?

2. The relationships between the governmental structure and the community's power relationships. What political ideologies are operative within the community?

3. How political leadership groups are formed in the community. Are they established with a strong organizational base? Are they integrated into the power structure? Are they based on interests or on political ideologies?

4. Shifts in the scope of government. Are local and national trends similar or different? Will they remain so?

5. The relationships between the socioeconomic system and the local political system. Are major economic decisions affecting the community made within or external to the community? What is the base from which the local political system is structured?

6. Relationships between the local political system and other political systems. Are county, state, regional, and national interests compatible with local interests? How much influence does each have on each other?

7. The manner in which issues are generally presented in the community. Do they dampen or arouse ideological competition?

The powers for influence and implementation that planners have available are generally channeled through organizational means, and the implementation of any new plans likely will require changes in the activity output of several community agencies. Thus it is important that a planning decision structure be formed to facilitate political decision-making processes. In comprehensive planning for health, three major constituencies need to be considered: the providers of services, whether they be organized through governmental or nongovernmental auspices; the users of the services; and the general society. Each of these constituencies can be subdivided into many subgroupings whose special interests require consideration. One device that has been built into many of the newer governmentally sponsored health service programs, such as the neighborhood health centers of OEO, is the requirement for the formation of consumer advisory boards. Additionally, in P.L. 89–749 the advisory board mechanism requires that the makeup of the board include at least 50% consumer representation. However, because of the almost innumerable interest groups that could be involved, the very makeup of such boards has created difficult political decisions in many communities and states throughout the United States.

Decisions as to the role and functions of such boards, as well as the spelling out of specific relationships of such boards to their parent organization, are also political decisions. In the past most coordinating and planning agencies, of which the councils of social agencies are a prototype, have been formed on a cooperative model. They are only viable if consensus about both means and objectives can be achieved. Since planning and its implementation will require a continuous series of transactions between outside interest groups and the agencies that provide health functions in the community, it seems likely that the cooperative model will not accommodate adequately the range of political decision-making and negotiation that will be required if planning is to be successful.

A health planning organization's major preoccupation should be that of creating and stating the community's health goals and objectives in such a way as to maintain contributions of effort. This is similar to the description Clark and Wilson give to the purposive organization in contrast to "utilitarian" organizations such as business firms and "solidary" organizations such as special interest groups: "Purposes become the basic instrument of unity; but at the same time they become the basic source of potential cleavage. Conflicts over purpose—in purpose oriented groups—will produce the most heated internal disputes. External actions will be efforts to achieve stated goals or to appear to be doing so."[34] It might be expected that the intensity of competition for resources (issues and causes, status, time, money, and effort) among health agencies would increase as resources become scarce and as the autonomy or domains of two or more organizations are questioned. Thus a health-planning organization should be structured in a way that provides a means for resolution of conflict and competition among interest groups by political decision-making processes.

To achieve this range of political decision-making will require some innovation in the form of an organizational model that serves to articulate the planning process. One suggestion has been to design an organizational structure that provides for a high degree of competitive activity within its structure.[35] It is argued that the competitive model might enhance the opportunities as well as the desires for all interested parties to enter into the planning negotiations. Figure 2 shows a general model for such a structure. The major innovation in this structure is the use of dual and competing policy committees, each charged with responsibility for policy in a particular dimension of the

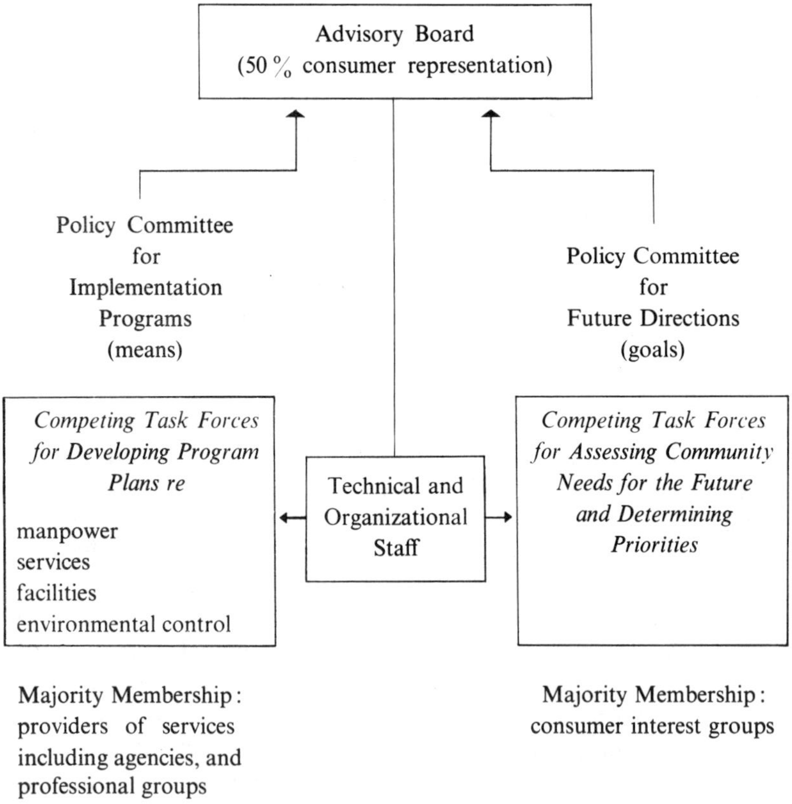

FIGURE 2. *A Competitive Model for a Health Planning Agency*

planning process. Resolution of incompatible policies would have to be achieved in the board as a whole.

Within such an organization, negotiation would be expected to occur between interest groups at each level of planning, between the two types of task forces, and between the two policy committees as well as at the board level. At the level of the task forces, if competing groups were to be formed purveyors would compete for the support of the different consumer interests and, alternately, consumer interests would have to secure support from providers of services to develop feasible directions and goals. Competition at every level of such a planning organization, hopefully, would provide motivation for participation by all parties and the opportunity for the communication processes and social transactions that would lead to a continual planning process in which all parties have a stake in the decision outcomes. Staff would not only have to have the technical skills of planning and analysis but also would have to be highly skilled in facilitating negotiations among the competing groups. Through such a mechanism or through the advisory board mechanism, inarticulate or relatively disenfranchised groups can be offered avenues of political mobility without the destruction of social integration so essential to the achievement of effective planning and implementation.

Although the technical aspects of planning are complex and require a great deal of skill, the true measure of whether comprehensive planning will become an accepted mode of social change in communities throughout the United States will be whether planners are able to develop an operational program that will take into account the articulation of the needs of the many interest groups within the community and provide the organizational context in which the several aspects of political decision-making can take place.

References

1. Britton Harris, "The Limits of Science and Humanism in Planning," *Journal of the American Institute of Planners*, XXXIII:5 (September 1967), 324–325.
2. Robert Dahl, *Who Governs?*, New Haven: Yale University Press, 1961, p. 1.
3. Floyd Hunter, *Community Power Structure*, Chapel Hill: The University of North Carolina Press, 1953.
4. C. Wright Mills, *The Power Elite*. New York: Oxford University Press, 1956.

5. Robert Lynd and Helen Lynd, *Middletown in Transition*, New York: Harcourt, Brace & World, 1937.
6. John Walton, "Substance and Artifact: The Current Status of Research on Community Power Structure," *American Journal of Sociology*, LXXI:4 (January 1966), 430–438.
7. Suzanne Keller, *Beyond the Ruling Class: Strategic Elites in Modern Society*, New York: Random House, 1963, p. 115.
8. Edward C. Banfield and James Q. Wilson, *City Politics*, Cambridge: Harvard University Press, 1963, p. 235.
9. See "Trigger for Community Conflict: The Case of Fluoridation," *Journal of Social Issues*, XVII:4 (1961).
10. Gabriel A. Almond and G. Bingham Powell, Jr., *Comparative Politics: A Developmental Approach*, Boston: Little, Brown, 1966.
11. Gabriel A. Almond and G. Bingham Powell, Jr., *ibid.*, p. 78.
12. Robert Dahl, *Who Governs?*
13. L. C. Freeman, *et al.*, "Locating Leaders in Local Communities," *American Sociological Review*, 28:5 (October 1963), 791–798.
14. Daniel J. Elazar, "Megalopolis and the New Sectionalism," *The Public Interest*, 11 (Spring 1968), 69.
15. Peter H. Rossi, "The Organizational Structure of an American Community," *in* Amitai Etzioni (ed.), *Complex Organizations: A Sociological Reader*, New York: Holt, Rinehart & Winston, 1961, pp. 301–312.
16. Paul A. Miller, *Community Health Action*, East Lansing; Michigan State University Press, 1953.
17. Aaron Wildavsky, "The Empty Headed Blues: Black Rebellion and White Reaction," *The Public Interest*, 11 (Spring 1968), 13.
18. Peter M. Blau, *Exchange and Power in Social Life*, New York: John Wiley, 1964, p. 22.
19. Sol Levine and Paul E. White, "Exchange as a Conceptual Framework for the Study of Interorganizational Relationships," *Administrative Science Quarterly*, 5:4 (March 1961), 583–601.
20. James D. Thompson and William J. A. McEwen, "Organizational Goals and Environment," in Amitai Etzioni (ed.), *Complex Organizations*, p. 186; reprinted from *American Sociological Review*, 23 (1958), 23–31.
21. James D. Thompson and Arthur Tuden, "Strategies, Structures, and Processes of Organizational Decision," in James D. Thompson *et al.*, *Comparative Studies in Administration*, Pittsburgh: The University of Pittsburgh Press, 1959, pp. 195–216.
22. James D. Thompson, "Decision-Making, the Firm and the Market," in W. W. Cooper, H. J. Leavitt, and M. W. Shelly, II (eds.), *New Perspectives in Organizational Research*, New York: John Wiley, 1964, pp. 334–348.
23. Robert Lane, *Political Ideology*, New York: The Free Press, 1952, pp. 14–15.
24. For a detailed model of ideological positions see Agger *et al.*, *The Rulers*

and the Ruled: Political Power and Impotence in American Communities, New York; John Wiley, 1964.

25. James S. Coleman, *Community Conflict*, New York: The Free Press, 1957.
26. See William V. D'Antonio, "Community Leadership in an Economic Crisis," *American Journal of Sociology*, LXXI:6 (May 1966), 688, for a case in which political ideology and operational decisions differed.
27. Lloyd A. Free and Hadley Cantril, *The Political Beliefs of Americans*, New Brunswick, N.J.: Rutgers University Press, 1968.
28. Paul Diesing, *Reason in Society: Five Types of Decisions and Their Social Conditions*, Urbana, Ill.: The University of Illinois Press, 1962, p. 198.
29. R. C. Wood with V. V. Almendinger, *1400 Governments: The Political Economy of the New York Metropolitan Region*, Cambridge, Mass.: Harvard University Press, 1961, p. 20.
30. William C. Wheaton, "Integration at the Urban Level: Political Influence and the Decision Process," in Philip Jacob and James Toscano (eds.), *The Integration of Political Communities*, Philadelphia: Lippincott, 1964, pp. 130–132.
31. James A. Robinson and R. Roger Majak, "The Theory of Decision-Making," in James C. Charlesworth (ed.), *Contemporary Political Analysis*, New York: The Free Press, 1967, p. 181.
32. Mary F. Arnold and Douglas L. Hink, "Agency Problems in Planning for Community Health Needs," *Medical Care*, 6:6 (November-December 1968), 454–466.
33. James A. Robinson and R. Roger Majak, "The Theory of Decision-Making," pp. 186–187.
34. Peter B. Clark and James Q. Wilson, "Incentive Systems: A Theory of Organizations," *Administrative Science Quarterly*, 6:2 (September 1961), 158.
35. Mary F. Arnold and Douglas L. Hink, "Agency Problems in Planning for Community Health Needs."

11

Effects of Community Power on Hospital Organization

L. Vaughn Blankenship & Ray H. Elling

The short-term, general hospital is generally viewed as a "community" institution as opposed to, say, a labor union, a fraternal group, or a professional association that has a more limited and specialized clientele group. In theory, at least, such a hospital is oriented toward the *community's* health and medical welfare, serves equally all segments of the population, and draws upon them for support; and decisions about which services should be offered, curtailed, expanded or reorganized are made at least partially on the basis of the "community interest."

In fact the hospital inevitably becomes much more differentiated vis-à-vis its environment and operates somewhat less ideally than such a model suggests. One hospital, for example, becomes known as "The Address" while another is characterized as for "the man on the street." Membership on the board of one hospital is a sign of one's arrival socially, and such membership becomes the prerogative of a semiclosed, self-perpetuating elite.[1] At another hospital certain informal understandings or pressures make it difficult for a general practitioner to get on the medical staff and, if he is on it, to find beds for his patients. Finally, the personal loyalties and institutional identification of certain doctors, nurses, board members, and even patients with the hospital may become so strong that the degree of objective rationality required to view the hospital and its needs from the point of view of the community at large is lost.[2] While there is some suggestive literature on the causes and consequences of such differentiating processes for organizations in general and hospitals in particular, there is still a great need for more study of this subject.[3]

One important aspect of the functioning of the general, short-term hospital that may be affected by this process of differentiation is its receipt of support from the community in the way of specific resources and more general expressions of favorable sentiments and attitudes. In an obvious and direct sense the goal achievement and, indeed, survival of the hospital depends upon its receipt of an adequate level of crucial resources which it cannot generate from internal sources alone, i.e., power, money, personnel, and cultural and technical artifacts and knowledge.[4] While the relationship between goal achievement and a favorable climate of community opinion seems less immediate and clear, it is reasonable to assume that the long-run growth and security of the hospital may well be enhanced by the favorableness of its general public image. Such favorable predispositions, from the point of view of a particular hospital, may become especially vital when it is challenged or attacked by other groups or organizations, including other hospitals, in the community. On the other hand, of course, the availability of such a pool of "good will" that can be mobilized in favor of the hospital may work to its eventual disadvantage if it enables the hospital to withstand pressures for change or reorganization from community leaders or those responsible for planning the community's hospital needs. In such instances, as the present study shows, the hospital may find itself ignored or bypassed by those in a position of power in the community.

In a multihospital setting the particular groupings of individuals and institutions with which different hospitals may develop differential ties potentially cut across a number of group interests: socioeconomic status, religion, profession, age, sex, and a number of others. One such group that may be of particular importance in affecting the ability of the hospital to get support from its community, as suggested above, is one distinguished in terms of power: the community leadership structure.

In the growing body of literature on the essential question of who governs in American communities, a great deal of effort has been expended in order to (1) develop reliable methodological tools for measuring power and (2) describe the shape and characteristics of the local power structure.[5] While there has been some disagreement about the validity of various techniques for identifying the community leadership structure and the interpretation of the results, one finding appears to be common to the various studies of the phenomena[6]: There are a highly restricted number of roles involved in making important community decisions and allocating community resources among competing uses.[7] By virtue of their key positions in the economic or governmental institutions in the community, it would be expected that those who fill such roles are in a particularly good position to influence the distribution of scarce communal resources to organizations like the community hospital. Furthermore, because of their greater knowledge of and contacts with authoritative bodies external to the community and their ability to "get things done" in the community, members of the local leadership structure are frequently able to determine the fate of local organizations such as hospitals when, as in the case of Hill–Burton or foundation aid, outside help is required to carry out some plan for maintenance or growth of the institution.

If there are, then, differential ties between the leadership structure and the various hospitals within a community, it would be expected that those which were more closely allied to the power structure would also be better supported by the community. That is, if it can be shown that the leadership structure in a community has or has had closer, more intimate connections with one hospital as compared with another, there should be some evidence that the former hospital has, in some sense, "done better" in getting support from the community than the latter. This chapter reports a study carried out in a large, multihospital community in upstate New York, which we will call Urban Center, in order to test this general hypothesis.

PROCEDURES

Data that had been collected earlier from all general, short-term hospitals in upstate New York (N = 136) had indicated that certain community variables such as size, income distribution, and proportion of professionals in the community were correlated with some of the indices we would be using in a test of the above hypothesis. For this reason we decided to focus on a single, multihospital community—in this case, Urban Center—as a means of controlling for the effect of such community variables.[8]

While there were more than ten hospitals in Urban Center, several of them were specialized, long-term institutions. These were excluded from consideration as were the governmentally owned hospitals in order to focus on those which were *formally* as alike as possible. Of the remaining seven general, short-term, voluntary hospitals in the community, four were selected for inclusion in this study. In 1959, when the study was carried out, these four hospitals accounted for 74% of the beds and more than 81% of all the admissions to this class of hospitals in Urban Center. One of them was Roman Catholic, and the other three were nondenominational. Of the three general, voluntary hospitals not included in the present report, one was primarily a teaching institution, one essentially a maternity hospital, and the third both quite small (60 beds) and relatively new.

One major problem with which the study was faced was to specify what was meant by community "support" of the hospital. This concept was defined broadly as a positive, consciously favorable orientation of the community toward the hospital. In an exploratory study of the type reported here it was believed to be desirable to be as eclectic as possible in selecting indices to measure the degree of community support received by a hospital. In the first place, there was little to be found in the way of previous work which indicated in any satisfactory way what measures might be used. Thus, reliance on one or two indices of support seemed a bit premature. Second, it was at best questionable as to whether we were dealing with some overarching, unidimensional variable when we talked about "support." Consequently, we spread the net wide and selected three different types of measures which, it was hoped, would allow us to talk about meaningful differences in community support for the four hospitals in study.

One group of indices was intended to catch the actual behavior of individuals in the community toward the hospitals. As indicated above, some of the resources which any hospital requires in order to achieve its goals includes funds, steady and reliable workers, and volunteers. While the latter "resources" appear, on the surface, to bear a different relationship to the achievement of organizational objectives than, say, funds, it was assumed that an active group of volunteer workers can (1) relieve some of the regular hospital personnel from more mundane tasks so that they may be used more efficiently elsewhere; (2) perform important public relations activities for the hospital so that people in the community are more aware of it and its needs; and (3) provide additional equipment, materials, and funds the hospital may desire. Furthermore, volunteers may provide certain services that help create the "hotel-like" characteristics of the hospital by which the layman tends to judge its quality and desirability as a place to go as a patient.

Information on the amount of money the four hospitals in Urban Center had received from all external sources, that is, money received from sources other than patient income, for the 10-year period of 1949–1958 was obtained from questionnaires filled out by each of the four hospital administrators and from annual reports filed with the

New York State Department of Social Welfare. This included funds from drives, donations, and contributions for current operations, bond issues, and other governmental payments. The data on volunteer services and activities were taken from the hospital administrator questionnaire, as was that for personnel turnover within the hospital for the years 1957–1959. The latter figure was used as an indication, albeit imperfect, of the steadiness of nonmedical, full-time personnel and the willingness of people in the community to work in a given hospital.

Two other indices were used as an indication of the general attitudes of people in the community at large toward the four hospitals. In a random sample survey of individuals in Urban Center and the surrounding metropolitan area (N = 280) conducted in the summer of 1959, respondents were asked to pick the hospital they would go to if they were completely free to choose for (1) a routine procedure, e.g., appendicitis or a fracture, and (2) a serious condition, e.g., neurosurgery or extensive diagnostic problems. In addition, they were asked to list all of the hospitals in Urban Center in order of their "general preference." The responses to these questions were used as an indication of how the general public in Urban Center evaluated the various hospitals in the community.

A final and more qualitative measure of the support these hospitals had received from their community consisted of an analysis of the history and development of the four hospitals during the decade of 1950–1959. This, it was felt, would give additional meaning to the other more quantitative indices used, i.e., help to avoid missing the forest for the trees and provide a backdrop against which the conclusions about community support of the hospital and its ties with the power structure could be drawn. The data for this phase of the study were drawn from various hospital, newspaper, and other written records as well as from lengthy interviews with hospital administrators, board members, community leaders, and other people in Urban Center who were in a position to be particularly knowledgeable about hospital affairs.

As far as the community power structure is concerned, there are three different though related measures that have been employed to date to identify this phenomenon in studies of community leadership.[9] One such method that has been used with success elsewhere is the so-called "reputational technique," which involves asking a panel of local citizens, "Who makes the important decisions around here?"—to paraphrase the question most frequently used. These nominations are then tabulated, a cutoff point is determined, and the resulting list of names is taken as representing the leadership structure.

Such a list of names was obtained from those individuals in Urban Center who had played an active role in one or more of a panel of 39 decisions that had taken place approximately during the five-year period from 1954–1959. A person was considered a decision participant if (1) he was so designated by at least one person formally responsible for any decisions included in the panel, (2) he was so designated by at least one other "in" person (formal or informal), and (3) he so designated himself. Most of the participants were interviewed and were requested to fill out and return a questionnaire that asked them, among other things, to "name the people in (Urban Center) whom you consider the most influential, whether they hold public office or not." A random sample of 80 out of the more than 500 questionnaires that were completed and returned by participants in these decisions was selected and the responses to this question were tabulated. After an empirical assessment of the number of people named and the number of nominations received by each, we decided that an individual had to receive five or more nominations to be considered a member of the power structure in Urban Center. As a final check, an additional 20 questionnaires were checked at random to see if any new names received the necessary number of nominations to be included on the list. In this random check no additional persons received five or more nominations so that the total number of "influentials" remained at 34.

In order to get a quantitative measurement of the connections these leaders had had with the four hospitals included in the study, it was decided to focus on less ambiguous, more direct contacts. Thus we examined (1) patient experience, i.e., had they ever been a patient in the hospital; (2) membership on the hospital board; (3) wife's membership on the hospital board; and (4) whether they had made donations to the hospital. To assess the more qualitative aspects of their relationships to these hospitals, we decided to ask them to list all of the hospitals in the community in order of their general preference and to indicate which one they would choose for treatment of a "major" and a "minor" medical problem.

Special questionnaires soliciting information on all of these items were sent to all of those nominated as "influentials" (N = 34) and 23 of them were returned that were either partially or fully completed. Since a number of these "influentials" also had been participants in the decisions referred to above, we had a check on their patient experiences in the four hospitals since one of the questions asked of all decision participants was whether they had ever been hospitalized and where. Finally, lists of all those who had been on the boards of the hospitals between 1955–1959 made it possible for us to find out if any of the "influentials" or their wives (or husbands) had been a board member during this period regardless of whether the special questionnaire was completed and returned.

RESULTS

There is little doubt that the community influentials of Urban Center have been differentially connected to and involved with the four general, short-term hospitals in the study. Whether we talk about board membership, donations, or patient experience, Crestview and St. Johns have been consistently favored by the members of the power structure over Central and Doctors' Memorial, as Table 1 shows. While running a hospital is generally considered a "man's" business, the Board of Crestview is composed exclusively of women and there have been several women board members at Central between 1955–1959. Between these two, only Crestview was apparently able to tap the wives of these community leaders for board membership.

TABLE 1. *Connections and Involvement of Community Influentials with the Four Major Short-Term Hospitals in Urban Center*

	Percentages by Hospitals			
Type of Connection	*Crestview*	*St. Johns*	*Doctors' Memorial*	*Central*
Board membership (1955–1959)	20.6	17.6	2.9	8.8
Wife's (or husband's) board membership (1955–1959)	11.8	0.0	0.0	0.0
Donated money or equipment (1955–1959)	17.6	26.5	5.9	3.9
Wife's (or husband's) patient experience (1955–1959)	29.0	16.1	6.4	3.2
Patient's experience	28.0	36.0	12.0	8.0

In conjunction with its female board, Crestview has an all-male Board of Councilors on which a little more than 20% of the leaders themselves served during this five-year period. Likewise, almost 18% of the leaders have been on the Advisory Board of St. Johns. As can be seen from Table 1, few of these influentials have had similar contacts with either of the other two hospitals in the study. In the case of

Doctors' Memorial this is particularly striking in light of the fact that its board more than doubled in size (from 7 to 18 members) in the period studied. Despite such a proportionately large increase Doctors' Memorial was, for some reason, either unable or unwilling to attract members of the power structure to its board.

Similarly, community influentials in Urban Center have discriminated among these four hospitals when it comes to making contributions of money or equipment. Less than 10% of them (9.8) report a donation either to Doctors' Memorial or Central in spite of the fact that the former hospital was the only one of the four to undertake a fund drive on its own behalf between 1955 and 1959. In contrast more than 40% (44.1) of these leaders report a contribution to one of the other two hospitals.

The pattern of hospitalization experience of the community leaders and their spouses is similar. Of these influentials who have ever been hospitalized locally (N = 25), well over one-third of them have been in St. Johns and 28 % have been patients at Crestview. In addition, all of those who reported a patient experience at Doctors' Memorial also reported that they had been patients in one of these two more favored hospitals at some time in their lives. Similarly, the spouses of these "most-nominated" leaders are most likely to have been patients in either Crestview or St. Johns with the former hospital clearly being favored over the other three.

As might be expected, these differential connections between the power structure and the four hospitals studied are associated with differences in the expressed preferences of community leaders for these hospitals. Each of these "most-nominated" influentials was asked to rank five hospitals—the four included in the study and one other, University Hospital—in order of their "general preference." As can be seen from Table 2, a majority (55.9%) ranked either Crestview or St. Johns first and only two community leaders (5.8%) selected one of the other two hospitals first. In addition, those who ranked either Crestview or St. Johns as first in their "general preference" tended to restrict their second choice to these same two hospitals. Less than 15% of these influentials ranked either Doctors' Memorial or Central as second and, while the table does not show this, none of them listed these hospitals first *and* second. If they ranked one of them first their second preference was either Crestview or St. Johns and vice versa.

Such a ranking in terms of "general preference" serves as a summary indication of their over-all feelings about these hospitals as they compare with each other. When these community influentials were asked about their preferences within a specific frame of reference—that of

TABLE 2. *The "General Preference" of Community Influentials for the Four Hospitals Studied*

	Percentages Favoring Hospitals			
Order of Preference	*Crestview*	*St. Johns*	*Doctors' Memorial*	*Central*
First	29.4	26.5	2.9	2.9
Second	26.5	17.6	8.8	5.9

hospitalization—their responses focused on Crestview and St. Johns, as Table 3 shows. When "the chips are down," medically speaking, only one of these leaders (2.9%) would pick either Doctors' Memorial or Central. Even when the medical problem was of a relatively minor nature—appendicitis, a fracture, influenza, etc.—few community leaders indicated that they would select Central and only one picked Doctors' Memorial if they "were completely free to choose any hospital [they] wanted."

It could be argued that these indications of preference for hospitalization are a simple reflection of the objective availability of better quality care in either St. Johns or Crestview. It is true that these two hospitals have put more emphasis on "high-powered" medicine and surgery than is the case for the other two. As the administrator at Crestview observed on one occasion, "The emphasis here, of course, is on serious cases. When somebody comes in with something, we give them everything we've got. We get to the TLC (Tender Loving Care) later." This

TABLE 3. *Hospital Preferences of Community Leaders in Urban Center for the Treatment of Minor and Major Medical Problems*

	Percentages Preferring Hospitals			
Type of Medical Problem	*Crestview*	*St. Johns*	*Doctors' Memorial*	*Central*
Minor (e.g., appendicitis, fracture, influenza, etc.)	23.5	20.6	2.9	14.7
Major (e.g., neurosurgery, extensive diagnosis, etc.)	29.4	26.5	2.9	0.0

being the case it is to be expected that these community leaders would prefer the "high-powered" hospitals when they were in real medical difficulty.

That something other than objective differences in the type and, perhaps, quality of medical care available is involved in these preferences is shown by the fact that these influentials also select Crestview or St. Johns (44.1%) for minor, more routine medical problems. There is no reason to believe that any of these four hospitals is substantially better equipped and staffed to handle such cases than any of the others.

At this point we can conclude, then, that these four hospitals are differentiated vis-à-vis the power structure in Urban Center. They are differentiated both in terms of the actual, direct contacts community influentials have had with them and in terms of the preferences, general and specific, of these leaders. A higher per cent of the "most nominated" influentials have had a greater number of connections with Crestview and St. Johns—as board members, patients, donors, etc.—than is the case for Doctors' Memorial and Central. Furthermore, when asked to rank order these hospitals in terms of their "general preference," only a small per cent of these influentials listed these latter two hospitals first or second. And when asked which hospitals they would choose for treatment of major and minor medical problems if they "were completely free to choose," these leaders were much more likely to pick Crestview or St. Johns than either Doctors' Memorial or Central.

The question remains, however, as to whether or not these differential relations with the power structure are in turn related to the ability of these four hospitals to get support from their community. Is there any indication that St. Johns and Crestview have, in some sense, "done better" than the other two hospitals? Part of the evidence necessary to answer this question is presented in summary form in Table 4.

Perhaps the most striking thing about the data presented in Table 4 is that the relationship between the various indices of community support and the extent of a hospital's ties with the power structure is not consistent. The two hospitals that have had the most numerous connections with community influentials are *not* consistently higher than the other two on the various indices of support.

Focusing for a moment on the first three indices of support—funds, workers, and volunteers—we see that Crestview was substantially ahead of the other three hospitals in terms of monetary support, having received more per 100 beds during this ten-year period than Doctors' Memorial and Central combined. On this particular index St. Johns is second. In terms of the turnover of full-time personnel between 1957 and 1959 the order of the hospitals is reversed with

TABLE 4. *The Relationship Between a Hospital's Connections with the Community Power Structure and Community Support for the Hospital*

	Hospitals			
Indices of Support	*Crestview*	*St. Johns*	*Doctors' Memorial*	*Central*
Funds, workers, volunteers				
Total funds received, 1949–1958 (per 100 beds)	$350,000	$250,000	$150,000	$150,000
Personnel turnover, 1957–1959 (%)	58.0	93.0	26.0	27.0
Volunteer service hours, 1957–1959 (per 100 beds)	550	350	700	350
Community attitudes				
Ranked *first* in "general preference" (%)	16.8	27.8	15.4	16.1
Preferred for treatment of *minor* medical problem (%)	12.1	25.4	13.2	13.2
Preferred for treatment of *major* medical problem (%)	13.6	22.8	8.6	7.1

Crestview and St. Johns both having considerably higher rates than those of the other hospitals. St. Johns is again at the lower end of the scale, this time along with Central, when we look at volunteer service hours per 100 beds. Doctors' Memorial ranks first on this item, while Crestview is some distance behind in second place.

When it comes to support of a more general nature as measured by certain expressed preferences of the lay community a slight pattern does emerge, though not one entirely consistent with the hypothesis advanced in this study. In terms of community attitudes St. Johns is consistently though not markedly better supported than any of the other hospitals. Almost 30% of those in the community sample ranked it first in terms of their "general preference"; a quarter of them said that if they were "completely free to choose" they would select St. Johns for treatment of a minor medical problem; and 22.8% also would choose it if they were in real medical difficulty.

As can be seen in Table 4, those in the community sample were about as likely to pick Crestview first in terms of their "general preference" as they were to pick either Doctors' Memorial or Central.

Likewise there was virtually no difference in the proportion of the sample that would pick one of these three hospitals for treatment of a relatively minor ailment. It is only when we come to the question of the need for major treatment that Crestview begins to edge out the other two hospitals.

The only one of these indices of community support consistent with the general hypothesis that a hospital's support position is related to the closeness of its ties to the community power structure is the monetary index. Both Crestview and St. Johns, the two hospitals that have had the most extensive ties with community influentials, are considerably above the other two hospitals on this one index. As far as the comparative willingness of people in the community to work in one of these four hospitals, however, both Doctors' Memorial and Central appear to be much better off than either Crestview or St. Johns, and the latter hospital has done no better than Central in terms of volunteer service hours. While all four hospitals enjoy a certain amount of loyalty and support in the community at large, only St. Johns stands out from the other three. Crestview, the other hospital that has enjoyed close ties with the power structure in Urban Center, does not appear to have any advantage over either Doctors' Memorial or Central when it comes to the expressed preferences of the lay community.

A brief summary of the hospital developments in Urban Center in the past decade or so should help to put some of these findings in perspective and aid in drawing conclusions about the relationship between a hospital's ties to the power and its success in receiving community support.[10] In 1950 these four short-term hospitals were in a relatively secure position, though each was very aware that key developments in the immediate future could affect this security in important ways. Twelve years later, in 1962, Central was on the verge of giving up its status as a general hospital to become a hospital for the chronically ill; Crestview had become an even more integral part of the Medical School complex in Urban Center; though it was having its difficulties with the Medical School, St. Johns was even more supremely secure than it had been a dozen years earlier; Doctors' Memorial, faced with the competition of a new 300-bed Community Hospital and a new University Hospital, was struggling hard just to remain open. Its future looked exceedingly bleak. Even as early as the summer of 1959 most people in the "know" in Urban Center were predicting a change of status for Central and the eventual demise of Doctors' Memorial. The events of the decade had been fraught with consequences for the four hospitals.

It had been apparent at the end of World War II that some substantial changes and additions would have to be made in the hospital facilities available in Urban Center. By 1948 they were high enough on the priority list so that Hill–Burton aid would be available to be matched with funds raised locally for the construction of new hospital space.

St. Johns had had a fund drive in 1947–1948 that enabled it to make a 100-bed addition to the hospital in 1950. This made it the largest hospital in Urban Center and in this respect put it one up on the other three. In addition, it had recently established a lay Advisory Board composed mainly of industrialists, bankers, and prominent lawyers—Catholic and non-Catholic.

Doctors' Memorial had been nursing its plans for renovation and expansion for a number of years, and it now prepared to submit them to the community. Of the four hospitals, its physical plant was in the most deplorable condition. Along with Central, Doctors' Memorial began to seek out influential figures in the community for board membership. Until this time the board of the latter hospital had been highly ingrown and was composed mainly of "second and third string" people, individuals who had developed an intense loyalty for and identification with the hospital. Between 1950 and 1955 the board was more than doubled in size (from 7 to 18) as a number of businessmen were invited to join it. Likewise, Central managed to get one or two of the more influential people in the community on its board while Crestview began complementing its socially exclusive female board with an all-male Board of Councilors composed of some of the "biggest people" in Urban Center. Though smaller in size, its general physical plant was the equal of St. Johns at the beginning of this period.

During the ten years that followed, three different Citizens Committees made studies of the hospital situation in Urban Center and submitted their respective reports to community leaders. The first of these Committees, headed by a junior law partner in the firm of the man who is known locally as "Mr. Urban Center," produced a series of recommendations that gave something to all the hospitals. It was a report in which desires of the hospitals predominated. When the probable cost of this list of goods was presented to community leaders, the plans were shelved as "unrealistic."

Where the hospitals' points of view had shaped the first report, the second reflected the thinking of community business leaders, particularly those who would have a major say in the fund drive which was necessary. The second Citizens Committee was handpicked and chaired by "Mr. Industrialist" who, as president of one of the large, national corporations in Urban Center, was reputedly able to control over "ten per cent of anything that's raised." The ethos of this report is conveyed by Mr. Industrialist's" later summarization of his committee's efforts: "We weren't emotionally involved. We got the best possible advice and carried out a thorough study. We simply sought the best possible facilities for what the community could afford to save lives. . . ." In brief, St. Johns was to receive over one million dollars for improving its nursing school and the other three hospitals were to lose their separate identities entirely and be sold to the Medical School. The proceeds from this sale plus the Hill–Burton aid and the balance of the funds raised in a community drive were to be used to construct a new Community Hospital according to the recommendations of this second Citizens Committee. Crestview, Doctors' Memorial, and Central were to be put out of the hospital business entirely as separate institutions. Unfortunately for Mr. Industrialist, this sale had to be approved by a two-thirds vote of each of the boards of the hospitals affected.

With a little wavering on the part of a few of the women on its board, Crestview fell into line and voted to approve the recommendation. The husbands of many of these women were both on the Board of Councilors with and business associates of Mr. Industrialist. Initially Central's board indicated that it would go along with the plan though it was with considerable trepidation. It was Doctors' Memorial, however, which laid the suggestion of this second committee permanently to rest. Only 11 of the 18 board members opted in favor of the proposed sale, one short of the legally required two-thirds majority. Following Doctors' Memorial, Central also reneged on its earlier position. The bitter feelings which these developments left behind were still apparent 5 years later in the summer of 1960. As one doctor was later to observe, "There was a line up of number two community forces against number one people."

With things still in a state of unresolved crisis, a third Citizens Committee, again under the chairmanship of another junior law partner in the firm of Mr. Urban Center, began a series of public hearings and, after an appropriate time lapse, issued another report. In the end these recommendations were adopted and more than 9 million dollars was raised in a community fund drive. St. Johns was given over one million dollars for its nursing home, Crestview was given a small part of the Hill–Burton aid to purchase a new cobalt unit and, in addition, its board negotiated a sizable loan from one of the banks in Urban Center that enabled it to make some needed renovations. Neither Central nor Doctors' Memorial received any money, though the latter was "allowed" to raise $300,000 among friends of the hospital. The largest bulk of the community's money and the Hill–Burton aid went for a new, 300-bed Community Hospital.

In retrospect, several things are clear. St. Johns, which started out with a new, 100-bed wing, was able to satisfy its additional needs for new nursing facilities without difficulty. In fact all three committee reports had agreed on one point: that St. Johns should be given funds for this purpose. Doctors' Memorial, which also had a nursing school in desperate need of new facilities, received nothing. As a prominent Catholic layman in Urban Center and a member of both the boards of St. Johns and Doctors' Memorial observed:

> There was politics in the money for St. Johns nursing home. When Doctors' Memorial earlier needed money for its nursing home, there wasn't any. But there was money for the St. Johns nursing home. Our good friend, the Monseigneur, was very influential with a lot of people, particularly "Mr. Industrialist." They had public hearings before the [third] report came out and Doctors' Memorial put forth its case but nothing happened.

Neither Central nor Doctors' Memorial were ever realistically close to receiving what they felt they needed from the community. They did not have the power to impose their view of reality on the community leadership structure or to enforce their demands for at least a share of either the community's funds or Hill–Burton aid. Because of their legal authority the boards of these two hospitals were able to veto temporarily the decisions of community influentials, but they lacked sufficient positive power to make their counterclaims effective.

DISCUSSIONS AND CONCLUSIONS

From the preceding discussion it is clear that the power structure in Urban Center has, in the past, had differential ties with the four hospitals in this study. Whatever else they might have achieved, it is certain that St. Johns and Crestview have received more than their share of time, attention, donations, and energy from community influentials. The consequences of these differential ties for these two hospitals and Doctors' Memorial and Central in terms of their receipt of support from the community in the form of certain important resources and more general community attitudes are somewhat more complex.

On only one quantitative measure of support, the monetary index, is the association between a hospital's ties with the community power structure and its support position in the direction predicted by the hypothesis. In terms of hospital developments in Urban Center during the decade of the 1950's, it is certain that Crestview and St. Johns, the two hospitals with the closest and best developed ties to the leadership network, did comparatively well while the continued existence of the other two—at least as general, short-term hospitals—is in considerable doubt. This was not the only possible outcome, however, as the description of these events makes clear: thanks to the intransigence of the boards of Doctors' Memorial and Central, Crestview escaped their subsequent fate. Once such a solution was ruled out by the actions of these two boards; however, only St. Johns and Crestview were given a share of the available financial resources.

Hospitals, even though they are located within the same geographical boundaries, have their separate, semi-isolated communities which they serve. Each is the hub of a network of loyalties, commitments, and values that are specific to it. All four of the hospitals in Urban Center had volunteers, staunch adherents in the community, loyal workers, and devoted doctors, nurses, and board members. This type of commitment and support stems from the day-to-day activities and operations of the hospital as it goes about the business of patient care. It is generated by the organization itself as a cooperative, purposeful system with minimum reference to the larger community and the leadership structure. How leaders A, B, and C feel and act toward a particular hospital is, in the *short run*, unlikely to affect how Citizen X feels about the kind of care he might get there or how Nurse Y feels about the hospital as a place in which to work. These are essentially private experiences that may be influenced only indirectly, if at all, by the actions of community influentials.[11]

Financial resources, however, are operative at a more general, community-wide level than is the case for other forms of support. In a limited sense this type of support also flows from the day-to-day operations of the hospital—patients leave bequests, doctors purchase a piece of needed equipment, and volunteers raise goodly sums by various means that are given to the hospital. Only in rare instances, however, would this be sufficient to sustain the hospital for any length of time. During periods of "crisis," when its very existence is called into question or when large infusions of new capital arc required if it is to grow or survive, the wider community including the attitudes and acts of influentials takes on a new urgency. Hospitals find themselves directly in competition with each other as well as with other community organizations for a share of the limited financial resources available, and one hospital's gain is another's loss. Ties with the power structure, which may be the gradual accretion of years, become critical.

Given the centrality of money as a resource in a capitalistic economy, it seems quite likely that the actions of community leaders in this regard will have a long-run effect upon the more mundane operations of the hospital which serve to generate other types of support.[12] While it appears that the power structure in Urban Center has only a limited ability and probably neither the time nor inclination to influence directly the day-to-day operations that result in other demonstrations of community support, their decisions vis-à-vis financial resources ultimately determine the face of institutional survival as well as the conditions of such survival. When the power structure in Urban Center defined Doctors' Memorial as a hospital that could not survive and used this as the justification for the withholding of funds, it may well have set in motion a chain of events that will result in its ultimate failure regardless of the other types of support it enjoys.

Close alliances between an organization and a group that is external to it—in this instance power figures in the community—appears, from the point of view of the hospital, to have potential disadvantages. Integrity maintenance and survival have been postulated as fundamental imperatives of formal organization.[13] To the extent that this requires drawing upon centers of power external to the organization, there is always the possibility that the "tail may begin to wag the dog." In exchange for the currency and perquisites of greater potential staying power, the institution makes commitments that reduce its flexibility in other respects. At the extreme, these groups that are external to the organization and its value system make decisions that threaten its very survival. Because of its commitments to these external power centers and subsequent loss of flexibility, the organization finds it difficult if not impossible to resist.

Something like this seems to have happened to Crestview following the recommendations of the second Citizens Committee. Precisely because it was so closely tied to the power structure, Crestview found itself in the position of being unable to resist the pressure to vote itself out of existence. Lacking such well-developed and long-standing connections with community influentials, both Doctors' Memorial and Central were in a better position to thwart the plans of the leadership structure. They were less beholden and committed to community power figures and, given the legal positions of the boards involved, could effectively veto the proposed solution. This exercise of negative power may have only postponed the day that these two hospitals will cease to exist, at least in their present form—though to have acted otherwise would have assured their early demise.

In the past, few studies of community power structure have attempted to ascertain the consequences of a particular type of structure or the actions of community influentials for the functioning of community organizations like the hospital.[14] To a large extent the interest has been in the other direction: How is one's role in various organizations—businesses, large and small, unions, civic "improvement" associations, and philanthropic institutions—related to one's position of power in the community. Similarly, many studies of behavior in complex organizations pay deference to the idea that the organizational ecology is important, but few have attempted to analyze systematically linkage points between the two and assess their impact on the organization.

With the recent growth of interest in the nature and structure of community power and the proliferation of studies on the subject, it seems likely that we soon will be in a position to begin characterizing communities in terms of their power structures. This will allow us to develop more sophisticated, quantitative techniques for analyzing the relationships between power structure, as an independent variable, and various aspects of community functioning including that of community organizations like the hospital.

References

1. Joan W. Moore, "Patterns of Women's Participation in Voluntary Associations," *American Journal of Sociology*, 66 (1961), 592–598. Philanthropic activity such as membership on hospital boards may also be a necessary part of the career pattern of the "successful" business executive, e.g., Aileen D. Ross, "Philanthropic Activity and the Business Career," *Social Forces*, 32 (1954), 274–280.
2. This process of overidentification with and commitment to a particular set of goals and a particular organizational structure for achieving them has been noted frequently in studies of relationships *within* bureaucratic organizations. See, e.g., Philip Selznick, "A Theory of Organizational Commitments," in *Reader in Bureaucracy*, Robert K. Merton *et al.* (eds.), New York: The Free Press, 1952, pp 194–202, and Herbert A. Simon, *Administrative Behavior*, *New York*: *Macmillan*, 1958, pp. 12–14, 198–219. In the present instance we are suggesting that the same sort of process may occur *between* a given organization and its larger "community."
3. Charles Perrow, "Organizational Prestige: Some Functions and Dysfunctions," *American Journal of Sociology*, 66 (1961), 335–341, and Ray H. Elling

and Sandor Halebsky, "Organizational Differentiation and Support, A Theoretical Framework," *Administrative Science Quarterly*, 6 (1961), 185–209.

4. For a theoretical discussion of the role of resources and the resource "mobilizing process" in organizations see Talcott Parsons, *Structure and Process in Modern Societies*, New York: The Free Press, 1960, pp. 22–27.
5. For a general review of these developments see William H. Form and Delbert C. Miller, *Industry, Labor, and Community*, New York: Harper & Row, 1960, pp. 517–549, and Robert A. Dahl, *Who Governs?*, New Haven: Yale University Press, 1961, pp. 1–8.
6. These disagreements revolve basically around (1) some very real methodological problems involved in identifying who has "power" in the community and (2) ideological differences in the interpretation of the data uncovered with some leaning heavily toward a pluralistic and basically optimistic viewpoint and others much more inclined to see the data as supporting an elitist theory. Among the host of articles on the subject see Raymond E. Wolfinger, "The Study of 'Community Power,'" *American Sociological Review*, 25 (1960), 636–644; Robert A. Dahl, "A Critique of the Ruling Elite Model," *American Political Science Review*, 52 (1958), 463–469; and William V. D'Antonio and Eugene C. Erickson, "The Reputational Technique as a Measure of Community Power," *American Sociological Review*, 27 (1962), 362–375.
7. The arguments of those who favor a more pluralistic interpretation of power in the local community and generally reject the notion of a power *structure* fail to be convincing. As Floyd Hunter recently observed in a review of Robert Dahl's book (see Reference 5 above), which purports to come up with a pluralistic answer to the question of who governs in New Haven: "I have no trouble in understanding that 'democratic pluralism' is at work in the upper reaches of the one-half of 1 per cent of the policy-making array of New Haven. The fact that Dahl finds no connection between this narrow band of civic democrats and the large body politic does not, as suggested, surprise anyone....

   "In spite of professed differences between New Haven and other communities and between Dahl's findings and those of others, it would appear that New Haven has a definable, small body of citizens, some of them politicians in an elective sense; some of them businessmen in a self-selected sense; and some of them in-betweens, who do call basic shots in major policy matters. The rest of the population is apathetic....

   "It would seem... that policies are set by narrow, sketchily defined knots of influence, or multiple pyramids of power, if you like, each acting on individual matters of policy in which the actors feel they have some expertise...." *Administrative Science Quarterly*, 6 (1962), 517–519.
8. In a comparative case study of two small single-hospital communities, it was found that relations between the hospital and the leadership structure differed considerably. The well-supported hospital was more closely tied into the

local power structure than was the case for the less well-supported institution. These differences in support were not found to be entirely attributable to socioeconomic differences between the two communities. Relationships with the power structure and certain important differences in the *structure* of power itself in each community appear to account for a large part of the substantial differences in the levels of support received by the two hospitals. See L. Vaughn Blankenship, *Organizational Support and Community Leadership in Two New York State Communities*, unpublished Ph.D. dissertation, Ithaca: Cornell University, June 1962, Chapters 6–8.

9. William H. Form and Delbert C. Miller, *Industry, Labor, and Community*, New York: Harper & Row, 1960, p. 517.
10. A much more detailed treatment of the events of this decade in Urban Center is present in Ray H. Elling, "The Hospital-Support Game in Urban Center," in Eliot Freidson (ed.), *The Hospital in Modern Society*, New York: The Free Press, 1963.
11. Robert K. Merton has reached similar conclusions in regard to interpersonal influence: "People ranking high in a certain kind of prestige hierarchy... may have little interpersonal influence upon all those who are not concerned with their particular spheres of activity and opinions.... Men with power to affect the economic life chances of a large group may exert little interpersonal influence in other spheres. The power to withhold jobs from people may not result in directly influencing their political or associational or religious behavior." See "Patterns of Influence: Local and Cosmopolitan Influentials," in Robert K. Merton, *Social Theory and Social Structure*, rev. ed., New York: The Free Press of Glencoe, 1957, p. 419.
12. On the fundamental importance of monetary resources to an organization in a capitalistic society see Talcott Parsons, *Structure and Process in Modern Societies*, and Max Weber, *The Theory of Social and Economic Organization*, New York: The Free Press, 1947, Chapter III.
13. Philip Selznick, "Foundations of the Theory of Organization," in *Complex Organizations*, Amitai Etzioni (ed.), New York: Holt, Rinehart & Winston, 1961, p. 25. Selznick puts forward this postulate as a fundamental tenet of structural–functional analysis. The same point has been made by others in different language, for different reasons, in a different context. See, for example, Peter Drucker, *The Practice of Management*, New York: Harper & Row, 1954, Chapters 6, 7; and Kenneth Boulding, *The Organizational Revolution*, New York: Harper & Row, 1953, pp. 55–57.
14. Some exceptions are L. Vaughn Blankenship, *Organizational Support and Community Leadership in Two New York State Communities*, Irving A. Fowler, *Local Industrial Structures, Economic Power, and Community Welfare: Thirty Small New York State Cities 1930–1950*, Ph.D. dissertation, unpublished, Ithaca: Cornell University, 1954; and C. Wright Mills and Melville J. Ullmer, *Small Business and Civic Welfare*, Report of the Special Committee to Study Problems of American Small Business, U.S. Senate

79th Congress, 2nd Sess., No. 135, Washington, D.C.: USGPO, 1948. To the extent that there have been discussions of the findings on community power structure and their implications for the communities studied they have focused largely on their relevance for democracy and democratic process at the local level, e.g., Robert A. Dahl, "A Critique of the Ruling Elite Model," and Floyd Hunter, *Community Power Structure*, Chapel Hill: University of North Carolina Press, 1953.

IV

PLANNING AS A MEANS OF RATIONALIZING THE HEALTH SYSTEM

ONE'S PHILOSOPHICAL BELIEFS ABOUT MAN AND HIS RElationship with nature seem far removed from the everyday pressures and demands that the administrator of a health agency faces; however, they are the underpinning of his decision-making and of what he sees ought to be done. Administration can be defined as those activities purposefully undertaken to enhance the rationality of an agency or organization in the achievement of its mission or goals. An administrator must make decisions under a wide range of constraining situations and under variable and uncertain conditions. He is limited in his problem-solving by the context of a particular organizational problem, by the pressures of time, by the availability of a technology and other resources, and by the type and quality of information available for making predictions about the future. He is limited also by the situations in which problems present themselves and by the organizational limits of his authority. Therefore, in order to enhance the rationality of his organization's decisions, he must understand, as far is possible, the total dynamic social context in which his organization is embedded.

The idea of planning implies that there is a rational element in what organizations do; that there is an opportunity for conscious choice among alternative goals and alternative means for achieving those goals—that man has some measure of control over his destiny. It is on the assumption that the outcomes of man's activities are not predetermined and that man is not necessarily subject to the whims of the fates that our ideas about planning and administration are based.

What we believe to be the range of control that man has over nature, however, will determine the extent to which we believe our conscious activities should be rationalized. If, for example, we believe that we can make choices only within very circumscribed organizational systems, such as fiscal management, then our planning will take place only within that narrow boundary. If, however, we believe we might have some control over the directions in which our society is going, then we extend the boundaries of the system of concern. The time dimension, too, has a bearing on our planning. The tyranny of the fiscal year reduces the opportunities for planning in the broader sense, although our uncertainty increases as we concern ourselves with more distant futures.

It was suggested earlier that by definition a health organization differs from other organizations in that its mission is expressly related to the achievement of health goals for the society. The health administrator, therefore, should expect to take into account the role, functions, and interrelationships of his particular agency in the broader system of the society. By virtue of this orientation to health goals, the models by which health administrators have evaluated the effectiveness of health organization activities have been shaped by the society's definitions of health and by its beliefs about the causes of illness. The biological model of Western scientific medicine generally has served as the central perceptual paradigm for our society's assumptions about the causes of health and illness. Man is perceived as a biological entity who is born, lives, and dies, and health is generally equated with biological life. (In a culture believing in reincarnation, this particular emphasis on the biological entity of man would not be of central interest.)

Although recent thought has begun to shift from the mere maintenance of biological life to a renewed questioning of the meaning and quality of that life, the scientific study of health has generally been approached from a biological model of reality. The ecological perspective to the study of man's health seeks to understand the complex, dynamic interrelationships between a living entity and its environment, and to discover how that entity changes and evolves in its transactional relationship with its environment in a time perspective. Thus the ecological perspective provides us with a broad model of man's relationships with nature.

There has been confusion in the health field about planning. The words "comprehensive health planning" mean different things to different people. If we mean, in the more narrow sense, planning for provision of comprehensive medical care services to an individual, then our concern is with the system of activities that relates to who does what in terms of the care of a patient within a particular organizational or interorganizational context. If, however, "comprehensive health planning" has a broader sense, then we look to a wider range of forces and activities that impinge on the health of the society. However, the phrase "comprehensive health planning" is bounded by the word "health," because comprehensive planning in the broader societal context would include planning of more than health or the meaning of "health" would be all-encompassing. This is not just semantic confusion; rather, the semantic problem is a symptom of a philosophical problem: Just how broadly can we plan?

The tools of planning often may be equated with the functions of planning. More tools are becoming available to us for the rationalization of our decisions, whether these are made in the narrow system sense or in the broad societal sense. Theories of prediction and decision-making, the development of an information technology, and theories of human behavior that aid us in making "more rational" decisions are crucial to our ability to plan, whether at the very specific operational level or at the broad societal level. The chapters in this part reflect all these concerns with what we know and how we shall use what we know to rationalize what we are doing.

-12-

The Ecological Perspective

Edward S. Rogers

Ecology is the science of relating a given something to its environment: an organism or species, in the case of biological ecology; a man or a human population, in the case of human ecology; or, in a wider sense, any biological phenomenon that has the property of interdependence with other, identifiable objects or events outside of itself (environmental components) and with which it engages in significant (determinative) interaction. Ordinarily the term "ecology" is not applied to the relationships within strictly inorganic systems. Thus we might speak of the ecology of fossil formation at a given geographical site, but we would not apply the term to the environmental sequences in the formation of the sedimentary rock, as such. The distinction is somewhat arbitrary, but it is not unreasonable in view of the unique role of the environment in the adaptive evolution of biological phenomena—which gives particular purpose to ecology as a field of study. In a broad sense, then, human ecology can be defined as the study of the structural and functional adaptive processes of man as a biological and social organism.

Conceptually, there are two approaches to ecology. The more common approach deals with an environment that is identified, intuitively or otherwise, in somewhat limited terms. For example, epidemiology is ecological in this sense when it inquires into the causation of a specific disease by studying its associations with, let us say, a half dozen or so of the more evident environmental conditions that are considered as likely factors in the causative system. The other approach, originally developed by the biologist Bews,[1] is holistic and seeks to detect every environmental relationship of possible consequence through an attempt to identify the larger system of interactions within which the event of particular interest may be expected to have occurred.

The first approach starts with the event and gropes outward to find the relevant environment; the other starts with the study of the whole ecosystem (to the extent that it can be identified) and moves in to focus on the event. If properly conducted, and if both seek to look at the same event, the findings of the two methods of study should converge. Nevertheless, the two methods may be expected to be differentially useful. The epidemiological approach may lead more efficiently to the discovery of the most immediate and accessible link in a causative chain, while the holistic approach should yield greater insight with respect to the total causative system and the range of probable consequences of a contemplated course of action. The holistic approach, therefore, should have the greater utility for long-range, comprehensive planning since it continually seeks to extend the boundaries of the system of concern in the direction of total reality.

Public health and medical science, without actually using the term ecology until quite recently,[2] have been ecologically oriented, in the epidemiological sense, for a long time. In fact, recognition of the existence of a relationship between environmental conditions, such as climate, and health appears in writings attributed to Hippocrates and probably has existed from the very earliest period of man. But the importance of systematic study of such relationships has been recognized only in the hundred or so years since Darwin. Darwin's analysis did more than pave the way to genetics and a new understanding of biological evolution. It also paved the way for advances in sociology through its documentation of the "web of life" concept as applied to the interdependencies of the natural world within which human activities now play such a major part.[3]

The early interests of public health in man's environment were focused largely on the detection and control of environmental conditions as the direct precursors of disease — e.g., with polluted drinking water, contaminated food, bacterial and viral agents and their carriers, isolation of infectious cases, protective immunizations, and the like. While it did not escape notice on the part of a few persons who were euphemistically considered ahead of their time, it was not until the mid-twentieth century that significant recognition was given the complemental roles of culture, attitudes, values, and institutionalized patterns of human behavior as determinants of man's health.

This widened view has added new perspective to the previous pattern in which man's contacts with his environment tended to be treated mechanistically. The new viewpoint is more dynamic in that it relates events to man as a thinking, choice-making social being. However, it has not altered the prior concept that the ultimate, determinative environment is physical and biological in character. The prevailing practice today, as seen, for example, in governmental programs dealing with man and his environment, is to treat the social-cultural factors as indirect agents. They are seen as sets of conditions which organize and influence man's use and contacts with the physical and biological environment (including his fellow man) rather than as possible direct agents in their own right. There is reason to believe, as will be discussed shortly, that they are both.

One cannot challenge the demonstrated utility of the new concept, even though it may be incomplete. It has, for example, brought about new and effective approaches in disease prevention since, in certain situations, the sociocultural antecedents of disease can be more easily brought under control than can the sources of direct contact between man and the disease-producing agent. For example, venereal disease is clearly more effectively controlled by information and education than it is by attempts to control prostitution. The new viewpoint also has focused increasing attention on political and organizational questions in the planning of public policy and the management of human affairs. We may not have solved the air pollution or population problems, but we are certainly aware of their complex nature and have abandoned faith in attempts to deal with them out of their broader social context—at least we have commenced to do so.

On the debit side, preoccupation with the novelty of this new viewpoint and overcommitment to its partial successes may be standing in the way of logical pursuit of the larger perspective that also should concern us. And, as is the nature of partial solutions, it may even be fostering new kinds of problems. For example, continued application of technology in "adding years to life" without balancing concern with "adding life to years"—and with precisely what that term implies—is fully as short-sighted and could lead to as many new problems as has our failure, during the past several decades, to match the application of our technology and organizational skills in world-wide programs of mortality control with an equivalent concern for their consequences. This failure was not for lack of prophets who foresaw the resulting population problem; it must be laid wholly at the door of what Jerome Frank[4] has aptly labeled the American addiction to the "quick fix"—too short-range vision and opportunistic incrementalism. We, as a society, appear to be intellectually and politically incapable of the self-discipline and imagination necessary to an understanding of contemporary problems in ecological terms, i.e., in terms of the total environment of relevance. Instead, we repeatedly commit our available resources to what, at most, can be only partial solutions based on partial analysis. Much of the massive, political effort expended in the Great Society programs may be identified in these terms. Again, we are well on our way to repeating this error in our attempts to deal with urban poverty. As important as it certainly is to remedy them, we do not really know the extent to which unemployment, inadequate education, and low living standards are fundamental causes, on the one hand, or symptoms of something still more fundamental, on the other.*

In order truly to come to grips with such a complex societal product as poverty, we should need no argument that understanding *all* the actors in the total environment of relevance is a necessary condition for the planning and implementation of sound social policy. If we accept this necessity, we should return our attention to the question of the nature of the total relevant environment of man.

It is clear that man, in contrast with other living creatures, is unique in the manner in which he thinks and in the role that cognition plays in his existence. He has developed a body of experience and knowledge that he communicates and stores in various ways and with which he interacts via the abstract processes of self-awareness, perception, learning, and reflective thought. To the extent that the outputs of these processes are externalized and made available to other human beings, through any of a number of ways of communication, they become part of man's environment just as truly as though they were material in nature. This, then, is a new kind of environment unique to man, created by him and yet powerfully active in shaping him as well. Recognition of the existence of such an environmental force appears increasingly in the writings of leaders in humanistic thought: the *noosphere* of Teilhard de Chardin, and of Vernadsky, and the *inner man* of Sir Geoffrey Vickers come to mind.[5] For descriptive purposes, and in order to fit the existing classification of environmental actors, it seems useful to suggest the term *cognitive environment.*†

Obviously, the cognitive environment is closely related to what is sometimes referred to as the cultural environment, but the two are not

* For example, in the most fundamental sense, all three might prove to be inevitable products of a culture which fails to reconcile the fact of individual differences among men, with the necessity of individual dignity, and to be incapable of effective resolution in the absence of correction of the root problem.

† The term "cognitive" as here employed embraces all processes of perception, knowledge, and thought. It includes symbolic forms, but is not restricted to them since perception and thought must certainly extend beyond the confines of such formal and informal structure.

identical phenomena. The identifiable culture, viewed as a system of artifacts, beliefs, values, and institutionalized behavior, mediates between man and its environment in terms of his survival and sustenance requirements and in terms of the more tangible needs of his ego and intellect. To the extent that culture, so defined, is stable enough to be identified, it is likely that it will be found to serve a largely homeostatic function—pattern maintenance in the Parsonian sense.[6] However, to the extent that man's apperception involves nontangible need forms (being unrecognized, how can one describe them?) and the nonsymbols of feeling–expression that also reach him from his cognitive environment, his behavior may appear to be idiosyncratic and even equilibrium-disrupting. At least these subliminal components of the cognitive environment would seem to have more to do with change than with pattern maintenance.

In other words, were there nothing beyond the precursors of the identifiable culture in the content of the cognitive environment, there would appear to be little occasion for innovation or change other than that made necessary by balance-upsetting alterations in the physical or biological environment of man, such as an ice age or a population explosion. Yet there is much evidence that culture change occurs quite apart from such necessity.

Thus man as a thinking, self-aware organism is involved in at least four sets of interdependent but separately identifiable environmental phenomena: the physical, biological, cultural, and cognitive systems. According to the holistic concept, these four systems presently constitute the relevant environment of man, the environment with which human ecology should be concerned.* However, such comprehensive inclusion is seldom practiced and most so-called ecological studies involve a more limited concept which, in the long run, may be a self-defeating process.

Despite logic and urgency, those who espouse the need for holistic analysis in the treatment of human problems in today's complex world should also recognize that neither the information sources nor the methods necessary to a true science of human ecology have been sufficiently developed.[7] Nevertheless, awareness of the need for a holistic approach seems to be increasing. There is cause for hope that the current interest in comprehensive health planning, and in the even

* If theological orientation can be expressed in rational terms, it can be linked with man's emergence as a thinking, reflective organism and encompassed quite satisfactorily within the concept of the cognitive environment. If, however, a vitalistic or metaphysical expression, is pursued, such theological consideration automatically must be excluded from scientific treatment, at least within the four dimensions discussed above.

more broadly based field of social policies planning, will draw constructive attention to the problems of ecological method that remain to be solved.[8]

HEALTH ORGANIZATION IN ECOLOGICAL PERSPECTIVE

Since a broader ecological approach is needed in order fully to understand man's relationships with his environment, it follows that many existing, well-intended organized patterns and programs which were formulated in the context of a more limited viewpoint are likely to prove inadequate, perhaps even dangerous, in the long run. Even though the concepts and methods for a holistic science of human ecology are not yet available in the guidance of everyday problem solving, the mere recognition of the existence of the need for holistic analysis must certainly have a salutary effect. Expediential decisions will always remain a practical necessity. But expediency as a way of life is quite different from expediency taken as a necessary, but recognized incomplete, interim measure. The wise health administrator will be he who can recognize incompleteness and attempt to make provision for it. The health leader will be he who can add to this an unquenchable drive to seek real and complete answers, and who can utilize the full potential for human betterment implicit in the concept of a "planning society."[9]

References

1. J. W. Bews, *Human Ecology*, London: Oxford University Press, 1935.
2. John E. Gordon, "Medical Ecology and the Public Health," *The American Journal of the Medical Sciences*, 235:3 (March 1958), and Edward S. Rogers, *Human Ecology and Health: An Introduction for Administrators*, New York: Macmillan, 1960.
3. Loren Eiseley, *Darwin's Century*, New York: Doubleday, 1961.
4. Jerome D. Frank, "Galloping Technology, A New Social Disease," *Journal of Social Issues*, XXII:4 (1966), 1–14.
5. Pierre Teilhard de Chardin, *The Phenomenon of Man*, New York: Harper & Row, 1959; and Geoffrey Vickers, "Ecology Planning and the American

Dream," in Leonard Duhl (ed.), *The Urban Condition*, New York: Basic Books, 1963, pp. 374–395.

6. Talcott Parsons, "An Outline of the Social System," in Talcott Parsons *et al.*, *Theories of Society*, Vol. I, New York: The Free Press, 1961.
7. Edward S. Rogers and Harley B. Messinger. "Human Ecology: Toward a Holistic Method," *Milbank Memorial Fund Quarterly*, XLV:1, Part 1 (January 1967); and Lawrence B. Slobodkin, "Aspects of the Future of Ecology," *Bioscience* (January 1968), 16–23.
8. Henrik Blum and Associates. *Notes on Comprehensive Planning for Health*, Western Regional Office, American Public Health Association, 1968.
9. See Chapter 13 in this volume.

13

Philosophical Dilemmas in Health Planning

Mary F. Arnold

The thesaurus and the dictionary can aid us in defining the word "planning," but a real understanding of the full meaning of planning is elusive. The following list of synonyms suggests that the term "planning" represents rather different kinds of concepts: "V. plan. scheme, design, frame, contrive, project, forecast, sketch; conceive, devise, invent; set one's wits to work; . . . lay down a plan; shape, mark out a course;... cast, recast, systematize, organize; arrange...."[1] One concept seems to infer the creation of a program of action; another, the problem of forecasting for the future; still another, decision-making; and another the process of enhancing rationality. All of these, however, imply that planning is purposeful and that there is intent to achieve a desired state of affairs.

If one thinks about planning as the ordinary language philosopher might,* it seems that the semantic problem of the meaning of planning might be resolved.

PLANNING AS A PROBLEM-SOLVING PROCESS

The term "planning process" is often used to denote the intellectual stages one goes through in logical problem-solving: identification

* "Recent work in philosophy suggests that, even if we know perfectly well how to use a word, use it unhesitatingly and correctly, and understand others who use it, we may yet be unable to define it completely and explicitly to say what we know."[2]

of the problem, analysis of the problem, identification and specification of alternative solutions to the problem, selection of alternatives for implementation, and evaluation. However, within this general problem-solving context are several more specific concepts of planning.

Program-Planning

Program-planning has been an important concept for health administrators. Essentially it means the development of a specific course of action for a circumscribed health problem, such as communicable disease control or maternal and child health. Typical normative prescriptions for this type of planning are found in the literature on health administration:

> [The good administrator] is familiar with methods, procedures, systems, the planning of schedules, the planning of budgets, and the establishment of standards of performance. He has learned that planning should be long-range; that it should permit flexibility; that it is a joint effort which must be done on a continuing basis and must be closely synchronized with review.... A skilled administrator tries his best, when participating in planning, to remember the value of asking himself on each project: Why are we doing it? What will it accomplish? Who is or should be concerned? How will it be done? Have alternative approaches been evaluated? When is the best time to do it?... Where is the best place to do it?[3]

Behind this model for program-planning lies the idea of preparing a purposeful course of action to be followed. This is analogous to the problem-solving process made explicit in John Dewey's *How We Think*.[4]

It is important, in order to understand today's confusion about the term "planning," to consider the underlying premises and assumptions behind this problem-solving process. In order logically to have a problem to be solved, it is assumed that with adequate knowledge man can control or at least meet nature on an equal basis. But since we are still in the process of teasing out the secrets of an orderly nature through scientific research, we face what Simon calls the principle of bounded rationality.

> The capacity of the human mind for formulating and solving complex problems is very small compared with the size of the problems whose solution is required for objectively rational behavior in the real world—

> or even for a reasonable approximation to such objective rationality. [Furthermore,] it is only because individual human beings are limited in knowledge, foresight, skill, and time that organizations are useful instruments for the achievement of human purpose; and it's only because organized groups of human beings are limited in ability to agree on goals, to communicate, and to cooperate that organizing becomes for them a problem.[5]

This logical positivism assumes that

> decisions can always be evaluated in a relative sense — it can be determined whether they are correct, given the objective at which they are aimed — but a change in objectives implies a change in evaluation. Strictly speaking, it is not the decision itself which is evaluated, but the purely factual relationship that is asserted between the decision and its aims.[6]

Thus, when program-planning is conceived as a problem-solving approach, the problem of the appropriateness of goals or objectives is an ethical or value problem, which is not amenable to rational analysis. Therefore, the choice of goals and objectives is left to the political process of obtaining consensus and resolving conflict or to specified agents of the social group (e.g., legislators, company executives, or agency administrators).

If follows, then, that goals will be relevant only to the mission of the organization as defined by its agents or to the more specific missions of the subunits of the organization. It also follows that programs, and organizations, will proliferate as attention is focused on specific problems that need solution and that the interrelationships and transactional effects among these problems are beyond the purview or responsibility of the problem-solvers. Lindblom argues that in our democratic, pluralistic society an adjustment process occurs as each decision situation impinges on another and that by a process of disjointed incrementalism the development of social change is coordinated.[7] This argument, however, implies that there is an implicit social determinism over which man has no control. Thus program-planning can be done only in segmental bits and pieces and can be of only a relative short-range character for the unit doing the planning.

Planning as Coordination of Effort

The above kind of planning obviously leads to a proliferation of segmented programs, hopefully coordinated within each planning unit by some sort of organizational planning. One often sees in the professional literature references to the problems of duplication of effort and of gaps in services rendered. These are the manifestations of the need for mutual adjustment as decisions of one group impinge on the decisions of others. Coordinative planning in this context implies that there should be coordination of the action of two or more organizations or units so as to increase availability of scarce resources (often stated as a need for efficiency) or to enhance the impact of the several organizations' actions. Thus there is an implied larger system consisting of the input and output constituencies of the particular set of organizations concerned with coordination. In this case, however, this larger system is merely the general arena in which a particular set of organizations operate and not the total social environment. This type of planning generally falls into an information exchange and mutual adjustment process, with occasional amalgamation of several agencies. The autonomy of each subunit of these sets of organizations is not questioned.

Warren, in his discussion of community decision organizations, emphasizes information exchange as a means of coordination.[8] Although this will reduce uncertainty in the organizational set, it does not follow that this will lead to any more rational planning for the community as a whole. Public Law 89–749, the Partnership for Health Program, is an attempt to develop coordinated comprehensive local and state plans for allocating resources to meet the health needs of each area, but there is no plan for the larger system planning that is tied directly to this. Additionally, the emphasis on facilities, services, manpower, and environment does not take into account basic consideration of the transactional environment in which health action occurs nor the transactional relationships with other systems of the society, for example, the economy. The segmental approach of this law's guidelines is further reinforced by the emphasis on geographic decentralization, restricting further the opportunity to plan for the larger system in the context of the future.

Coordination reduces uncertainty for agency decision-makers, but in so doing it also reduces the field of operations and the innovative alternative actions that might evolve if the larger system were considered.

Planning as Decisions About Allocation of Resources

Another concept of planning that is based on the problem-solving assumption is that of making rational allocation decisions. In this case there are two kinds of problems: allocating resources among alternative means of achieving a specific desired outcome and choosing among different desirable outcomes. In the first case there is a specific desired outcome with several potentially effective means of achieving that outcome. The problem is that of distribution of a given amount of resources in order to optimize the probability of achieving the outcome at the most efficient level. Here cost–benefit analysis and other rational decision-making tools of management are used. The quantitative tools of the systems analyst provide a rational calculus for decision-making. Once again the application is one of bounded rationality, and there recently have developed a great many tools that depend upon mathematical models, probability theory, information theory, and game theory to aid the decision-maker. The slang expression for this type of analysis is "how to get the best for your buck."

The second problem, allocating resources among several program areas, is quite different, and it once again faces us with the problem of whose values should be enhanced. Assuming a constraint on the availability of resources, the choice becomes an ethical decision for the logical positivist—or for the monist, a problem of finding a common utility measure against which disparate outcomes can be measured. The management tools depend upon a strong assumption that utility or benefit is a measurable commodity and that all aspects of the system can be transformed into the same measure. This is the point at which many of us, unfamiliar with the logic, become disturbed: "You can't measure pain in dollars. How can you make a choice between programs that will save children's lives and those that might relieve the chronic disability of the elderly?"

The Pan American Health Organization's monograph on health planning discusses these dilemmas:

> Because the resources available are in short supply, the health authorities cannot escape the problem of assigning priorities or preferences to health activities according to the age of individuals.... Generally, it may be said that there are two views on the social importance of the health of individuals:
>
> (a) that one person's life is of the same importance as that of any other; or
>
> (b) that the life of certain persons is more important to the community than the life of others.
>
> If the first view is adopted, decision on health would logically follow the corollary of the basic thesis, i.e., to reduce to the utmost every obstacle to health with the resources available, regardless of the age of the beneficiaries. Highest priority would be given to the diseases whose reduction required the fewest resources.
>
> If the second view were adopted, it would be necessary to establish

> a yardstick for defining how much more one life was worth than another... this would be represented by the additional contribution which saving a given life would make to life expectancy and YPC (years of potential productive capacity)....
>
> If this purely economic criterion were adopted then health activities would be chiefly aimed at reducing health hazards for persons in the age group 15 to 55 years.[9]

Here the utility measure, the social value of individuals, has opened the door to the larger system. The very logic of the systems approach presents a problem of what are the boundaries of the system. Thus, if planning is considered only as rational decision-making about the allocation of resources within a narrow system, how can we assure that this suboptimization is not shortsighted and even potentially detrimental to the larger system? For example, we are now facing the problem of a rapidly increasing population, to a large extent due to the health measures imposed in the past to control the diseases of early infancy and the epidemic diseases.

PLANNING AS THE CREATION OF A PLAN

The view of planning as the creation of a plan is not so much concerned with the process of decision-making or problem-solving as it is with the creation of a blueprint of action. Almost every major city in this country has some kind of administrative unit that concerns itself with the creation of a plan for the physical development of the community that is expected to guide governmental operations. Some of these are clearly defined as departments or boards of planning, while others such as zoning boards may not be recognized as a planning unit. Housing, zoning, industrial development, tax structures, and transportation are the usual areas of concern.

The general method of operation of these units is to study trends and projections for various demographic and economic characteristics of the community and to prepare and later administer, once adopted, a plan for where industry or multiple dwellings may or may not be located, how transportation can be facilitated, and how, when appropriate, urban renewal and governmental housing shall proceed. Such planning generally serves the goal of maintaining and enhancing the tax base for the community or of maintaining certain desired and valued characteristics of the community.

Peterson calls this kind of planning "deductive planning" in that "the planner draws up a blueprint on a flat surface or in Latin *planum*, and the design is completed before the first steps are taken toward its realization."[10] The process by which the plan is created may be based on the rational problem-solving model, and it is assumed that this is a skill of the professional planner, but scientific logic is not a requisite of such planning. Too often planning groups or legislative bodies may revise a carefully developed plan for political or other considerations and the plan as finally administered is no longer based on a rational analysis. Every one of us is all too familiar with the situation where a planning group or a program administrator will start with the solution to some vague or implicit problem without actually specifying explicitly the objectives or goals to be served.

The creation-of-a-plan concept implies a reasonably stable environment in which the plan is to be implemented. An excellent example is that of the Bay Area Rapid Transit System in California, where a master plan was created and presented to the voters for approval. But unforeseen delays, such as suits, political maneuvering, and inadequate consideration of rising economic costs in the original plan, by the fall of 1968 created a monstrous situation wherein the implementation of the plan threatened to come to an ignominious halt with gaping holes in major urban arteries. Consideration and forecasting of changes in the environment may be considered in the development of a master plan, but this blueprint type of plan has a prepackaged quality about it. It is a common joke that office buildings, built for particular organizations, are never designed or perhaps finally built to accommodate for the changes in space requirements that will occur during the period of building. The difficulty is that the present in which the development of the plan occurs immediately becomes the past and, unless the changing present has been accounted for and forecast, the plan becomes obsolete as it is implemented. The longer the time between plan development and plan completion and the more uncertain the environment, the more likely is obsolesence to occur. Thus a plan per se, unless change mechanisms are built in, is often static rather than dynamic.

Standard Operating Procedures as Plans

When a master plan is designed for general and vague goals, there is no way to evaluate whether the action is achieving the goals it is designed for. It becomes easy, then, for these behaviors to become valued in themselves. Without concrete evidence that the action is or is not successful, the only kind of evaluation available is based on social norms of behavior. These surrogate criteria become standard operating procedures. The health field is prone to this problem, since in many public health program areas the goals are broadly stated. One set of criteria that have developed are standard expected behaviors. Thus, in health agencies one often finds a great deal of conflict around who should take action and the rights and obligations in professional roles.[11] Professional organizations spend much time in developing standards of practice, and these are substituted for missing effectiveness criteria in program evaluation.

For example, maintenance of the health of all children of a particular health jurisdiction at maximal capacity—a typical mission of child health programs in health departments—is incapable of evaluation since it is an ever receding, as well as an unattainable, goal—given our present state of knowledge and the scarcity of resources. Any plan of action to achieve such an objective will be general in scope and will have to rely on social criteria for evaluation. (See Chapter 16 for a discussion of this type of evaluation.) Procedures become standardized, unquestioned, and often incapable of adaptation.

PLANNING AS THE CREATION OF A UTOPIAN WORLD

The foregoing discussion has suggested that deductive planning leads to segmental attention to problems and does not allow consideration of the larger system. But a holistic approach to social order also leads us into the dilemmas of utopianism, because in order to plan for the larger system we have to have an image of what we wish the world eventually to become:

> The boundaries need not be demarcated with nice precision. It is moreover not the literary form that established the universe of discourse ... but the intent to evoke a vision of man in an earthly paradise that would be radically different from the existing order and would presume to render its inhabitants happier in some significant sense of that ambiguous yet unavoidable word.
>
> The utopia should perhaps be distinguished from the religious millennium because it comes to pass not by an act of grace, but through human will and effort.[12]

Manuel's analysis of the utopian visions of current times suggests two opposing images: one of a spiritual man, and the other of a world of greater sensate satisfaction.[13] The social planner, when concerning himself with the larger system, must face what shall be the measure of the "good life" before he can deal holistically with the larger system. Over the past several decades we have begun to recognize that what constitutes the good life is defined quite differently by people in different life circumstances. The present worldwide challenge of current system values by the youth is a case in point.

Thus the dilemma of the monist is that of what values are to be optimized for the system as a whole.

PLANNING AND SOCIAL CHANGE

Often planning and social change are discussed together as if they were recent phenomena. The modern problem, rather, is that of an awareness that there seem to be fewer persistent patterns of action today than in the past. Change occurs in sequential events, and since today there is a rapidly accumulating technology, worldwide instant communication, increasing specialization, and an expanding population, the directions of social change that affect more and more people seem to be less and less certain. This high degree of uncertainty in our social environment makes us more conscious of social change.

Theories of social change stem from our philosophical beliefs about nature's order and man's relationship with nature. The social Darwinians emphasized society's progression from the simple to the complex; the functionalists assume an essential state of equilibrium; while others see society as a tension management system.[14] These explanatory theories are theories of how change occurs within society, of what initiates change, of what determines its regularities and its discontinuities, and by what rules change comes about. Obviously, if there is an inevitability to the character of social change, it is incompatible with the idea of planning, because planning assumes that there is a potential of control. To plan requires an assumption of goal or purpose and the creation of desired outcomes that differ from what would be expected had planning not occurred. Moore's definition of social change is helpful in seeing where ideas of planning and social change are related: "Social change is the significant alteration of social structure (that is, patterns of social action and interaction), including consequences and manifestations of such structures embodied in norms (rules of conduct), values, and cultural products and symbols."[15] Therefore, another meaning for planning is that of guided social change.

A PLANNED SOCIETY VERSUS A PLANNING SOCIETY

The preceding discussion has raised two philosophical dilemmas inherent in the various concepts of planning we use. One has to do with the fact/value dilemma of the positivists—that the "ought-to-be's" are ethical or value choices and, therefore, given man's diversity planning only can proceed segmentally and in a short-range time perspective. It is further assumed that the aggregate of these segmented islands of planning will create a mutual adjustment process that in the long run is socially rational. But this disjointed incrementalist approach leads us to an underlying assumption of social determinism over which rational individual thought has no control. If this is true there is little logic for doing even segmental planning.

The other dilemma is that of the monist who sees the problem of planning as the problem of how to take into account the goals of the larger system. But his dilemma is his recognition that in order to take the larger system into account one must be a utopian or be all-knowing. The utopian view is unacceptable unless it can account for man's individualism and diversity, and we certainly are not all-knowing:

> How is it possible to judge systems without looking at the consequences of our system changes to the generations to come? Of all the principles of ethics that men have been able to devise, none is so fundamental as the ethical postulate that we are morally obliged to meet the demands that the coming generations would have imposed on us were they able to speak to us today.
>
> In the context of the problems of large systems that include not only the world of today but also of tomorrow, it is clear that no person or group of persons—scientist, politician, or whatever—can honestly say that he understands enough to guarantee by his decisions and recommendations an improvement of even a small sector of society. We are all suboptimizers, perhaps prone to the most dangerous kinds of suboptimization.[16]

The Planned Society

There is a genuine fear in our society of centralized planning because it brings to mind a totalitarian way of life:

> Man retains a self-directing capacity that defies any attempt to treat him as a simple reactor to stimuli. We are reluctant to undertake social planning because we know that man cannot be influenced as readily as the physical environment. We cannot really predict results; we cannot feed in stimuli and get simply direct results. Thirdly, the

> political costs of attempting social planning are extremely high, and we fear the loss of other planning opportunities as we attempt social planning.[17]

A planned society conjures up images of "big brother" and of repressive action, because most of us could not imagine ourselves in the position of being the society's planning agent, of being the ultimate decision-maker; and, therefore, we cannot trust those who believe they might be. Too, we have had recent historical experience with planned societies, and they are an anathema to our values and beliefs about individual freedom.

We therefore are caught between the recognition that segmental planning that does not consider the larger system has detrimental and sometimes irreversible effects and the knowledge that man's present capacity for prediction and forecasting the future is inadequate for the task of planning for the larger system. We do not like the unplanned consequences of segmental planning, and we do not want the constraints of a planned society.

A Planning Society as an Alternative

There is another alternative open to us if we have the innovative capability to achieve it: the development of a political structure and the social capacity to make ourselves into a planning society. A planning society would differ from a planned society in many ways:

1. The directions and goals for the future would be explicit but always subject to continual evaluation and revision.
2. There would have to be a concentrated and continual effort to keep the citizens of the society aware, on a probabilistic basis, of current goal priorities, of potential alternate goals, and of the ways in which each can be achieved.
3. At the most general planning level, the issue of the relevance of current goals to the future should be the primary policy decision problem.
4. At the more specialized levels of planning, the system of control and coordination should be based on assessment of the role each plays in the achievement of the general goals to be served.

A planning society would require an informed citizenry, able to cope with uncertainty and continual change, and even more importantly it would require a future-oriented society. This is a large order. It would require major changes in our educational system, although we are beginning to see a move toward teaching by self-discovery and by logic rather than by rote prescription, which hopefully will begin to prepare a citizenry more able to cope with uncertainty and change. It would require revision of the roles of our decentralized political jurisdictions. But most of all it would require a recognition of the primary immediate satisfactions of society's values over individual's values.

STEPS TOWARD A PLANNING SOCIETY

To think about how a planning society might be achieved a picture comes to mind: It is an illustration in *Gulliver's Travels* of Gulliver awaking to find himself tied down by thousands of little threads with which the Lilliputians had secured him. There he was, a huge giant, struggling to release those tiny bonds. Is this not what we are experiencing in our society today? There seem to be the random convulsive movements of the end of a sleep and, as we become awake, we are finding ourselves tied down with many minuscule threads, each of which is easily broken but, in the aggregate, they prevent us from getting up and on with the new day's work.

Our Lilliputian bonds are the bonds of past ways of thinking and acting in our social enterprise. So our first step is that of casting off the old ways that are holding us back—to release ourselves from these bonds.

Ideas about Cause and Effect

One of the most difficult changes in our way of thinking is manifest in our relatively recent recognition that our previous models of nature have been overly simplistic. The germ theory of disease led health workers to believe that application of isolated, specific treatments to individuals or to the environment would be the answer to our health problems. If we only learned enough we could apply this knowledge and wondrous things for mankind would occur. The relatively simple addition of chlorine to water stopped great epidemics since the application of heat or chemicals in a specified way could destroy pathogenic organisms, but we were unaware then of the ecological role some of these organisms played. The simple triadic model of epidemiology was neat and orderly and made logical sense. The host, the agent, and the environment became the focal points for a chain of causal events, and public health efforts were bent to "break the chain of infection." With wonder drugs and chemicals we could foresee the eradication of tuberculosis, venereal disease, and malaria.

These relatively simple initial successes reinforced support to biomedical research in its search for single, causal relationships, and even today the public, as well as many health workers, strongly believes that science can tease out from nature the simple secrets that will solve our health problems. However, scientists have begun to recognize that nature is not that simplistic and that some of our cherished control measures may have had some undesirable consequences.

In spite of the fact that at least twenty years ago there was a beginning recognition by health professionals that problems might be the result of a poorly understood interaction of several causative factors (e.g., accidents), we have continued to apply an assumption of single causation to much of our program-planning and problem-solving. It is not so very long ago that we attacked a complex of health problems by eliminating a common symptom, poor housing, and found to our dismay that the problems were not solved.

Thus one major change that is occurring is in our way of thinking about causation, recognizing today that life is much more complex than we ever dreamed. Playing into this has been the accumulating information and theories from the social sciences that the behavior and motivation of individuals and groups are also highly complex. Some years ago the social sciences were fighting the battle of scientism because of the imprecise nature of their data and measurements. Today even the so-called hard sciences have begun to embrace the idea of interaction and transaction among variables. So one of the Lilliputian threads we are now breaking is the simplistic model of cause and effect; instead we are beginning to think in terms of causal systems.

Changes in Ideas About People and Organizations

Just as our ways of thinking about solving disease problems are changing, we are finding changes in our thinking about how to organize our efforts. If one feels that problems can be approached segmentally, then it follows that one has to organize segmentally. We have been in an era of differentiation of function and of specialization to serve our segmental problems. As society has become more differentiated, organizational forms have been adapted to meet this need.

One very strong theme that has developed over the centuries about the way to organize is apparent in our concepts of hierarchy and of the bureaucratic scalar model of organization to serve the needs of integration and coordination. Although the scalar model of authority was invented in Roman times to aid in the control of vast territories,[18] this model has been adapted and developed until by the 1930s the so-called "principles of administration" articulated by Mooney and Reiley[19] were accepted popularly as almost immutable.

The descriptive model of the logic of a bureaucracy by Max Weber[20] indicated a shift in thinking from the logic of the military model where units were formed like a group of chessmen—each carrying out similar functions and all controlled and coordinated at the top by a master player—to an incorporation of the idea that each unit might perform different functions, but each still to be coordinated by a hierarchical form of authority. This is essentially a machine model.[21] Today there is a general, popular belief in the logic of coordinating discrete units of action by a hierarchical authority system. There is some suggestion that this belief has so permeated the society that it is a cultural trait.[22]

In the health field we have worked from this assumption of a machine model for organization partially because we have segmentally selected problems to be solved (e.g., communicable disease control, environmental control, short-term care, or long-term care) and, particularly, because this was a culturally defined normative organizational form. Playing into this is the direction of scientific and technological specialization, the professionalization of specialist groups, and so on. But, as specialization has proliferated, we have found that the mechanistic model of organization becomes increasingly difficult to support.

Therefore, another Lilliputian bond we are struggling to break is our belief about how our efforts should be organized. Recently, with the stimulation of studies of human behavior in organizations and the development of a technology and models for consideration of systems, new models of organization are developing. These, for the most part, are still merely gleams in the theorists' eyes, but we are finding experimentation going on in industry[23] and in government.

Some of the greatest opportunities for experimentation have come to the health field with the passage of Public Laws 89–749 (Comprehensive Health Planning) and 89–239 (Regional Medical Programs) and with the development of the neighborhood health center concept of the Office of Economic Opportunity. The opportunities for experimentation are available, but it may be too soon to expect enough of a sloughing of our strong beliefs in hierarchical authority to develop new organizational forms.

Changes in Ideas About the Future

De Jouvenel suggests that we are able to consider only a future that is imaginable and plausible (called by him a futurible) and able to work only with a futurible over which we think we have some mastery (a conditional futurible).[24] The future stretches out before us like a red carpet that we are weaving from the past and the present. What we have done in the past and what we are doing today is creating our tomorrow. However, we can only surmise what this future will be from our knowledge of the past. The difference today in our thinking about the future is our greater recognition that it is the transaction of the past and present that creates the future. Most of the problems we have attempted to solve in past times have been based on our view of the present rather than our view of the future. We looked to past trends and possible causative factors and assumed that only by intervening in the current system could we change the current directions of these trends of the past. For example, we assume trends in demographic characteristics will persist, and we make decisions based on these ideas of persistence of trends. Because of this present orientation, social action has taken the form of putting out fires and of relieving stresses as they occurred.

To develop a planning society, one of the most difficult bonds we will have to shed is that of our orientation to the present in our problem-solving. We must begin to think of an evolving, conditional future. Recently groups such as the Commission on the Year 2000 have formed to develop tools for a future orientation. Techniques, such as the Delphi technique, and the use of alternative scenarios are being developed.[25, 26]

The experience of a class in looking at the trends for the year 2000 and their implications for health is an example of how a future orientation can change how one thinks about planning. The students were divided into task groups: one to look at technical and scientific development, one to look at physical environment, another to pursue projections for changes in social values and life styles, and a fourth to look at economic and political development. As they presented the differing projections from each perspective, the class discovered that there were some major conflicts in their projections. At this point they were able to go back and look at the validity of the assumptions that led to each projection and to begin to develop probable alternative futures.

It is this kind of probablistic analysis of the future that will enable us to plan more rationally for the future we desire. There is no reason why comprehensive health planning groups, or other social policy-planning groups, could not proceed in this way to provide information about alternative futures that could be the basis for a dialogue with the general citizenry of the community and the nation.

SUMMARY

The concept of planning has evolved to the point where it presents us with some basic philosophical dilemmas. If we accept the idea that man should have some control over his fate, then we are faced with the problem of how the goals for the larger societal system shall be determined and how their implementation can be continuously made relevant to an ever changing future.

The suggestion has been made that the development of a planning society may provide a solution to the above problem. To move from our current segmental approach to planning to that of a planning society will require changes in our conceptions of cause and effect, in our beliefs about how work should be organized, and in our orientation to time. These changes are beginning to occur but can be accelerated if those agents of social change in professional guidance roles—such as educators, community organizers, planners, and administrators—accept and incorporate these requisite concepts of a planning society. Only then will we be able to form a political structure that will allow the citizenry to participate in a meaningful way in planning for the future.

The health field has been handed a challenge in our society, the extent of which was perhaps not even recognized by Congress. The challenge is one of developing a method of social planning whereby a pluralistic democracy can plan for the future it desires. At no other time in the history of the world has such an opportunity been mandated to a subsystem of the society to transform a set of conflicting ideals into a viable reality. In our society we have had two somewhat conflicting philosophies about how things should work. The individual and the business firm have ideally been expected to plan ahead to defer gratification in the interests of future success. The Protestant work ethic placed a value on working hard for rewards in the future. However, our ideal of individualism also implied that this should operate in an open society, and the public sector should take a minimal planning role. But with interesting inconsistency, government is often compared with the business firm in the interests of efficiency. However, efficiency means rational planning and control, which are inconsistent with the idea of autonomy in the private sector of the society. In a democracy some way must be found to bring all segments and interests of the society into the planning process. The word "comprehensive," whether attached to planning or to health services, spells out the challenge to the health system.

It is my contention that we are fast coming to the crossroads whereby the choice will be between a planned society and that of a planning society. In the arena of health the opportunity is here to develop a model for other sectors of the society. Can we set the stage for a planning society before it is too late?

References

1. Peter Mark Roget, *Thesaurus of English Words and Phrases*, New York: Grosset & Dunlap, 1933, p. 218.
2. Hanna Fenichel Pitkin, *The Concept of Representation*, Berkeley: University of California Press, 1967, p. 6.
3. Harold M. Graning, "Major Aspects of Administrative Theory," *Health Education Monographs*, No. 7 (1960), p. 22.
4. John Dewey, *How We Think*, Boston: D. C. Heath, 1933.
5. Herbert A. Simon, *Models of Men*. New York: Wiley, 1957, pp. 198–199.
6. Herbert A. Simon, *Administrative Behavior*, 2nd ed., New York: Macmillan, 1957, p. 49.
7. Charles E. Lindblom, *The Intelligence of Democracy*, New York: The Free Press, 1965.
8. Roland Warren, "The Interorganizational Field As a Focus for Investigation," *Administrative Science Quarterly*, 12:3 (December 1967), 396–419.
9. Pan American Health Organization, *Health Planning: Problems of Concept and Method*, Scientific Publication No. 111, April 1965, pp. 5–6.
10. William Petersen, "On Some Meanings of 'Planning,'" *Journal of the American Institute of Planners*, XXXII:3 (May 1966), 133.
11. Mary F. Arnold, "Perception of Professional Role Activities in Local Health Departments," *Public Health Reports*, 77:1 (January 1962), 80–88.
12. Frank E. Manuel, "Toward a Psychological History of Utopias," *Daedalus*, 94:2 (Spring 1965), p. 294.
13. *Ibid.*, pp. 293–322.
14. Wilbert T. Moore, *Social Change*, Foundations of Modern Sociology Series, Englewood Cliffs, N.J.: Prentice-Hall, 1963, pp. 1–21.
15. Wilbert T. Moore, *Order and Change*, New York: Wiley, 1967, p. 3.

16. C. West Churchman, *Challenge to Reason*, New York: McGraw-Hill, 1968, p. 16.
17. Cyril Roseman, *The California State Development Plan—Issues Related to Social Organization and Interaction*, paper given at First Policy Conference, California Chapter of American Institute of Planners, September 30–October 1, 1966, Monterey, California, mimeographed.
18. Mason Haire, "The Concept of Power and the Concept of Man," in George B. Strother *et al.*, *Social Science Approaches in Business Behavior*. Homewood, Ill.: Dorsey Press and Richard D. Irwin, 1962, pp. 163–183.
19. J. D. Mooney and A. C. Reiley, *Onward Industry!*, New York: Harper & Row, 1931.
20. Max Weber, *The Theory of Social and Economic Organization*, trans. A. M. Henderson and Talcott Parsons, New York: Oxford University Press, 1947.
21. Lewis Mumford, *The Myth of the Machine*, New York: Harcourt, Brace, & World, 1967.
22. Herbert G. Wilcox, "The Culture Trait of Hierarchy in Middle Class Children," *Public Administration Review*, XXVIII:3 (June 1968), 222–235.
23. Tom Burns and G. M. Stalker, *The Management of Innovation*, London: Tavistock, 1961.
24. Bertrand de Jouvenel, *The Art of Conjecture*, trans. Mikita Lary, New York: Basic Books, 1967.
25. Olaf Helmer, *Social Technology*, New York: Basic Books, 1966.
26. Herman Kahn and Anthony J. Wiener, *The Year 2000*, New York: Macmillan, 1967.

14

Why We Need to Plan

Richard M. Bailey

An economist's perspective on developments in the field of health—or the health industry, as it is frequently called—may be compared with analyses that economists make of business organizations and other industries in our society. The rationale of the economist for viewing the production of health services as an industry is based largely on the observation that medical services are produced and sold in our society in a manner not very different from the way in which other goods and services are sold. Specifically, though health professionals like to talk about the "need" for medical care, by and large our health organizations and institutions are structured to respond only to an expressed demand. Need is a nice professional concept, but the kinds of health services traditionally produced are typically those that can be sold in the marketplace. They are medical services designed to meet the test of the marketplace: services the public is willing to pay for because of a reasonable expectation that they will be visibly beneficial to them.[1]

THE PRODUCTION OF MEDICAL SERVICES

Historically, medical services generally have been produced in a relatively small scale of medical practice or, one could say, a medical firm, to make the business analogy even stronger. In this typical medical firm the physician has been the key factor in the production

This paper is based upon a speech delivered before a conference on "The Planning Process: Physician–Consumer Involvement" sponsored by the California Medical Education and Research Foundation, San Francisco, California, July 18–20, 1968.

of all health services. Traditionally these services have been highly personalized and have led to many discussions about the sacred and close physician–patient relationship. These physician services have been tailored to what the physician interprets as the patient's requirements—what kind of care he may require. To put a little more perspective on this analysis, by backtracking forty or fifty years to a time when medical knowledge was much more limited than it is today, we would probably have to admit that much of the physician's service contained a large component of tender, loving care and human concern—and a relatively small amount of scientific data or information. Typically, the physician saw the patient only when the patient was quite ill and suffering from obvious physical discomfort. This pattern of seeking medical care remains prevalent today: Most patients do not buy services from the physician unless they feel some real discomfort. Problems defined as minor by the patient are cared for in a multitude of ways: with home remedies, neglect, or what have you. The important point is that the patient typically comes to the physician only when he feels ill.

On the other hand, how has the physician responded to the patient? Initially, it should be recognized that the physician is cast in a role somewhat different from that of most producers: The physician–patient relationship may be more properly conceived of as agent–principal rather than producer–consumer. The patient is analogous to the principal in law. He employs an agent, the physician, to do something for him, to act in his best interest. So the transaction between patient and physician can hardly be regarded as a straight across-the-table bargaining activity in which the patient asks about which services will be produced and what price will be charged. Rather the patient asks the physician to provide services that the physician believes will contribute to the patient's well-being. Because the physician has taken on this kind of agent or trustee responsibility, the medical profession over time has conceived of this process of medical services production as unique. It has openly opposed attempts to conceive of the transaction as involving a common production process. Much emphasis has been placed upon the "tailor-made" aspects of the transaction. To use commercial terms, we might say that the services typically produced by the physician have been of a job-order type. They have been specially packaged to meet a particular patient requirement for services; they are not mass-produced. Medical services simply are not discussed in terms that refer to a high volume, standardized way of production, as is done in most other goods and service industries.

Another interesting thing about medical services is that those typically produced are primarily only those deliberately sought by the patient. There has been no great promotion effort on the part of the medical profession to sell *more* or *different* kinds of medical services. In fact, a whole body of medical ethics has prevented advertising, prevented the creation of demand, and prevented the encouragement of people to seek more medical services. Indeed the emphasis has often been placed on discouraging more demand. It is also apparent that the services made available by physicians have been largely curative. Curative services can be sold.[2] Curative services derive from a felt need on the part of the patient. When the patient is ill, the encounter with the physician holds forth some real prospect of being beneficial to him. In this instance it becomes rational for the patient to go to the physician and buy medical services. This is the way our health service system is largely organized today—on the basis of providing only those services that can be sold in a free market setting. But note that this is a limited bundle of services! It may not begin to cover the spectrum of services that professionals should make available.

Much concern is expressed today about the distribution of medical services. This problem is closely related to the traditional way of selling medical care like other goods and services. Where demand is strong, where incomes are high, where people are educated sufficiently to have high expectations from medical services, there we find most of the physicians. Of course, an adequate population base is necessary, but even within a community such as San Francisco or New York or Atlanta the density of physicians and the quantity of services provided are definitely centered in a few geographic areas. Physicians are located where the demand for their services are strong. We likewise find other medical facilities grouping around these sources of strong demand—hospitals, convalescent homes, and related establishments.

CONSUMER DEMAND FOR HEALTH SERVICES[3]

Given that the purchase of most medical services has traditionally been in a market setting wherein the consumer has selected and paid for these services just like he has when buying other goods, attention now turns to the way in which this market has functioned. A fundamental point to be made in this context is that the consumer has demanded only those medical services that have appeared to be rational for him to buy—services from which he might reasonably expect to receive a visible payoff. In the order of things, we might classify these demands for medical services by order of urgency and, hence, the priority in which medical care has been sought. They are:

1. Demand arising from an emergency/serious situation—where life and death are the alternatives.

2. Demand for treatment of not-so-serious conditions—acute problems where life is not threatened or chronic illness where management of the problem is needed. In all of these examples it is likely that physical or mental discomfort are present.

3. Demand for medical services to detect developing medical problems early—prevention of illness or disability or early detection that may make proper management of the condition more efficacious.

CONSUMER DEMAND FOR LIFE-SUSTAINING HEALTH SERVICES

Economists refer to the concept of utility as meaning the benefit that the consumer expects will be forthcoming from his purchase of this or that good or service. Applying this concept to the three types of demand for medical care mentioned above, one might say that the consumer could expect the greatest utility to be derived from a medical service that is life-saving in nature; less utility from the alleviation of an acute condition or chronic pain; and perhaps exhibit an ambivalent attitude of either very small or even negative utility regarding the purchase of preventive medical services. As concerns the prevention of death or serious disabilities, it might be expected that the great majority of people have a strong taste for services of this type—few have a fervent death wish or like to see others die or be in great pain. Is there any doubt why consumer demand has been strongest (and public expression of urgency greatest) for services that prevent quick death or serious disabling consequences? We see evidence of this demand expressed in the supply of the many acute-care hospitals that dot the countryside and in the large number of hospital-oriented medical and surgical specialists who are concerned with repairing bodies broken either physically or by damaging disease. Moreover, we even see this expression of demand in the predominant types of health insurance policies that are marketed in this country with their principal emphasis upon hospital care for acute conditions with payment being for quite limited duration and the illnesses or accidents covered being those requiring surgery or intensive medical treatment to avoid death or permanent disability.

CONSUMER DEMAND FOR HEALTH SERVICES TO ALLEVIATE ACUTE OR CHRONIC CONDITIONS

The demand for medical services intended to alleviate acute problems that are not life-threatening has been growing rapidly in recent years as the result of numerous factors. Among these factors are increased patient awareness of the physician's ability to treat such problems (largely related to better drugs and medicines), higher incomes, and availability of services. Patients visiting physicians for such complaints often make up what is known in the trade as the "bread-and-butter" work of medical practice. These are medical services with which the physician has become quite familiar, and though he personally may not receive as much psychic satisfaction from producing such services as he would from participating in the more dramatic act of saving lives, he is familiar with this role. Thus, as medical demand has grown in the aggregate—and many of the earlier killer diseases such as smallpox and polio have been brought under control by vaccination—most physicians have found demand for this type of service growing more markedly than any other.

Economists frequently engage in sharp debates over the nature of certain goods and services in their attempts to classify them as investment or consumption goods. Investment goods are often regarded as those which generate a payoff to the individual or society over a comparatively long period of time and may, in fact, be necessary prerequisites to further productive work. Consumption goods are assumed to yield short-run benefits to the purchaser and in one way or another produce some pleasure for the user while being consumed. Applying these investment/consumption criteria to medical services is fraught with problems, but a gross example might be to say that the purchase of an appendectomy could be called an investment expenditure while the purchase of an office visit to a dermatologist for removal of a wart on the hand could be called a consumption expenditure. The former operation may be essential to the preservation of life; the latter, to make one's hands more beautiful. It is quite probable that the utility of the first operation exceeds by a wide margin that of the second. Yet it is this latter type of demand for medical services that is growing very rapidly in our generally affluent economy—a type of demand that seems to be more influenced by the income level of the patient than anything else.

As noted above, insurance companies have found the demand for health insurance coverage greatest in those instances where life is at stake. Barring a major catastrophe, demands for medical services of this type are reasonably predictable—they are not services that are willingly sought and thus subject to the personal fancy of the patient. The demand for medical services to alleviate relatively minor problems or self-limiting conditions, however, is subject to widely different and highly unpredictable influences. It is for this reason that insurance companies are reluctant to write policies covering such services unless there is a substantial self-insurance clause in the contract requiring the patient to pay the first $100 or $200 of claims each year. (Both Titles 18 and 19 of the Social Security Amendments of 1965 recognize this problem and require that initial costs be borne by the patient each year, normally the first $50.) Since demand by consumers for these services are high and growing, we find physicians and medical institutions organized to produce these services in large quantity. However, just as we find individual patients according lesser priority to these services than to those of a life-threatening type, so also we find hospitals and physicians ranking these services similarly. They are, in a sense, less important. They are more likely to be consumption goods than investment goods.

CONSUMER DEMAND FOR PREVENTIVE HEALTH SERVICES

Turning finally to the demand for medical services that emphasize early detection or the prevention of illness, we are confronted by a situation that illustrates most clearly the problems created by consumer ignorance. Economic theory grants that the consumer is rational in making purchases. He considers the various products and services that his tastes dictate; he weighs the expected utility of possessing one or another of the goods or services, taking into account his income and the relative prices of each alternative; and then he makes his decision with the view of maximizing total utility. All of these decision-making activities presuppose that the consumer is well-informed about the choices at hand. Now we find him presented with a new medical service—a service that may detect a disease in its incipient stages or prevent future illness. How is he to evaluate its utility? How can he express a level of effective demand that will lead to the production of the service?

If the consumer is rational he will not buy preventive health services unless he can be convinced that the marginal utility of the service will exceed the marginal utility derived from purchasing some other goods or services. But who can be so convinced?—perhaps a person who is aware that he is in a high risk group. Perhaps a preventive service can be urged upon a patient who is already in the physician's office or hospital for some other reason. In such a case the marginal cost of the preventive service may appear to be low (or even zero if the service can be disguised as part of the total bill covered by insurance). But how can the demand for preventive services be self-generated when the consumer is so often unaware of their existence or, if aware, finds it literally impossible to evaluate how beneficial they may be to him personally? In decision theory terms, the potential consumer is being asked to evaluate a purchase decision problem filled with uncertainty. There is little opportunity to measure the size of the risk that is undertaken by failure to purchase the service. The data do not exist in most instances. Thus the purchase of preventive services presents a case of consumption under a high degree of uncertainty leading to what appears to be a rational decision on the part of most consumers: a decision *not* to purchase such services!

THE EFFECT OF INCOME ON THE DEMAND FOR HEALTH SERVICES

Since our focus is upon consumption theory, let us now turn to a discussion of the influence that purely economic factors—income and prices—may have upon the decision to purchase various kinds of medical services. To do so we will use graphs to present such relationships since hard data are not available. In a sense these are the author's hypotheses about the effect of income and price upon aggregate medical demand—the way that the population as a whole may behave in its demand for health services.

The effect of income on the demand for medical services to treat serious illnesses falls along a spectrum ranging from high to low. We say that the income effect is high if an aggregate increase in income leads to a more than proportional increase in the demand for these services. Conversely, if there is slightly any increase in demand with an increase in income, the income effect is low. Using a chart whose vertical axis measures income (Y) and whose horizontal axis measures the quantity of these services demanded (Q), the demand curve for life-sustaining health services probably looks like Figure 1.

The demand curve DD reflects a relatively slight effect of income on the demand for services to treat emergency/serious illnesses. That is, level of income may not play a major role in the quantity of such services demanded except in the sense that the higher one's income, the greater may be one's access to the institutions and personnel

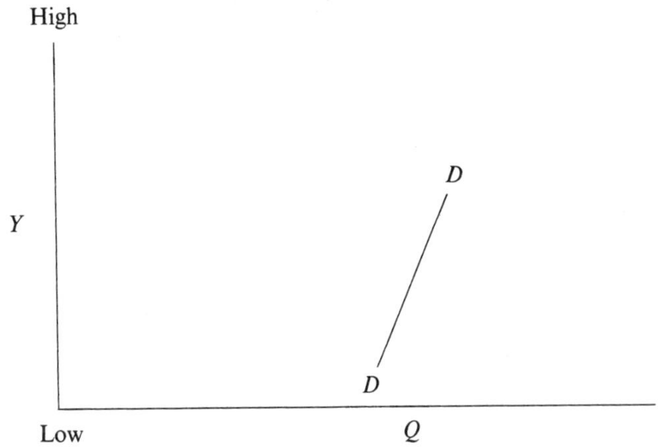

FIGURE 1. *Consumer Demand for Life-Sustaining Health Services as a Function of Income*

producing such services. But heart attacks, cancer, automobile accidents, strokes, and appendicitis strike the rich as well as the poor with approximately equal frequency. Moreover, the health care delivery system rarely closes its doors on people who need such services even through they may not have the income with which to pay for the services. People with emergency or life-threatening medical problems are usually able to enter the medical care delivery system in one way or another without first considering if they have the means to pay. They have a vital and immediate need, they are accepted for treatment, and their income is considered later. This opportunity to receive some care coincides with the section of medical ethics that says that no patient will be denied access to medical care if he is in real need. Surely the care that the poor receive may not be equal in quality to that received by the more affluent—but generally some care is available. Of course, as time passes and the population grows, we may see an increase in demand for the treatment of emergencies or serious illness. But such demand is not usually a direct function of individual income at any particular point in time. Demand for these services, then, is not seen as being particularly sensitive to the income of the patient.

Turning to the effect of income level upon the demand for curative services to treat problems of a nonlife-threatening type, we might envisage a set of relationships as shown in Figure 2. The demand curve *DD* reflects a strong income effect on the demand for these services. The explanation advanced for this relationship is based on two

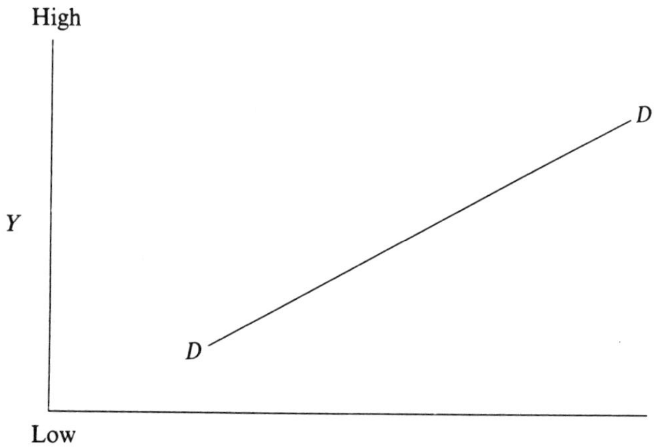

FIGURE 2. *Consumer Demand for Health Services to Alleviate Minor Health Problems as a Function of Income*

points: (1) the superior nature of medical services vis-à-vis most other goods and services and (2) the fact that, with higher incomes, the marginal utility of other goods or services that might have been very high when incomes were low now diminishes rapidly and medical services yield relatively higher utility. Of course, we also find the linkage between education and income level to be very strong. Hence, other factors explaining the increased demand for services to alleviate these acute but not-death-inducing illnesses may be related to a different set of tastes or the possession of more information that leads to greater rationality in the allocation of one's income.

It bears note that coverage of these services under either public programs or private insurance contracts results in a subtle increase in the individual's income—an increase, however, that can be spent in only one manner: for the purchase of medical services. Small wonder why third-party payment for such services is viewed as a "bottomless pit" into which a very substantial amount of expenditures may be rapidly absorbed.

Our final concern is with the effect of income level on the demand for preventive health services. Conceptually, this demand might be pictured as in Figure 3. In this case we find the total quantity of such services demanded to be low at all income levels (the curve is close to the vertical axis), with perhaps some slight increased propensity to consume these services at the highest income levels. Here we return to the issue of consumer rationality: Why does the demand for these

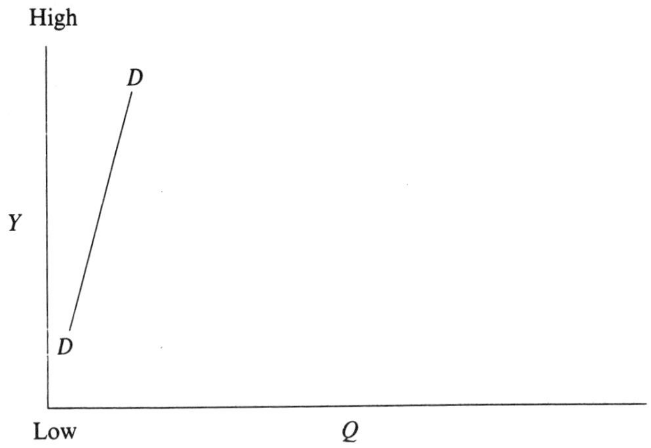

FIGURE 3. *Consumer Demand for Preventive Health Services as a Function of Income*

services appear to be so small? The apparent answer is found in the very uncertain knowledge that the consumer possesses about the value of such services from a medical viewpoint. Spending $100 for a series of tests that are interpreted by the physician as indicating that the patient is in good health may merely confirm what the person already believed to be true. With higher incomes, $100 may seem to be a small price to pay for such assurances. However, greater utility may be attached to the purchase of other goods or services that provide more immediate gratification.

THE EFFECT OF PRICE ON THE DEMAND FOR HEALTH SERVICES

The three diagrams that follow show the effect of price (P) upon the aggregate quantity demanded (Q) of certain health services. Applying this concept to the demand for emergency/serious services results in a graph like Figure 4. Here, we find the quantity demanded relatively insensitive to the price of the service. The reason, again, is that these services are generally not consumed under what might be called "pleasant circumstances." Hence, price may act neither much as a deterrent or incentive to use. It would be wrong, of course, to assume that there is no effect of price on the demand for these services: witness the effect of hospitalization insurance coverage on the use of hospitals. Insurance, in this case, acts to reduce the out-of-pocket cost of the

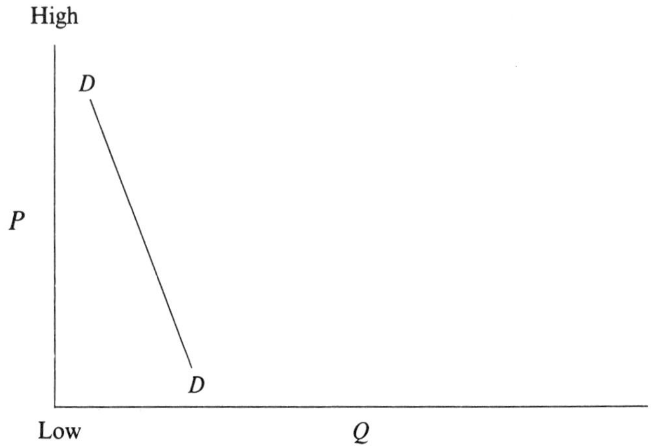

FIGURE 4. *Consumer Demand for Life-Sustaining Health Services as a Function of Price*

medical and hospital services to the patient below the going market price. A lower price may then result in a shifting of marginal utilities among various alternative goods or services. But confusion abounds here too. If the medical problem is truly serious, the possession of hospital insurance may merely accelerate the use of the service—the transaction may not be delayed until there is no alternative but hospitalization. It also may be true that many of the medical reasons for hospitalization are not for the treatment of emergency/serious conditions. Some misclassification of the medical problem may arise so that the cost of care can be shifted from the patient to the insurance company. In summary, casual observation of the effect of price on the demand for emergency medical services may indicate a rather close relationship, but if one examines more closely the nature of these services and what they are for, it becomes doubtful if price is as important a factor as assumed.

The effect of price upon the demand for nonserious, curative medical services probably is quite strong, as depicted in Figure 5. The lowering of price in this instance results in a substantial increase in demand. Several explanations can be offered:

1. A lower price makes a given service more attractive vis-à-vis other alternative purchases. There are many substitute products that compete with medical services when the consumer seeks alleviation of a nonserious problem: various proprietary drugs and medicines, home remedies, alcohol, nonprofessional advice, and so on. Lowering the price of medical services makes these alternatives less desirable and hence more medical services are demanded.

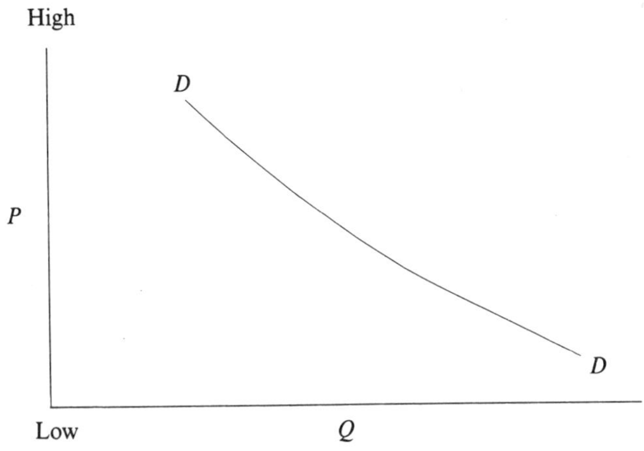

FIGURE 5. *Consumer Demand for Health Services to Alleviate Minor Health Problems as a Function of Price*

2. Insurance coverage may, in essence, lower the price of a given service literally to zero which removes any economic barrier to use.

3. Lowering price makes the service available to a broader market so that consumers who would never have considered the service as a possible purchase now enter the market expanding total demand. As mentioned above, some of these services may be provided to the patient while in a hospital, although options generally exist for producing the services in an outpatient setting.

Finally, we consider the effect of price on the demand for preventive medical services. Figure 6 illustrates this relationship. The segment of the demand curve *DD* indicates that few consumers buy these services at high prices and only a somewhat larger number buy these services as price decreases. In the aggregate, there is a relatively small amount of demand. As with our explanation of the effect of income on the demand for these services, it appears that if the price of preventive services is high, very few consumers will find the purchase rational—uncertainty of benefit (or perhaps even fear of learning something one does not care to know)—will serve to make the high cost a deterrent to use. With lower prices a somewhat larger demand for preventive services may be generated as the price of uncertainty decreases. But unless the price is lowered almost to (or at) zero, it is doubtful if demand for these services can be stimulated much through regular market (price) incentives. Rather, a problem may still exist in increasing the consumption of such services because in addition to monetary cost, some pain and certainly the expenditure of several hours of patient time is inevitable. To shift the demand for these services even further

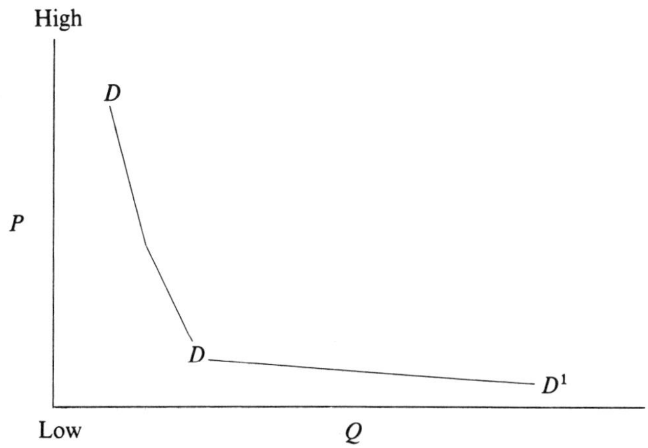

FIGURE 6. *Consumer Demand for Preventive Health Services as a Function of Price*

to the right (to increase total consumption), as represented by the DD^1 segment of the demand curve, probably would require a substantial educational effort and improvements in the techniques of practice to reduce the uncertainty attached to the value of such services. Reducing prices substantially (moving down the *DD* curve) might bring a one-shot increase in demand by people whose tastes incline in this direction. Beyond that, special efforts to increase consumption would probably be needed (DD^1 curve).

To summarize this section on consumer demand for medical services, it should be emphasized that with the exception of demand for emergency, live-saving care—which is not very responsive to either price or income — the demand for other curative services is quite responsive to purely economic factors. Demand for preventive services shows some relationship to income and price levels, but to generate any substantial increases in demand, educational efforts coupled with price changes would be required. Accepting the thesis that consumers are basically rational in their decision-making about prospective expenditures (limited primarily by their knowledge of benefits to be derived from various medical services), we may better understand why some services are widely sought even though they may not be highly regarded by physicians—and other services are not purchased although health professionals might give high priority to such consumption. Uncertainty is a very important element in consumer decision-making, and when it is present individual calculations of utility to be derived from a given expenditure may result in purchases that do not optimize the person's best interests. But can the consumer be blamed for such lack of knowledge? It may be that most health services are not like other goods and services. Hence reliance upon market processes to generate an optimal level and mix of demand can lead to some undesirable resource allocations.

THE MEDICAL MARKETPLACE

The prior discussions of the traditional market for medical services and what seem to be the major economic factors influencing the demand for various kinds of services leads us now to focus upon some private market strengths and weaknesses. Specifically, where does the private market do a good job of allocating resources and where may it be inadequate? In our country the underlying concept of the value of producing goods and services in a free market setting is based upon the belief that the market is an efficient allocator of resources. By this it is meant that if one accepts as given the income distribution existing among various groups in society—or within any given group, for that matter—then if a good or a service is demanded by an individual who is willing and able to pay for it, producers will respond to provide these services. In this context we believe that the market is an efficient allocator because it provides the individual with the opportunity to spend his income to attain maximum satisfaction. But this opportunity to spend is always subject to his ability to spend—his income. If one person has an income of $20,000 a year, he may spend that income differently from the way someone else might spend $20,000 a year—and that is well and good. We further believe that having this freedom to spend and to select from a wide variety of goods and services in the market is very important to maintaining other individual freedoms. A quite different pattern of expenditures also may be expected when consumers have vastly different levels of income, say, $20,000 per year and $2,000 per year. Even here economic theory posits that each consumer will have the greatest opportunity to satisfy his desires if markets are free and consumer choice is broad.

The point that needs to be stressed is that for this market to work effectively and to distribute goods and services to various consumers at low prices, it is important that the producers be highly competitive. It is important that the consumer has many options to buy various kinds of goods or services at various prices, at various levels of quality, and in a variety of combinations. If the market is to work effectively.

the consumer also must be sufficiently knowledgeable to discriminate in his choices, to know what he is buying, and to be able to discern the relative value of particular goods or services. If we find that producers are competing, and if the consumer is informed, then we can take another step: We can say that in this kind of market setting, consumer well-being will be maximized by encouraging producers to organize their activities to maximize their own best interests.[4] Consumer and producer interests harmonize in a competitive marketplace because strong competition among producers leads to providing a variety of services at low prices. Another way to say this is that the self-interest both of consumers and of producers is served when producers are highly competitive. This leads to the rationalization of profit maximization among producers because, in a competitive market, the producer is able to maximize his profits only by offering services at low prices. If consumers are not satisfied with the producers' prices or services, they will refuse to buy his output and will soon put him out of business. Someone else who responds to the consumers' demands will get the business.

The purpose of this discussion about the marketplace is to lead up to a focus on the medical service industry. In the field of health, many physicians have traditionally held somewhat fallacious beliefs about the degree of competition existing in medicine. One of these beliefs is that medicine is highly competitive. Economists, on the other hand, are quite inclined to downgrade the free competition explanation of medical practice and to describe the industry as a distinct form of monopoly. The reasons given by economists are these: (1) In a highly competitive industry, prices are set by the forces of supply and demand as they interact in the marketplace. In the case of medical practice, prices are set by individual producers who possess a high degree of discretion to discriminate in pricing as they see fit. (2) In a competitive industry, price competition is used between producers as a means of attracting a greater number of consumers. In medical practice, the use of price as a competitive instrument is frowned upon and declared to be unethical. (3) In a competitive industry, the product or service that is offered for sale generally is homogeneous. In medical practice, the service offered is conventionally treated as heterogeneous (individual health care) with considerable differentiation occurring in both the mix and number of services produced. (4) In a competitive industry the consumer has the opportunity to be well informed and is able to bargain among the producers to obtain the best terms of sale. In the market for medical services the consumer is not well informed: He selects his physician on the basis of highly subjective criteria and, after the selection is made, is in a relatively weak position to bargain on price, other services to be purchased, or to whom referral for additional attention will be made since advertising is unethical. (5) In a competitive industry there is ready ease of entry into the industry. In medical practice there are numerous barriers to entry. Nationally these barriers are erected through the educational process. At the state level the barriers are maintained by the licensing of physicians. At the local level medical societies and hospital staffs act as barriers to entry into practice.[5]

By the very way in which medical services are provided, we are saying implicitly that these services are no different from other goods and services. Those who want to buy medical services and have the income to purchase them can have them (subject to being informed as to what is purchased). We have assumed that there is competition and, therefore, as the consumer enters this marketplace to buy medical services, he does so in a setting where the resources supposedly are allocated effectively. Many statements in medical publications are based upon these ideas. Accordingly, physicians are encouraged to act in their own best economic interest, feeling that consumer well-being also will be served well.

Personally I do not believe we can say that if the physician acts in his own economic interest this will benefit the consumer. Of course, there is much conflict in the language here, even within the medical profession. What needs to be recognized, though, is that if you accept statements about problems of competition in medicine and about the lack of consumer information or education concerning medical services, it becomes almost impossible to say that the typical market setting for the provision of medical services can solve all the problems in this field today. Some services are not bought because of lack of income; some services are not purchased because the price is too high; and some services are not even produced because physicians do not see much of a market for them. Overriding all these matters is the lack of competition in the industry.

In summary, an overview of the medical practice industry reveals that the producers are in a very strong bargaining position relative to the consumers. Over the last twenty to twenty-five years, as demand for medical care has grown for a variety of reasons, the power of the physician–producers in the marketplace has been strongly evident. Because consumers have not been in a good bargaining position, the physician–producers have not been subjected to pressures to be more efficient in their productive activities. This strong demand, moreover, has made it easier for physicians to raise their prices rather than increase efficiency. If the industry were more competitive, such price increases would not be possible because the competitive incentives to increase efficiency and to reorganize the production process would work to the consumers' advantage, not to the advantage of the producer.

GOVERNMENT'S ROLE IN THE MEDICAL MARKETPLACE

Recently the medical profession has felt itself besieged by all sorts of pressures from the federal government. Why does government intervene in the marketplace to change certain ground rules? Economists hold that there are three justifiable reasons:[6] One reason is to supply services—often called pure public goods—that simply cannot be provided in the normal market setting. We could not maintain a very good army if different persons decided to buy one day per month of a soldier's time, or one tread for a tank, or one life preserver for some ship, etc.

Market transactions are also inadequate for the purchase of police and fire protection and a number of other goods or services where we know that production would not occur if they were sold only in a market setting. Economists say that these goods possess externalities—benefits that accrue to many individuals without their paying directly. As an example, if I hired my own army to help protect the city in which I live, all other people would get a free ride on my army: They would receive benefits without sharing in the costs. Moreover, there probably would be an underpurchase of defense services. To provide adequate "essential" services, we recognize that they must be purchased by the public so that everyone who benefits from the externalities shares in the cost.

A second reason why government intervenes in economic affairs is to affect the income distribution. Typically, in this country such intervention is designed to benefit only those persons who suffer the grossest inequalities of income. Hence, we have social security programs and welfare programs that tax the more affluent and redistribute resources to the poor.

The third area of government intervention is in purchasing goods and services where the market operates less than full time. These quasi-public goods are such things as highways and research. Certainly highways and bridges could be private ventures, and we could pay each time we drive over them. Research also could be purchased privately. There is the general feeling, however—because of externalities—that not enough research or highways or bridges would be produced to meet the public need. Therefore, government intervenes and produces, or pays to have produced, some of these goods and services.

I submit that this is the position in which we find health services today. There is a belief in the public sphere that the market does not work part of the time and does not provide an adequate quantity of medical services. For various reasons medical services are considered important—more important than certain other kinds of services and goods whose production is left purely in the private market. There is the feeling that these services should be made available to more people. In essence this is what is being said in the declaration that medical care is a right and not a privilege. The statement implies that medical services should not be denied because of income considerations. Moreover, we are recognizing that many externalities of medical care make this a unique service. We have witnessed actions by government to stamp out communicable diseases. Here the idea of externalities comes across very strongly. That is, if in trying to eliminate a highly communicable disease we left it solely up to each individual to purchase a vaccine, we would soon have some very difficult medical problems on our hands. This could occur because some people would purchase the services and get some benefits and others would not. Those not able to purchase the services for a variety of reasons (poverty, ignorance, because they are children, and so forth) would be exposed to the disease, and the problem of externalities would become very evident. Thus public policy concerned with communicable diseases and sanitation indicates that these problems are so important to large numbers of people that they must be dealt with outside of the market setting.

Another point needs brief mention: The rationale regarding health services has changed over time. Part of today's basis is the new concept of the significance of human beings in matters of economic growth. In the past most growth in the economy was attributed to an increasing abundance of material capital. Now we find that the balance has shifted, and human capital turns out to be relatively more important—and scarcer.[7] Increasingly we look at health expenditures in part as investment and in part as consumption. From a national economic policy point of view, it appears to be a wise investment to pay today to obviate some medical problems tomorrow. Prevention today may keep the recipient from becoming totally dependent on society in ten, twenty, or thirty years. These public expenditures for specific kinds of personal health services may be viewed as part of a national investment policy.[8] Justification for public investment in personal health is that healthy people are more productive in the long run.

Typically, we consider health services to be consumption goods. This concept fits in nicely with the various demands for health services mentioned earlier. We usually fail to consider that if a youngster does not get adequate medical care (either because his family neglects his physical needs or has inadequate income to pay for medical services) this neglect may impose a burden on society at some later date if he suffers a serious disabling illness. So for all of these reasons—problems of the market setting and problems of the nonavailability of certain services—government has found a rationale to enter the marketplace and to say that medical care is a right, not a privilege.

Defining medical care as a right and not a privilege implies a number of long-run and serious changes in the organization of our delivery system for health services. Assuming government is serious in its purpose, there are several options opened for action. The first is for government to set itself up as a major producer of medical services. The rationale to be employed is that there is something wrong with the way these services are provided today, that there are not enough of them, that they are not adequately distributed, or that there is not enough variety. The government could then move in and become a new, large producer of these services. As a second option, government might shun the production route and become a new, large consumer, acting in the consumer interest both for services purchased directly and for production of medical services in general. Government seems to have selected the second option and is now moving rapidly and forcefully to enlarge its role as a consumer of health services. In fact, government seems to be anxious to be rid of the producer role that it has had, in part, in the past. Public production of health services traditionally has occurred in city health departments, county hospitals, and city clinics. The passage of various pieces of legislation in the last few years has literally worked to destroy many of these governmental health services-producing institutions, and government now is oriented to creating incentives for private producers to replace these public organizations.

Let us consider some of these incentives for private production. First, we have the establishment of the Regional Medical Programs. This is a direct governmental attempt to affect the production of medical services at the regional level. Three years ago the Group Practice Facilities Act was passed, based upon public reasoning that there should be more large comprehensive group medical practices.

Incentives—subsidies, if you will—are provided to private physicians to encourage them to form new kinds of organizations for the production of medical services. In 1966, Comprehensive Health Planning legislation was passed by Congress. The focus of this legislation is very broad, but its intent is clear: to place the responsibility for careful planning and organization of the health care delivery system at the local level. All parts of the community are encouraged to consider what is desirable and necessary to make health services broadly available. The federal government views its role largely as offering seed money to assist the planning process.

Government acts as a major consumer in the sense that it specifically purchases services for some population groups under both Medicare and Medicaid legislation. The major point that should be made here is that government is concerned with the market setting, the distribution, and the availability of various kinds of medical services. Government is concerned that the market cannot resolve these problems by itself, especially if we define access to health services as a right rather than a privilege. In this way the government behaves like a collective consumer—one which either creates incentives for production of new services or provides funds for people to buy services where and as they will.

Not only is government thus defined as a collective consumer, it is a considerably better informed consumer than the average person—in part because it employs many professionals. As an informed consumer, government is now asking many new questions about the whole organization of the medical industry: about the kinds of services being produced, whether they really accomplish anything or whether they improve health. These questions have a great bearing on the mix of medical demands. As an economist, I see an interesting situation developing. Within the medical profession specifically, and within the whole health industry generally, there are many monopoly powers—powers with which the individual consumer has been unable to cope in the past. But now government is entering the scene in its new role of collective consumer. In the process government is starting to behave like a monopsonist, a very powerful purchaser. Some conflict is inevitable: It is a natural result when any powerful producer meets any powerful consumer head on. The situation developing in the health field today is analogous to a large retailer's treatment of its suppliers: "Meet certain standards, or we will buy elsewhere." Government, as an informed consumer with many dollars to spend, is beginning to ask questions not only about the availability of services but about their application at a point in time in the development of a disease when the services will be most effective. In so doing, government's attitude is to create positive financial incentives to encourage private producers to make these services available.

For an example in the health field, let us take a given disease—measles. For many years the treatment of measles was largely in the private sector. People who had the disease, or who sought to purchase an effective vaccine when it became available, were the ones who received care. And so parents subconsciously or consciously made decisions for their children—either to catch measles and then seek treatment or to take the child for a vaccination and effectively eliminate the problem. In this setting measles continued to be a very large problem nationally, even after the vaccines were developed, because many people did not have their children vaccinated. Now government as a collective consumer is looking not only at measles but at many other kinds of diseases with one question in mind: What is the best point in time to confront this disease? And it may very well be said, as with the measles example: Eliminate it at its source: Make sure that vaccines are provided for everyone, and back up the availability with strong efforts to get everyone vaccinated.

The focus and organization of our medical system in the past have been to deal with problems after the patient has contracted an illness; to deal with problems when the individual sees it directly beneficial for him or his child to see the doctor; and to repair damage that has already occurred. As an informed consumer, government has questioned this approach and accordingly has conducted a number of studies in recent years on cancer, heart disease, kidney disease, automobile accidents, and so on.[9] The answers that keep coming to the fore would warm an epidemiologist's heart: To be effective in caring for most of these problems, intervention must come early.

If government continues with these analyses and concludes—as an effective, informed consumer—that the best way to obtain these services or to have these illnesses or diseases treated properly is to tackle them early, then several actions are likely to follow: government may begin to create financial incentives to encourage the private production of these medical services—many of which are barely produced today and many of which are not produced at all because they have not been salable in the private market. This may mean simply that we are going to see increasing emphasis placed upon the production of preventive services—not only preventive services in the form of annual examinations but preventive services that carry many implications in terms of changing the whole nature of the medical services production process. Physicians have been reluctant to talk about mass production. All medical services are seen as job-ordered—tailored to the individual patient. In looking after the individual patient, though, physicians too often neglect society. But if you say that instead of buying individual services at the moment the individual feels a "real" need and you start asking questions about buying services at the time when they will be most effective for large groups or people, it may mean that physician involvement ultimately will be minimal or the production process will be markedly different from that we now experience.

SUMMARY

This discussion provides a preface for why we need to plan. It is strongly evident that the economist's approach is to ask the direct question: How does one get goods or services produced that are in line with society's needs? Generally the economist does *not* say, "Go start a new governmental firm to produce these services." Rather he encourages the private production of these services by making it profitable. The analyses that we have covered, which deal with attacking diseases early in their development, can be transferred into specific goals. If government wants to achieve these goals, it may do so by rewarding those producers who respond to these goals. Conversely, the public attitude may make it financially difficult for those who do not respond to meet this kind of demand.

The implications of these changes—for the medical profession, for all the health professions, and for the traditional production process—are great. It means taking a new look at what needs to be done and what services need to be produced in the future. We are saying that individual market demand criteria are not the *only* existing criteria. Increasingly, government seems ready to funnel funds into areas where the payoff to society seems higher. This may be in producing services in ways quite different from those we are accustomed to today. It may mean the complete reorganization of many of the institutions of health. But I do not see government anxious to use force to bring change. Rather, I see government using financial (economic) incentives to make things possible that have seemed only idealistic before. As a society we are searching for objectives and exploring ways to make them financially attractive for producers to respond accordingly. The changes that are occurring in the health field need to be viewed in this over-all context. The simple phrase that medical care is a right and not a privilege implies tremendous changes in the kinds of medical services that need to be produced, how they will be distributed, how the professions will interact with one another, and how various organizations will respond to meet the needs.

If the marketplace were really adequate, if consumers were really informed, and if there were not powerful professional interests, then we could sit back and say let the market solve the problem. But I think we must admit that none of these conditions hold very well today. As we focus more on the problem of the provision of health services, where they are most effective, and how they can be produced, it is to be expected that government will increasingly create incentives for physicians to change and to respond to these new markets. And they will be *new* markets! This must be kept in mind when we talk about why we need to plan. By so doing we may be able to surmount any philosophical bugaboos that are carry-overs from the days of pure laissez-faire medicine and realize that both health personnel and institutions now need to respond to a new set of market demands in our society.

References

1. An interesting discussion of the "need" versus "demand" controversy as applied to the health field may be found in Kenneth E. Boulding, "The Concept of Need for Health Services," *Milbank Memorial Fund Quarterly*, XLIV:4 (October 1966), 202–223.
2. A number of the factors affecting patient demand for medical care are included in Paul J. Feldstein, "Research on the Demand for Health Services," *Milbank Memorial Fund Quarterly*, XLIV:3 (July 1966), 128–165.
3. The following sections discussing consumer demand for health services draw heavily upon materials published recently by the author in "The Microeconomics of Health," included in Henrik L. Blum and associates, *Notes on Comprehensive Planning for Health*, Western Regional Office, American Public Health Association, San Francisco, California, 1968.
4. James Quick and Rubin Saposnik, *Introduction to General Equilibrium Theory and Welfare Economics*, New York: McGraw-Hill, 1968, p. 137.
5. One of the best articles documenting the market power of organized medicine is Payson Wolff *et al.*, "The American Medical Association: Power, Purpose, and Politics in Organized Medicine," *The Yale Law Review Journal*, 63:7 (May 1954), 938–1022.

6. Robert Dorfman (ed.), *Measuring Benefits of Government Investments*, The Brookings Institution, 1965, p. 4.
7. See such studies as Edward F. Denison, *The Sources of Economic Growth in the United States*, Suppl. Paper No. 13, Committee for Economic Development, New York, 1962; Theodore W. Schultz, "Investment in Human Capital," *American Economic Review*, 51 (1961); or Gary S. Becker, *Human Capital*, New York: Columbia University Press, 1964.
8. This view is the fundamental theme of *Estimating the Cost of Illness*, U.S. Dept. of Health, Education, and Welfare, Public Health Service, Health Economics Series No. 6, 1966.
9. These studies have emanated from the Department of Health, Education, and Welfare, Office of the Assistant Secretary for Program Coordination, and are titled *Program Analysis: Disease Control Programs*, 1966.

15

Tools for Planning

Mary F. Arnold

The skills and knowledge that are used in planning are an integral part of the process of planning, whether one is planning at the societal or community level or carrying on specific agency program planning; and there is an artificiality to a discussion of the tools of planning when the context in which the tools are to be applied is removed. Although planning as a process requires the application of creative insight and intuitive logic, there are some special tools available that, if skillfully applied, can aid in achieving greater rationality in the planning process. If one describes planning as those activities required to organize and implement an intervention in current patterns of activities with the purpose of achieving a different outcome or set of outcomes than would have occurred if there had been no intervention, there is an assumption that planning is a deliberate and conscious effort to create a desired effect. It is a process of reason—of rational decision-making. It is important, however, to understand this underlying assumption of rationality in the process of planning before one can understand how the tools of planning are used. Planning involves making decisions about problems, values, desired outcomes, activities, and feasible action with the expectation that these will be wise and reasoned decisions for solving problems and achieving desired outcomes. Decision-making in planning is expected to be consciously rational.

There are, however, different kinds of rationality, depending upon the kind of problem that is involved. Diesing[1] has suggested that there are five kinds of reason that are functionally necessary in society. The first of these is logical rationality that concerns the logic of cause and effect. Much of problem-solving depends upon the knowledge (or beliefs) we have of how problems we wish to solve are caused. Most disease control programs, for example, are dependent upon a logical rationality. We attempt to alter specific factors in the host, the agent, or the environment in order to prevent or ameliorate the effects of the disease. The more knowledge we have about causation of the disease, the more we should be able to find ways of dealing with the problem.

The second kind of rationality is economic rationality. In this case the decisions are not about causes of the problem, because these causal relationships are assumed. Rather, the decisions involve efficient allocation of resources to achieve multiple outcomes. The problem of limited resources, whether they are people, money, technology, or time, underlies economic rationality. Knowledge about cause and effect is assumed. It is necessary, therefore, to order the outcomes or objectives in some sort of preference scale if economically rational decisions are to be made. Once there is knowledge of the probabilities of effect of various alternatives and their order of preference in terms of some common scale of preference (utility), calculations can be made as to the "best" way to allocate resources to achieve the maximum utility. Under the premises of economically rational decision-making, for example, one might order disease problems in terms of costs to the society or costs to the individual or some other order of preference and then determine the best mix of resources for achieving the greater gain. Problems of priority and resource allocation are problems of economic rationality.

Before one can make either logically or economically rational decisions, however, there are three other reasons that must be served. These often underlie what are called "people problems." They have to do with the reason of social behavior. The first of these Diesing calls social rationality, and it involves the maintenance of social interaction and social integration, because without at least a minimal base of common values, expectations, and norms, action would occur on an individualized basis—on each individual's perceptions of what is logical and economically rational. Concerted actions of people could not occur. The second kind of rationality that serves as a social base is what Diesing calls legal rationality. These decisions function to define the parameters of social rationality—of what is morally acceptable. It is illegal, for example, to use physical punishment in the control of personnel in an organization except under carefully and legally spelled out conditions or special situations, such as certain physical restraints in the treatment of mental patients or in institutions of correction. Thus legal rationality focuses on the limits that might affect other people.

Finally, Diesing suggests a fifth kind of reason—political rationality—that articulates the values in the society about authority and responsibility through organized forms for the achievement of all other kinds of rationality. Essentially, the question resolved in political rational decision-making is "Who shall make what decisions for whom and under what conditions?" (See this volume, Chapter 10.) Olson makes the point that economic ideals and sociological ideals "are not only different, but polar opposites; if either one were attained, the Society would be a nightmare in terms of the other,"[2] and he further suggests that "the choice of a position along the continuum between the economic and sociological ideals must be made by the political system."[3] Thus the problems of planning differ in terms of the kind of rationality that is operating.

Even in the early stages of planning, when potential alternative selections to problems are being sought, limitations are considered, either implicitly or explicitly. For example: Is the suggestion legal? Is it moral? Is it practical? Is it acceptable? These limitations are the manifestation of different dimensions of social reason.[4] In this chapter major attention is placed on tools that can aid the planner in making decisions more rational in relation to logical and economic rationality. However, occasionally reference is made to the social, legal, and political dimensions of the use of these tools.

TOOLS FOR PLANNING

One way of characterizing the tools used in planning is to think of them in terms of the stages of problem-solving: problem identification, assessment and problem analysis, determination of alternate courses of action, decision for action, implementation, and evaluation. Thus, we have tools that

1. Aid in the description and definition of the situation, now and in the future, and in defining the parameters of the problem and the desired outcomes to be achieved.
2. Aid in the prediction of future states and the consequences of various strategies for action, as well as in making optimal decisions about strategies for achieving desired outcomes.
3. Aid in the implementation, guidance, and control of action.

Conceptual Tools and Models of Reality

As our scientific and technical knowledge has expanded, we have learned many ways of organizing this knowledge. Each different scientific discipline, for example, attends to different aspects of reality. To be sure, each society has certain common ways of organizing its general knowledge, for example, Eskimos have many more words in their language to differentiate different kinds of snow than are found in the English language. Every person during maturation learns to pay attention to certain stimuli and to disregard others that are not relevant. Thus, to define problems for planning purposes or for assessment of the present and the possible future, we bring together data that fit a particular model of reality that is useful for the purposes of the moment. As Bruner states it:

> [A theory] entails, explicitly or implicitly, a model of what it is that one is theorizing about, a set of propositions that, taken in ensemble, yield occasional predictions about things. Armed with a theory, one is guided toward what one will treat as data, is predisposed to treat some data as more relevant than others. A theory is a useful way of stating tersely what one already knows without the burden of detail. In this sense it is a canny and economical way of keeping in mind a vast amount while thinking about a very little.[5]

The various sciences have given us a variety of ways of categorizing and identifying phenomena of reality. Different models or theories about reality attend to different kinds of data. Molecular biology, for example, uses one kind of data and political science uses a different set of data and the problems that each would identify would be completely different, even though each provides important ideas about the world around us. Thus the deliberate use of different conceptual models for describing problems in health planning is useful in problem analysis. For example, there are many ways to describe "health." A *biological or physiologic model* emphasizes data that describe the way in which physiological processes function; illness may be described in terms of biochemical (e.g., blood electrolytes), mechanical (e.g., pressure or temperature), or biological (e.g., genotype) properties and changes. Diseases may be defined by the organ systems most involved or by the agent responsible, such as the tubercle bacillus. But we also define "illness" through descriptions of behavior. *Behavioral models* define disease or illness in the ways people act. For example, alcoholism is defined more from a behavioral than a biological base. *Social models* for describing health and illness come from sociology and socioanthropology. Social characteristics are the descriptor data. The deviance model, for example, pays attention to the social role that is expected of the well person and how illness behavior changes these expectations. *Demographic models* are another way of focusing on particular phenomena of health. Attention to prevalence, incidence, rates of disease by population groupings, vital data, and broad descriptors such as age, sex, occupation, and geographic location indicate different "theories" about what is relevant in defining health problems. Thus different conceptual models produce different kinds of questions about a problem and its solution.

Similarly, there are a variety of ways that phenomena about the organization of social behavior can be perceived and analyzed. For example, *structural models* give us a mechanical view of social organization. Sets of positions are described and integrated by authority or some other organizing force. The organizational chart is the best example of a structural model: It emphasizes the differences among parts of an organization and the location of certain responsibility and authority, such as who is in charge of what. Obviously this is not a complete description of an organization, although it is useful for certain purposes. *Economic models* emphasize allocation of resources, costs, and utility measures. The budget is an example of an economic model of the organization. *Political models* focus on the phenomena of power, and *interpersonal models* focus on the personal actions and feelings of people in interaction.

The most recently popular model is the *systems model* that attends to the interrelationships between component parts—on dynamic change and flow processes.

These and other conceptual models come from many sciences and disciplines and represent many theories about the relationships of different kinds of phenomena. For example, in Table 1 the different kinds of questions one might ask in describing the problem of alcoholism and in finding solutions to the problems have been indicated in terms of the probable conceptual models underlying the questions.

Different conceptual models, or theories, provide insights about problems that aid in predicting or hypothesizing potential ways of finding effective solutions. As we have come to realize that there is usually no one way of looking at a problem, we can begin to recognize that there may be a variety of alternative paths that can be taken for solving the problem.[6]

General Models

The acceptance of the idea that we define our world on the basis of our theories about the phenomena of the world has led to the construction of general models or analogues using mathematical symbols. A model, as mentioned earlier, is a shorthand description of the

TABLE 1. *Questions Elicited from Different Conceptual Models in Planning for Alcoholism*

PLANNING PROBLEM	*Characteristic Questions*	*Probable Conceptual Model*
Identification of the Problem	How many deaths from cirrhosis of liver due to alcoholism?	Physiological
	How many accidents due to drunken driving?	Behavioral
Definition of the Problem	How many people are affected? Where are they located? Age, sex, socioeconomic characteristics?	Demographic
Causative Factors	What personality characteristics are associated?	Behavioral
	With what drugs can the alcoholic be treated?	Physiologic
	Can the alcoholic and his family be helped to work out problems?	Behavioral
Program Alternatives	Should alcoholics be arrested? What action should the courts take?	Legal
	What effects would clinics and counseling have problems?	Physiological and Behavioral
Program Implementation	Where should the alcoholism unit be placed? in the health department? in vocational rehabilitation? in welfare? in mental health?	Structural
	How much public health nursing time should go to alcoholism? What is the expected payoff?	Economic
	Will the legislature support a program?	Political
	How can an alcoholism unit be introduced in an ongoing program? How will staff react to need for additional training?	Interpersonal
	What parts of the alcohol program are carried out in public health, in education, in welfare, in police and highways, in mental health, etc.? How does each affect the other?	Systems

relevant attributes of reality. The most general model is the mathematical model. This is a description in symbolic terms of characteristics of phenomena that can be manipulated with the logic and rules of mathematics. Where one is dealing with complex, dynamic, multiple variables, mathematical models are extremely valuable. For example, in a system where something lines up randomly for a certain processing, the queuing model can be used. The same mathematical logic can be applied whether we are figuring how to service cars efficiently, how many tollgates to use on a bridge, or intake policies for a rehabilitation unit.

Tools for Prediction and Forecasting

Successful planning depends upon how well we can predict what is likely to occur in the future, and this ability in turn depends upon our certainty about the causes and effects of phenonema. The tools of prediction are generally statistical in nature, but qualitative data can be used. Bross lists five kinds of predictions we can make:

1. *Persistance prediction:* Stable characterstics that do not change over time. The disadvantage or limitation of this type of prediction is that it assumes minimal change and depends upon continuous stability.

2. *Trajectory or trend prediction:* This includes change, but there is an assumption that the rate of change is stable.

3. *Cyclic prediction:* This assumes that there is a cyclic character of events that is stable, as one might find in seasonal variations in disease and illness patterns.

4. *Associative prediction:* This assumes a stable relationship between two events.

5. *Analogue prediction:* This assumes a somewhat mirrored correspondence between two sets of events where one can be observed and used to predict the other.[7]

In discussing the predictive system, Bross suggests that in order to have predictability the information used should be both "valid" and "sharp." Validity is dependent upon measures of the relative frequency of the occurrence that is said to have a specific probability. Previous experience, or experience with samples, can provide an estimate of validity. In other words, are there enough data available to be reasonably sure that the assigned probability of occurrence is to be expected in the future? Sharpness has to do with the necessary or essential discrimination of categories. For example, birthrate is calculated on the base of the total population. However, if we used this probability figure for predicting the number of babies that will be born in a particular and specialized population group, the prediction will not be very sharp.

Statistical predictions can be either deterministic—i.e., a precise prediction about how each observation will occur—or stochastic—i.e., a prediction of a proportion of observations that will turn out in particular ways in the long run. For example, one can estimate the probability distribution of accidents from various causes but cannot predict specifically to whom they will occur.

Recently some new methods of prediction have been used in forecasting for the future. Khan and Weiner[8] use the method of scenarios, wherein events of the future are predicted on the assumption that there will be no substantive change in present trends. Then they superimpose one, and then another, possible change in current trends and finally predict effects. Another method, called the Delphi technique, uses a group of experts not in contact with each other to make predictions about social and scientific change, and the differences in their predictions are then resolved through a process of analysis.[9] Another method of forecasting is that of building a model and simulating what may occur under various kinds of circumstances. There is much information that is not amenable to quantification, yet it may be important for predictive purposes. Much of our knowledge about social change and of macropolitical processes is based on careful objective descriptive analysis. For example, although every community is different, a careful historical analysis of past patterns of change can aid in predicting future change. Such predictions cannot be made with statistical measures of certainty unless special techniques as above are used; nevertheless, they can be valuable if carried out objectively and carefully.

Decision-making Tools

Decision-making is defined here as the determination of an appropriate action from among alternatives, because unless there is a choice among alternatives, there can be no decision. In planning there are several kinds of decisions that must be made:

1. *Decisions about the desired states of the future: What are the goals or objectives to be achieved? What is their order of preference?* These are the most difficult decisions to be made since they are value decisions. In order to make this kind of decision one has to have information that defines the parameters of the problem and the alternative futures that are feasible and possible. There are several methods

available, however, for eliciting the preference order of the decision-makers, whether these be the administrators of a program or the general public. One method is to look in the past at where resources have been allocated. Marvin Frankel shows how analysis of federal budget figures for health over a time period can point up changes in priorities.[10] By reviewing where resources have been allocated and how these allocations change over time, a picture can be brought out of the way priorities have been set in the past. Resources might be personnel time or money, and allocation categories might be in terms of populations served, functions performed, and other such categories. However, underlying this type of analysis is the assumption that in the long run organizational allocative decisions are economically rational. In fact, Lindblom makes this case in his justification of his disjointed incrementalism model for decision-making.[11] Another method is suggested by Churchman and Ackoff, wherein the decision-makers are presented with a series of potential objectives and through a logical process of comparisons are asked to examine and re-examine their choices until there is a logical consistency in the order of preferences.[12]

The difficult problem in determining goals or objectives is determination of who are to be considered as the decision-makers in the situation. This is a political question that must be resolved through some sort of political decision-making process. The health field has developed as a major part of our economy under conditions where ever receding goals have been accepted. Because of the development of technology we began to realize the potential of our goals of reduction of disease and death, as for example, in the case of eradication of particular diseases, we have been able to justify expenditures on the basis of reducing death and disability. However, today we are just beginning to be able to foresee the broader social consequences of carrying health goals to completion. In reducing certain deaths we are increasing chronic disability and the other attendant problems of old age. Reduction in infant death rates and other death control has led to a burgeoning population. Today, in most of our health programs the utilities to be sought are closely related to what might be defined as the "good life." Health, illness, and disease are intimately intertwined with socioeconomic status, education, geographic location, occupation, family patterns, etc. What constitutes the good life for some is not even in the realm of conjecture for others; and even our personal definition changes as our circumstances in age, economics, or other statuses change. Therefore, decisions about goals will require the resolution of conflicting value preference scales of many interest groups and clarification and identification of these different value premises. Until there is a means of dealing holistically with the problem of system purpose (see chapter 12), when we can take an ecological approach to goal setting, such conflicts of necessity will be resolved on a political basis.

2. *Decisions about strategies for achieving desired goals.* If there is knowledge about what objectives are to be accomplished and it is known what means are available for achieving the outcomes desired, then the decisions about strategies for achieving goals or objectives are computational in nature. Here the tools of logic and of economic rationality serve in the decision process. Scientific research provides us with the knowledge about cause and effect or, based on the accumulation of information from the past, we make predictions about the probability of effect of various alternative actions. Statistical analysis is the basic tool to be used. However, when faced with decisions about the optimal uses of resources to achieve objectives, the tools of the management sciences and the economists can be used.[13]

3. *Decisions about program implementation, guidance, and control.* Once a plan of action has been decided upon, there are the problems of implementing this plan. As mentioned earlier, consideration is given to the problem of implementation when alternative solutions to problems are first considered, but the data and tools used are different for these types of problems. Here the problems are social action problems—getting people or organizations to act in a particular way, deciding who does what when, and assuring that the plan proceeds as expected. There are, however, some management tools that can aid in the decision-making. One group of tools is called network analysis. Program Evaluation Review Technique (PERT) and the Critical Path Method (CPM) are examples. These are graphic ways of describing what events must take place in a logical sequence to reach a particular outcome. The analysis includes determining the activities required to reach each event stage and the resources and timing involved. Although these were originally developed for operational control purposes, PERT has been used successfully in the planning and coordinating of action in health programs.[14]

Another set of tools that are useful in the implementation process are the skills of organization. For example, the location of a particular program in an organization may affect what activities can or will be undertaken. For example, accident prevention in a maternal and child health unit would likely consist of quite different activities than in an environmental control unit. Location of a program predetermines the social relationships between people in the program, the type of leadership and concepts that may be used, and the expectations of others about what should be done. The structure of an over-all planning unit will affect what kind of planning is done. If, for example, a planning unit is organized on a geographic or political basis, then particular interest groups such as local governmental units will be relevant. If, however, the planning organization is set up on a functional basis, a different set of interest groups will emerge. As part of the organizational structure, a system of authority is necessary for action to take place. There are different ways of achieving this. Authority may be hierarchical in nature or may be shifted into different patterns for different types of functions.

Skills of Influence

In analyzing a series of community programs some years ago, Miller identified what he called "skills of influence."[15] The following list includes Miller's, but others have been added:

1. *The skill of expertise or knowledge*: For special problems the knowledgeable advice of an expert can influence behavior. For example, an attorney can influence our actions based on his advice about the legality of an action.
2. *Skill in manipulation of symbols and of communication*: Unless there is understanding of what action is desired, it is difficult to influence another to carry out that action.
3. *Skill in providing access to special and needed resources*: This is more than having power and authority. Rather, it includes a knowledge of where resources can be obtained and how they may be tapped.
4. *Skill in legitimating action:* This is a skill in making the desired action seem to be the right thing to do.
5. *Skill in organizing and arranging people and resources*: This is done in a way that makes the desired action occur.
6. *Skill in engendering enthusiasm and trust:* or in reducing fears that there will be detrimental consequences to the action.
7. *Skill in bargaining and in conflict resolution:* Often action cannot proceed until there is a resolution of conflicts of values or competition among several groups.
8. *Skill in predicting the effects of action or of nonaction:* The skills of prediction also can be skills of influence in that they aid in defining the parameters of action.

Each set of conditions wherein action is desired requires a different mix of these skills but, to the extent that we can apply these skills, we will be able to effect program implementation.

Information and Intelligence as a Tool of Planning

Information, as intelligence, is essential to every aspect of planning, of program implementation, and of evaluation and thus deserves a special section as a tool of planning. Information theory and the theory of cybernetics have brought new insights to the use of information.

General information theory as developed by Shannon includes three aspects to the problem of information-processing: *The technical aspect*—How accurately can the symbols of communication be transmitted? *The semantic problem*—How precisely do the transmitted symbols convey the desired meaning? *The effectiveness problem* — How effectively does the received meaning affect desired action?[16] Until recently the technical and semantic problems of information-processing were neglected in the consideration of communications. But Shannon's mathematical model of the technical problem and the increasing use of computer technology have taught us that there are technical limits to the information-processing that occurs in an organization. For example, there is a risk of error, which increases with speed of transmission; thus time must be allowed for information transmission. Because of noise and other factors in the receiving system, not all information is received and, therefore, it is essential that redundancy be built into any information system. Additionally, information loss is inescapable in any communication system.[17]

Information is needed to maintain control of the information-processing system itself. This is the idea of feedback as discussed in Chapter 16. Thus the core of any planning process is its information system. What kinds of information are needed, how often, under what circumstances, and for what kinds of decisions are questions that must be answered in building a viable planning system.

In summary, the tools of planning are varied and require both conceptual and technical skills for their application. They may aid in problems of logical and economic rationality and be statistical and analytical in nature, or they may be more related to organizational and motivational concepts, as the problems of social, legal, and political rationality enter into the planning process. If one views planning as a dynamic social change process, it must call on the concepts, skills, and knowledge of all the sciences to be effective.

References

1. Paul Diesing, *Reason in Society*, Urbana Ill.: University of Illinois Press, 1962.
2. Mancur Olson, Jr., "Economics, Sociology, and the Best of all Possible Worlds," *The Public Interest*, 12 (Summer 1968), 114.
3. *Ibid.*, p. 117.
4. Criteria of limitations are discussed in James L. Bemis, "Problem Solving Through the Process of Specification," in Mary F. Arnold (ed.), *Health Program Implementation Through PERT*, Western Regional Office, APHA, San Francisco, Continuing Education Monograph, No. 6, 1966, pp. 24–29.
5. Jerome S. Bruner, "The Perfectability of Intellect," in P. H. Oehser (ed.), *Knowledge Among Men*, New York: Simon & Schuster in cooperation with the Smithsonian Institution, 1966, p. 26.
6. Amitai Etzioni, "Shortcuts to Social Change?," *The Public Interest*, 12 (Summer 1968), 40–51.
7. D. J. Bross, *Design for Decision*, New York: The Free Press, 1953.
8. Herman Kahn and A. L. Weiner, *The Year 2000*, New York: Macmillan, 1967.
9. Olaf Helmer, *Social Technology*, New York: Basic Books, 1966.
10. Marvin Frankel, "Federal Health Expenditures in a Program Budget," in David Novick (ed.), *Program Budgeting*, Washington, D.C.: U.S. Government Printing Office, 1965, pp. 155–187.
11. Charles E. Lindblom, *The Intelligence of Democracy*, New York: The Free Press, 1965.
12. C. West Churchman and R. L. Ackoff, "An Approximate Measure of Value," *Operations Research*, 2 (1954), 172–181.
13. Abe Suchman, *Scientific Decision-Making in Business*, New York: Holt, Rinehart & Winston, 1963.
14, Mary F. Arnold (ed.), *Health Program Implementation through PERT*.
15. Paul A. Miller, *Community Health Action*, East Lansing: Michigan State University Press, 1953.
16. Claude E. Shannon and Warren Weaver, *The Mathematical Theory of Communication*, Urbana, Ill.: University of Illinois Press, 1949.
17. F. deP. Hanika, *New Thinking in Management*, London: Hutchison, 1965.

~ 16 ~

Evaluation: A Parallel Process to Planning

Mary F. Arnold

Planning, the process of determining how desired outcomes can be achieved for the future, is dependent upon information from the past. No matter how well planning is done, the future reaches forward fraught with ambiguity. But because it is possible to learn from the past and because the future can be forecast on the basis of the present and the past, we are able to plan for the future. Even so, the future is only to be conjectured and predicted, because it has not yet occurred and, therefore, is uncertain. One major way of reducing this uncertainty about the future is through the use of information about both the past and the present. For planning purposes, information is needed about the effects of past activity, about whether previous plans were actually followed, about occurrences in the environment that may have affected the outcomes of action, and about new scientific and technical discoveries that may affect how much can be achieved. There are many kinds of data that can be used for the purpose of making predictions and for determining how much mastery is possible over what is to come. Thus planning depends upon having available a means of systematically generating and collecting these many kinds of information so necessary for a continually changing future.

Evaluation is best considered to be that systematic planned feedback of information needed for guiding future actions. In a sense evaluation is the mirror image of planning in that it is the process of looking back upon action and making a judgment about it in order to provide the necessary information for planning for the future. There is a cycle of evaluation–planning–implementation–evaluation that is a continual forward-moving process along a time continuum.

In this way of thinking about evaluation, it is a rather specialized kind of information-processing by which relevant data are sought and judgments are made about the meaning of the data to guide decisions about future action. Both planning and evaluation necessitate understanding the nature of information and the tools of prediction and of decision-making, as well as the character of the kinds of decisions about action that will be made. (See chapter 15.)

THE WHY OF EVALUATION

Most people will say that evaluation is necessary in order to know what has been accomplished and whether past action was effective. Such knowledge may give personal satisfaction, but it does a bit more. It gives confidence that previous decisions about action were in fact wise decisions. It gives those supporting or financing programs confidence in their judgments about giving such support; it provides the supporting information that increases trust in one's competence to make decisions about the future.

It is also important, however, to ask whose actions will be guided by the evaluation. When Congress or a legislative body of the state or local agency asks for evaluation of a governmental program, the action that will be guided is theirs—the allocation of funds for the future or of new legislation. If the evaluation is to guide the program administrator, quite different kinds of action will follow. Thus, whose actions and what kinds of action for the future are being guided are important considerations in determining what information is needed for evaluative purposes.

What happens in the situation when it is found that objectives have *not* been accomplished? In reality, it is extremely difficult to admit lack of success, and it is often difficult to change or adapt what is now being done even without evidence of success. However, knowledge of the effect of a program is essential information if rational planning is to be achieved. But it is also necessary to know why the program was not successful. Was it due to an unknown situation in the environment that was overlooked in the planning stages? Was it due to incorrect assumptions or beliefs about the potential effects of the program's activities? Was it due to an unrealistic plan, an inability to carry out the plan as originally conceived? Was it due to lack of knowledge (the uncertainty in the situation) or poor judgment? Although it may be pleasant, or unpleasant as the case may be, to have knowledge about accomplishment, it is not intrinsically good in itself; rather, its value lies in the use of this new knowledge as a guide for action.

Building-in Evaluation

The idea that evaluation should be "built-in" means that planning should include arrangements for the concurrent and continual collection and review of information to guide the program's activities, as well as to review periodically the program's effects. What these special kinds of guidance information consist of, how often they are obtained, and when and how they are used are the evaluative problems of planning. To understand these information needs in some detail, it is useful to consider the questions one asks in the assessment phase of planning.

TYPES OF EVALUATION

There are several levels of evaluation, each one more complex than the next. The first and most simple level—that of program management control—assumes that activities under way are appropriate and effective for reaching the expected objective. It is assumed that there is a stable input of personnel, money, and technology from the environment and that there is a stable demand for the program activities being performed. The decision and control center indicated in Figure 1 represents the person or persons responsible for maintaining these activities. Figure 1 represents routine management control of program activities. There is usually a set of program plans with standards for operating, and the program activities are adjusted on the basis of these operating criteria. This is analogous to a thermostat. When the temperature gets to a certain point, the control center turns off the furnacc; then, when the temperature drops to a certain point, the control turns on the heat.

The next level of evaluation relates to efficiency of operations. The question changes from "Are activities being performed as expected?" to "Are activities as efficient as they could be?" Again neither the objectives nor the general type of program is in question, rather the concern is how best to make use of the resources available.

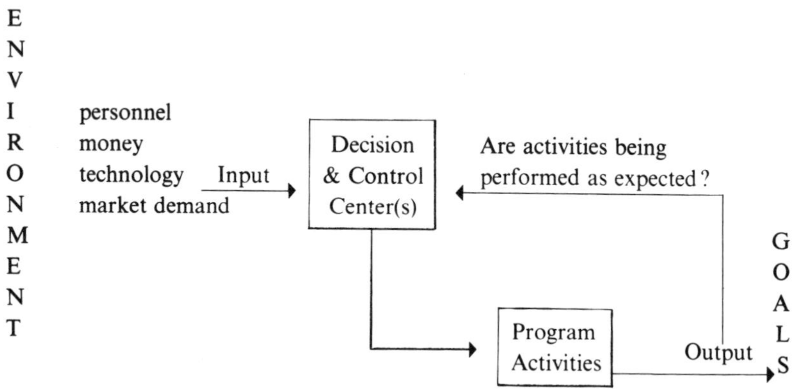

FIGURE 1. *Management Control of Program Activities*

At this level of evaluation, ways of changing the program activities to increase efficiency must be available. Analysis of various parts of the system and comparison of alternatives are used. For example, in a clinic program one might consider changes of work schedules, shifts of personnel functions, different record and reporting systems, and change of intake policies to increase efficiency. But the general program is not questioned in terms of its effectiveness in achieving its goals.

At the third level of evaluation the problem is more complex, because the question of program effect is asked. The memory unit holds information about cause and effect of program activities. Information about changes in the environment are assessed and program activities are evaluated in terms of achieving the desired objectives.

Finally, there is an evaluative question that asks whether the program is still appropriate for what the future is expected to be. In Figure 4

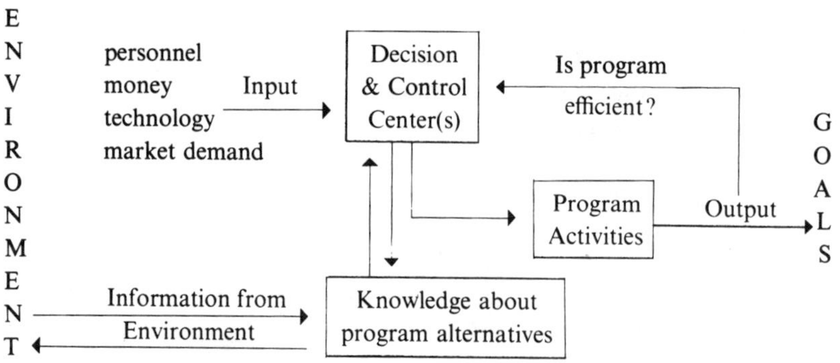

FIGURE 2. *Evaluation of Program Efficiency*

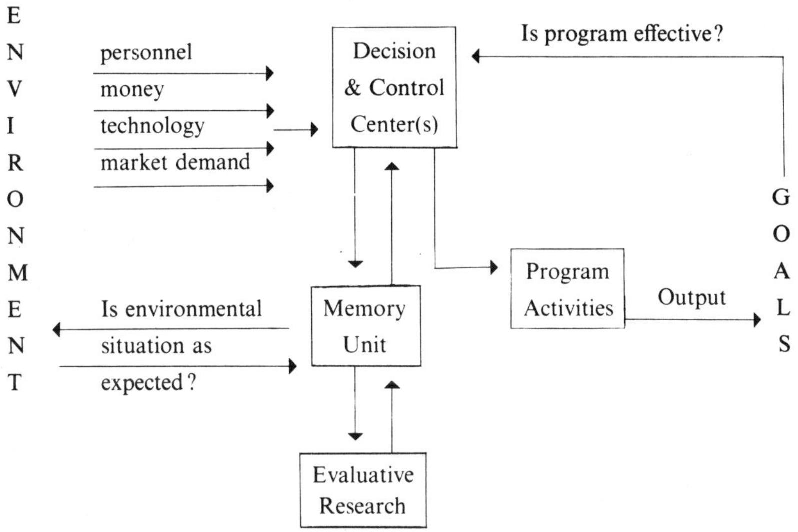

FIGURE 3. *Evaluation of Program Effect*

two additional stages have been added: consideration of the future and assessment of the capability of the program for achieving possible new goals. This level of evaluation is also the assessment phase of planning.

In Figure 5 all levels of evaluation have been brought together to illustrate the complexity of questions that can be asked for evaluative purposes. In a sense every aspect of what is being done should be continually evaluated. Probably the most important aspect of evalua-

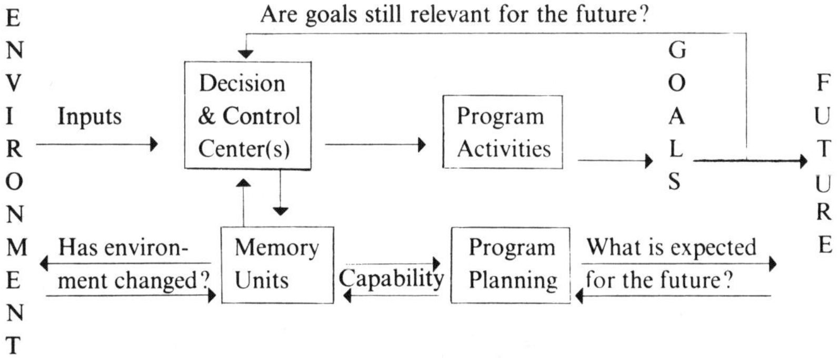

FIGURE 4. *Evaluation of Goals for the Future*

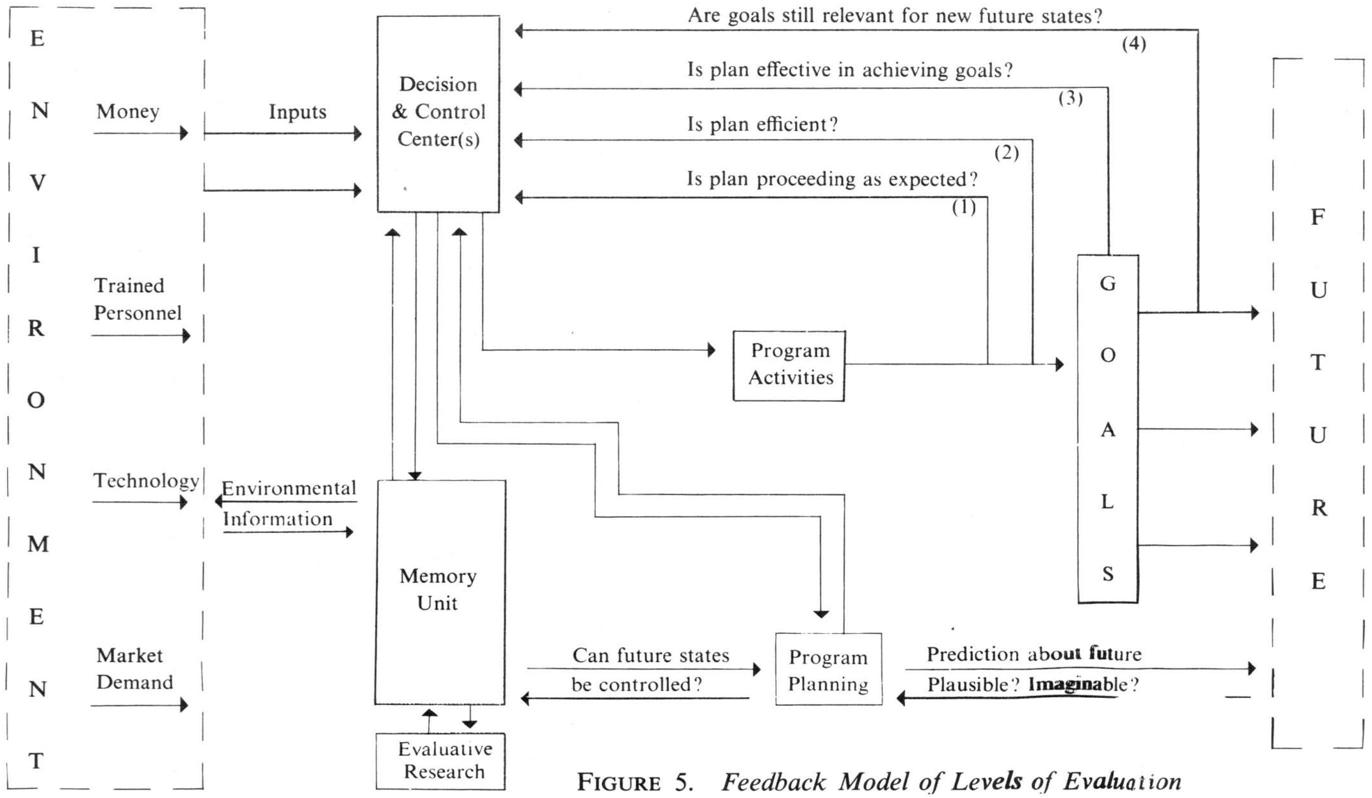

FIGURE 5. *Feedback Model of Levels of Evaluation*

tion is maintaining awareness of the assumptions made in each aspect of planning, because these are the criteria that must be used for making evaluative judgments. In planning many assumptions are made: about cause and effect of relationships (what causes the problem and what can be done about it?); about the environment (what can be influenced and what cannot?); what support and resources can be expected; what else is going on that may affect the outcome; and particularly, what value has been assumed for the outcomes to be achieved in comparison with alternative uses of resources. These assumptions are based on knowledge from the past and are the baselines against which judgments are made about current action.

Because of the wide range of evaluative decisions to be made, it is important to understand the sources and kinds of information that should be used at all levels of evaluation.

INFORMATION NEEDED FOR EVALUATION

The assessment phase of planning is actually an evaluation of the current situation. Is there a problem that should be tackled? Or will there be a problem if some action is not taken? Once there is awareness of a problem, then attention moves to the future and what new objectives could be achieved. To understand this new future it is necessary to make predictions based on all available information about the problem. Descriptive data about the problem are reviewed; the available technology for solving the problem is considered. But most important, priorities begin to form based on what is predicted about the problem in the future. For instance, infant mortality is high and it could be lowered: Is this worth undertaking? Chronic illness creates a great deal of disability and is of high cost to the community: What can be done about it? Does this have equal, higher, or lower priority than doing something about infant mortality? These values or priorities are not always explicit. The health professional, for example, tends to consider all health problems that have a high frequency of death or disability attached to them as having high priority, while others may not even perceive this as a problem.

In assessing problems adequately, various kinds of information are essential:

1. *Descriptive information:* Definition of what constitutes the problem; where it occurs; in what populations; in what geographic

areas; what the trends are; what has happened in the past; and what might be expected in the future.

2. *Scientific information about the causes of the problem*: What is known about the causes of the problem; what probability is there that a certain cause has a specific effect on the problem? What other factors enter into the causation? Epidemiologic data supply information on causation of health problems, but are there other factors to be taken into consideration, such as community attitudes and beliefs about the problem?

3. *Technical information about how these causal factors can be changed:* What is known about the possible effects of particular actions? What probability of success would there be if a particular set of actions were to be carried out? How much staff would be needed? How much would it cost? How many people would be affected?

4. *Technical information about the chain of effects necessary to achieve a solution to the problem*: What series of activities would have to be performed to achieve the estimated effects? For example, it might be estimated that infant deaths could be reduced by 10% if all mothers not now receiving prenatal care were to receive it by the second trimester; but it was also known that facilities must be available and that the mothers must use the facilities. Thus there are a series of things that would have to be done before achieving the final effect. Probability estimates can be made for achieving each of these subgoals or precedent events.

5. *Estimates of the probability of changes in the environment outside program control:* Most estimates about the future are based on an assumption that the situation will stay reasonably the same as it is, but this, too, is an estimate. Therefore, it is important to identify likely occurrences that might change estimates for the future. For example, the passage of new legislation may change many assumptions, as did Medicare. It is often possible to predict possible changes in economic and social trends and to prepare contingency plans if a careful environmental* surveillance is maintained.

6. *Information about relative values and risks of potential outcomes:* What utility measure is to be used? Which values will have priority over other values? Currently, for example, programs that aid in the reduction of poverty have a high priority. And every potential program

* Environment as used here implies all factors outside the control of the system decision centers.

has undesirable consequences as well as desirable ones. What effect will the other consequences have on the priority given to a particular action?

Only when as much of this information as possible is gathered can a clear-cut estimate be made of what can be achieved by a particular program. This estimate becomes the criterion by which the effect of the program is later measured. But in the process of planning, information is identified that will be needed for all four levels of evaluation, because it is on the basis of these assumptions and estimates that criteria for evaluating later action are developed. The need for information can be seen at each level of evaluation.

Is the Program Proceeding as Expected? The information gathered at this level of evaluation is used for guidance and control of the operating program, as well as for future information about how realistic the plan was. In this case no question is asked about the assumptions of cause and effect nor of the relative value of the objective; rather the interest is in what is actually happening within the program itself. For instance, assumptions were made about what activities would be needed to achieve the expected result, and from this information a plan of action had been devised. Also, expected parameters of the environment had been previously estimated; for example, availability of staff and other resources and also what else might be occurring outside the program's control. Some estimates of performance have to be available—such as the amount of time to carry out a specific task, the most efficient ways of carrying out the tasks, and performance criteria or standards of performance built from these estimates. At this first level of evaluation, performance is measured against certain standards expected to be performed. Often it is necessary to develop performance standards during the program operations, because data may not be available for making good predictions. In such a case it is essential to evaluate whether performance standards that are developed are within the range of the expectations held during the planning phase. In this kind of evaluative situation the only concern is with guidance of the programmed plan: Are the deadlines set being met? Is money being spent at the expected rate? Are personnel doing what is expected of them? These are the standard operating procedures every organization needs to maintain coordination and stability.

Is the Program Proceeding Efficiently? At this level of evaluation several kinds of performance criteria are used:

Efficient use of resources. Given an expected outcome and a given amount of resources, the desire is to use the resources to their optimal potential. Efficiency is related to the costs of achieving an outcome. What is the optimal use of personnel and money? It is important to recognize that the cheapest way may not be the most efficient way of achieving an objective. Efficiency is the ratio of cost to benefit. For example, it may be more efficient to buy good quality paper stock at a higher price if it will save secretarial time. Efficiency always should be related to the outcome of the total process. Time studies, periodic reviews and sampling, or performance budgeting are tools for calculating efficiency. Averages of performance are generally inadequate, because they tell nothing about the expected range of variation. It is important to know the range of variation that can be expected in order to estimate differences in performance from the expected. Only then can a decision be made about correction of the situation.

Subgoal criteria of performance and proximate criteria. In many programs there is a sequential chain of events that must occur for the final achievement of a program goal. For example, in educational programs it can be measured whether needed information is made available through a variety of means; but this is not a criterion of effectiveness, it is merely a measure of performance. If in the initial assessment phase of planning the sequence of events necessary to achieve the expected outcome has been identified with clarity, then it is necessary to know whether these performance criteria are being met. *Lead time* should be estimated. In many programs a long period of time is required before expected program activities can be expected to pay off. It becomes necessary then to use performance criteria as proximate criteria for future effects. Thus, for programs with long-term effects, some criteria for performance for the short-term review must exist, even though the effect may not be immediately measurable. For example, utilization rates or increases or decreases in case loads are proximate performance criteria used to indicate that something is different from what was expected. But standards of performance need to be established to give a base against which current performance is compared.

Questions about performance are asked to decide whether to continue action, whether some adjustment needs to be made in the program activity, or whether it is time to stop and look at the expectations held of the plan and possibly to change them. To answer these questions we move to the third level of evaluation.

Is the program effective? To make such a judgment it is necessary to have clear-cut, predetermined, measurable criteria of effect. It is also necessary that the specific activities of the program have an estimated effect on the outcome to be measured. Finally, it is necessary to estimate whether factors outside the control of the program have had an effect on the outcome. Since the evaluative question—Is the program effective?—is asked, a judgment is to be made about program activity because there is a question whether to continue the program as planned or to make some minor changes.

If it is found that the criteria of effect have been met, there is still not enough known about the situation to make a decision about next steps. So it must be asked, even with a successful program: Why has the program succeeded? Was it because of what was done in the program (and did the program proceed as expected)? Was it because something changed in the environment? How did that change the original estimates of potential effect of the program activities?

In planning it is necessary, as stated before, to make assumptions about the effects of other factors in the environment on the outcome to be achieved. But it also needs to be understood that over time and in the dynamics of the real world these things are never stable. If these assumptions have been identified and made explicit, then it is possible to provide for continual surveillance of changes that would effect either the program activities or the estimates about the effect of the program. For example, if a new drug becomes available or is in testing stages and looks promising, it is necessary to assess the potential effects on the expected outcome of the program. When chemotherapy first was considered in the treatment of tuberculosis, it was obvious that a building program for hospitals for tuberculosis patients should be reviewed in the light of the potential effect of the use of chemotherapy. Similarly, a new law may affect what can be done in a program. This in turn will effect the estimates of potential outcome. These examples seem obvious, but many programs or activities continue in spite of new information that changes the underlying assumptions about a program.

Information about changes in the environment may be new scientific information, new technical information, changing demographic and social conditions, financial support and potential resources, or factors affecting the program either within or outside its control. For the assessment of ongoing programs and for evaluation of effect, an intelligence system should be provided that is related to the assumptions previously made about those things that may affect the program outcome. This is evaluation of assumptions about cause and effect.

Three actions can be taken if a program is successful: (1) continue the program as planned, revising the criteria of effect for the next time period (relevant only if the program is of a continuous nature); (2)

revise the plan to meet a new criterion of effect (relevant if the program was a pilot or demonstration or if the major effect has been completed); or (3) complete action, wind up the program, and store information gained for use in future, similar situations through reports, publication, or other information storage (relevant only when the program is a one-time operation).

If, on the other hand, it is found that the program does not meet the expected criteria of effect, there are new sets of questions to be asked that relate to an analysis of why the program was not successful. It is then necessary to refer to the assumptions made during the analysis of the problem: Were the assumptions about causation valid? Were there unexpected changes in the situation or the environment? Did the program proceed according to plan? This process of analyzing why effect was not accomplished might be called evaluative research. To do this well one must know what the expectations were in each of these areas and how they were or were not met during the course of the program. Following analysis of lack of success, there are four alternative actions for the future: (1) adapt the old program in the light of the new information (relevant for a continuing program); (2) establish a new method or program for accomplishing the objective (relevant if the objective still has the same priority for action); (3) establish a more realistic objective and continue the old program (relevant if the problem still has high priority); or (4) shift resources for the achievement of another objective, end the program, and store information for a future similar situation. Figure 6 shows this process in diagram or flow-chart form.

Evaluation of effect is post facto; however, many programs are of such a nature that there is a time span between what is done and the outcomes expected to be achieved. Thus careful analysis has to be made of the questions asked at the first levels of evaluation: Did the program proceed as planned? Was it realistic in terms of the environment? Causal factors are but one part of a decision to choose a certain course of action. The other aspect is the preference held for one set of outcomes over another. This leads back to the fourth level of evaluation or to a new assessment of the situation.

Is the outcome expected to be achieved still relevant for the future and worthwhile in comparison with other benefits that could be achieved with these resources? Objectives and goals shift and change depending upon whose they are, whether they are short range or long range, with what other goals they are being compared, and what additional consequences may be expected as a result of the program. At one point of time and under a particular set of circumstances a particular goal may be agreed to be desirable; but with technological and social change or even with initial success, the program objective may no longer have high priority when weighed against other potential objectives. One tendency in the health field has been to give priority to life itself rather than to the quality of life. Today, although an increasing proportion of the gross national product goes into health, there is increasing dissatisfaction with the way priorities have been placed on the use of resources. Thus one important kind of evaluation is that of the review of the relative value of goals.

In this case the information needed is attitudinal and political in character. Decisions may involve many people, and the priorities given are the culmination of the resolution of differences among a plurality of interests. However, these decisions are also dependent upon the breadth of choice available to the decision-makers. Studies of search behavior show that there is always a tendency for people to look for the solution closest to past activity. Thus, to extend the range of choice there should be a planned, predictive analysis of future trends to be evaluated against current programs. And at this point a new planning process has started.

PROBLEMS IN EVALUATION

Evaluation is a complex series of processes for feeding back information to guide action. It is a mirror image of planning in that it is the process of reviewing what has occurred against criteria of expectations that are developed in the planning process. To plan without making explicit these many kinds of criteria by which a program is to be evaluated leaves the planner the problem of evaluating post facto without adequate information. In the previous discussion it was shown that there are at least four types of evaluative criteria that can be used: (1) Outcome or benefit criteria for evaluating effect. (2) Performance criteria for evaluating efficiency. (3) Assumptive criteria about cause and effect for analyzing effect. (4) Value criteria for assessing previous determined goals. To build-in evaluation to any program, all four criteria should be specific and explicit. Only then can the worthwhileness of a program be assessed. Also, the timing of each evaluative process should be planned. This is, however, a highly rational approach to evaluation. It assumes that cause-and-effect relationships either are known or can be determined with the application of adequate research

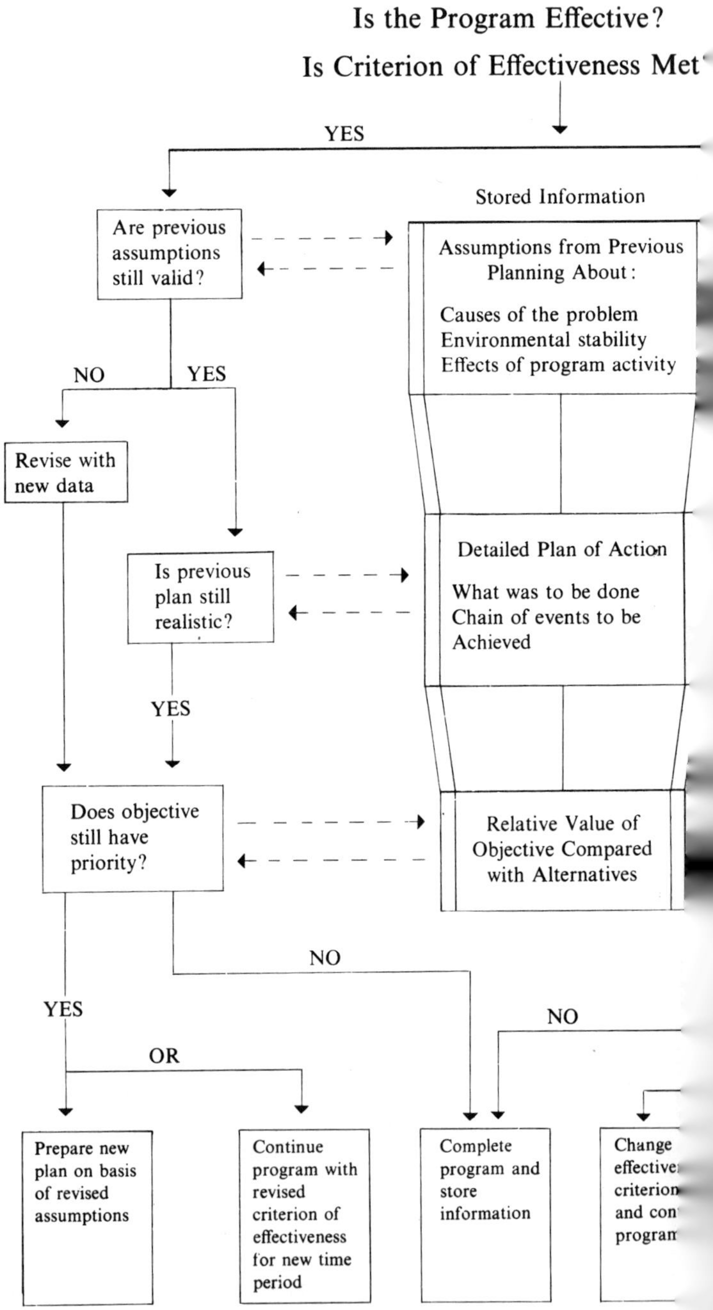

FIGURE 6. *Flow Chart of Proced*

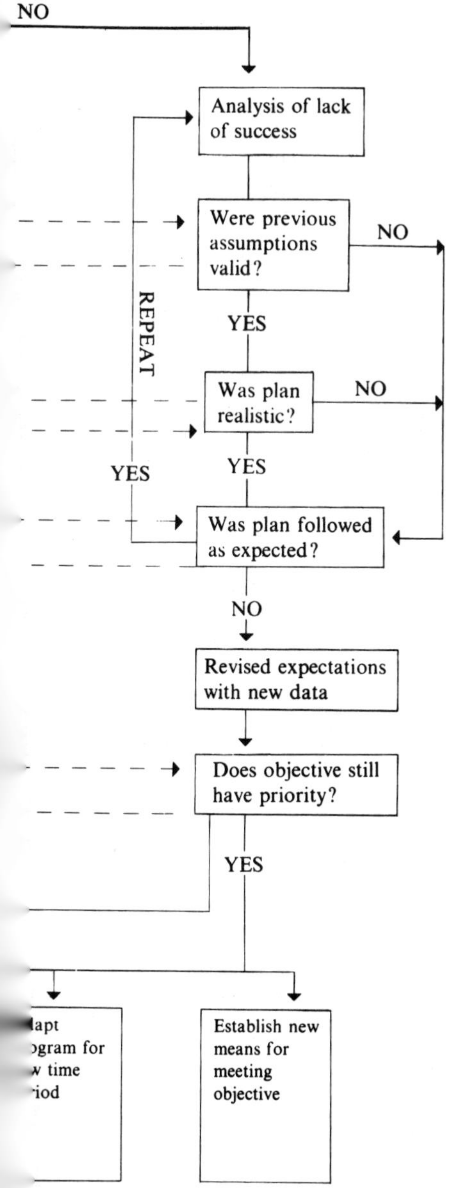

ation of Effect

techniques. It assumes that there always can be an agreed-upon scale of desirability for goals and objectives. It assumes that it can be known ahead of time what information needs to be collected to make the evaluative judgment. In reality, these latter assumptions seldom can be completely fulfilled in an operating program. What can be done then?

Thompson* has suggested that where assumptions about cause and effect are not questioned and when criteria for outcome are clear-cut, the efficiency level of evaluation is adequate; if there is a question about cause and effect but there still are clear-cut criteria for outcome, effectiveness is the major problem. But if clear-cut criteria for meeting objectives are not available, then it is necessary to fall back on social judgments about program activities. Figure 7 shows this model with types of information that can be used in each situation.

For illustration, the following four evaluative problems will help to identify the evaluative problem and what can be done:

1. A home health aide program is initiated, and after the initial period the administrator wishes to evaluate the performance to establish a reasonable budget for the following year.

This is essentially efficiency evaluation, but it can be done only if there is a clear-cut measure of performance. Probability costs to the community could be used and an estimate of savings or benefits made as a result of the program. (For example, hospital days might be saved by the use of the program.) Data would be needed on performance costs in comparison with benefits saved. Costs of alternative personnel patterns could be estimated, and only once an estimate was available for activities to be performed could utilization rates and variation of costs by activities be assessed. In this situation the value of the program is not questioned, nor the actual program.

2. A voluntary agency has funded a program to develop new methods for reaching a particular target population and wishes to know whether the program was successful.

This is a type of effectiveness evaluation that is based on a measure of performance: Did the project develop new methods that reached the "hard to reach"? In such an exploratory situation external variables are not predictable, since the program is somewhat a trial-and-error kind of action. Therefore, the evaluation would be historical and descriptive. It might include some hypotheses as to cause-and-effect relationships, but it would be unrealistic to expect to be able to test assumptions about cause and effect. A running account of the major decisions made during the program, including the assumptions that were made at each time period about the situation, would be the data

* James V. Thompson, *Organization in Action*, New York: McGraw-Hill, 1967.

Assumptions About Criteria of Desirability for Outcomes (Ends)	Beliefs or Assumptions About Means of Achieving Outcome (Cause and Effect): *Highly Certain*	*Uncertain*
Clear-cut	*Evaluation on Basis of Efficiency* Performance budgets Cost benefit Work-flow analysis Cost-effectiveness Work-load ratios Analysis of performance variance & cost variance	*Evaluation on Basis of Effectiveness* Time or historical comparisons Evaluative research (cause-effect) Descriptive reports of completion of objective Measurement of surrogate effects (proximate criteria)
Diffuse	*Evaluation on Basis of Acceptable Performance* Activity reports (no. visits) Comparison of performance rates (e.g., utilization) Comparison with past performance Accomplishment of predetermined subgoals Judgment of experts Comparison against professional standards	*Evaluation on the Basis of Acceptable Surrogate Criteria* Professional standards (e.g., accreditation, training) Acceptance by general public or financing group Judgments by expert opinion

FIGURE 7. *Examples of Evaluative Procedures by Certainty of Assumption*

needed for final evaluation. However, final evaluation would be based on continual assessment of each previous subdecision. Change from the past would be used as the criterion for effectiveness.

3. A health service has been introduced in a ghetto neighborhood, and the funding agency wishes it to be evaluated.

There are several kinds of evaluation inferred here. The question is probably related to the use of funds that might better be used in some other way; but unless clear-cut measures of effectiveness had been determined in the beginning, it would be difficult to know on what basis the evaluation is to be made. If the evaluation is to be made on a criterion such as a change in the health status of the population, then the change should be measured in both the user and the nonuser populations of the neighborhood served by the health service. This probably would require periodic surveys on a sampling basis of both populations. If this specific kind of criterion cannot be used, then it becomes necessary to fall back on the judgments of certain experts: the clients, the nonclients, the professionals, peer groups of the professionals, etc.

Efficiency evaluation of internal staffing patterns would depend again on having a clear-cut criterion of effectiveness or benefit against which alternative patterns of staffing, or of procedures, could be compared on a cost basis. If such a criterion is not available, then performance would have to be compared against similar programs or against performance standards provided externally. Performance budgeting with analysis of variations beyond an expected range would have to be used.

4. A health officer believes that a restaurant sanitation program is using resources that could be better used elsewhere, and he wishes to evaluate the program.

The problem here is one of evaluation of goals in addition to efficiency and effectiveness. Assuming that information from technology and science suggests that the process of inspection has a low probability of affecting any possible disease transmission, the problem is one of whether the criteria for desirability for this program are to be taken in terms of scientific values or social or political values. Restaurant inspection may have a high priority in terms of public demand in spite of its low priority in terms of its effectiveness for preventing disease.

In each of these cases, all four kinds of evaluation can be applied; however, unless the necessary data are readily available and previously built into the program, evaluation for efficiency or effectiveness can be more expensive than continuing the program. Although efficiency is important, because it may release resources for accomplishing something else, and an understanding of effectiveness is important, since it tells whether the resources could be used to better advantage elsewhere, both depend upon having built-in criteria for evaluation. When these are not available there is the practical question of when to commit new resources for program evaluation.

WHEN SHOULD RIGOROUS EVALUATION TAKE PLACE?

Before resources are committed to rigorous and precise evaluative procedures it is wise to consider what decision will be made if the program does not stand up under such an evaluation. Since evaluation is a means of guiding action for the future, serious thought should be given to alternatives to action that might occur. There are a number of situations in which it may not be wise to commit a large amount of resources to evaluation:

1. When the cost of carrying out a rigorous evaluation is higher than the cost of the program.

This requires some assessment of the cost of evaluation and the cost of not evaluating. In the neighborhood health center example, the cost of evaluation for effectiveness, as well as for efficiency, probably would be quite high if it entailed a periodic sample survey of the area population. However, if this were done for one area, the information might be extremely valuable to the country as a whole and such an evaluation might be considered well worth the cost to guide future national planning. If every such center were to be evaluated in this way, fewer services could be provided, because such evaluation would use scarce resources. Thus the costs of such evaluation not only should be considered in terms of the particular program but also should be assessed in terms of the larger system benefits that might be provided by such evaluative information.

2. When the current program is the only strategy available, and there is evidence that it may be having some effect.

This situation is tricky because it should not be used as a rationalization for not evaluating. First the analysis prior to evaluation should include what would occur if the program were to be discontinued. Second, there should be some definitive search for other alternatives before an attempt is made to evaluate. The very act of searching for other alternatives usually will start the evaluative process.

3. When the program is obviously desired by the community regardless of its effectiveness.

The example of restaurant inspection is of this type. There are often certain legally required programs that by any logical analysis would not stand up under a true efficiency or effectiveness evaluation. Perhaps the first question then is: Can the law be changed readily? There are other programs that, were they discontinued, would be so disruptive to other activities that it might be wiser not to put them to the scrutiny of a rigorous evaluation.

4. When change of program activity would be too disruptive to other programs.

It may be obvious even without a rigorous evaluation that a more efficient use of resources could be found by the reallocation of personnel; but this could create such dissension that it would damage other necessary programs. If, for example, a strike were to be called because of such a change, serious consideration should be made of the potential costs of the change in comparison with the gains that might be made through change of the program.

SUMMARY

Evaluation has been shown to be a complex cycling, iterative process that parallels the planning process. Although evaluation looks to past performance, as planning looks to future performance, both are dependent upon skilled use of information in making decisions. Clarity and specificity are desirable, and they depend upon the skilled and knowledgeable use of many kind of data, as well as upon the ability to use these data in making reasonable and relevant predictions. To build-in evaluation means to build into our thinking an analytic approach to what we are doing; it means building into our programs an information system that will provide the means of evaluating decisions and actions; and it means continually asking the simple but pertinent question about every program action: "Why should this be done?"

17

Agency Problems with Community Health Planning

Mary F. Arnold & Douglas L. Hink

Under the stimulus of recent legislation—Public Law 89–749 (Comprehensive Health Planning) and Public Law 89–239 (Regional Medical Programs)—efforts are under way throughout the nation to start planning for a more rational allocation of health resources. If effective planning is to be achieved, the many interests of the consumers of services, of the distributors of services, and of the general public will have to be woven into the fabric of the plans. If a more rational allocation of health resources is to be achieved, the varied institutions and agencies relevant to the health system will have to find new ways of coordinating their efforts. Studies of community action indicate that community-wide planning for the coordination of services, particularly in the larger urban areas, has only been sporadically successful. In a study of Jewish community agencies in Boston, Morris showed that, if agencies were jointly experiencing crises in financing or in manpower, there was a better potential for effective cooperative planning.[1] Myerson and Banfield, in their Chicago study, showed that diffusion of power reduces opportunities for coordinated action.[2] In the literature a variety of factors have been identified as obstacles to community planning: threats to agency domain, diffusion of power, pluralistic decision-making, and centralization of corporate and governmental authority.[3, 4, 5, 6, 7]

As an ideal, coordination is not new to health professionals and, in the professional literature, emphasis often is placed on goodwill and a cooperative spirit to achieve willingness to conform voluntarily to community plans. Incentives are proposed to offset the problems of autonomy and conflicting interests by reducing the unattractive aspects of the potential loss of agency autonomy often inherent in interagency planning.[8] It is our thesis that a cooperative spirit does not necessarily lead to the implementation of coordinated plans and that, even where there is a strong desire and willingness to work together on the part of community agencies, there are some major obstacles in the very structures of the organized community that militate against the implementation of cooperative efforts.

It seems important at this time of change in the health-planning structure of many communities throughout the country that these additional barriers to cooperative planning be identified so that newly developing planning organizations will have a greater potential for success in adapting to changing health and social needs than in the past. The following analysis of interagency planning problems stems from reports of agency experiences in one community, but the frustrations and difficulties these agencies encountered have relevance for other similar communities in that they provide clues to planning problems in addition to those that have previously been reported.

REPORTED EXPERIENCES FROM ONE COMMUNITY

During the conduct of an exploratory study of health service needs of the chronically ill that might be met by voluntary agency programing,* six health agencies in a rapidly expanding metropolitan community were contacted and intensive interviews were conducted with nine administratively responsible persons affiliated with these agencies. The agencies contacted were the city and county health departments, the visiting nurse association, a local voluntary health agency, the social service unit of the county hospital, and the community's social planning council. Data were obtained on the history, the general administrative structure, the budget and mission of the agency, and its activities with particular reference to programs for the chronically ill. The greater part of the interview with each administrator was devoted to his perceptions of community health needs and how they might be met, on the assumption that the administrator represents the agency's general perspective.

* In the study from which these data come, patients and their physicians were interviewed as well as agency administrators.[9]

Each administrator interviewed reported that coordination was a major problem in providing services for the chronically ill, yet other information obtained showed a probably better than average situation among the agencies in this community. The monies expended per capita, the professional caliber of the agency personnel, and the reported interrelationships among agency staffs would compare favorably with any other similar community in the United States. The administrators interviewed were well known to each other; they sat on each other's agency committees, cooperative working relationships had been developed between agencies, and a great many formal and informal contacts were reported.

Although only six agencies were represented in the interviews, the data showed that they were part of a highly interrelated organizational system. The *Directory of Health, Welfare, and Recreational Services*, published in 1965, listed 116 different agencies, of which 63 provided some kind of health or personal care services (social, vocational, and recreational services were not included in these 63). Eight coordinating groups were listed in the directory, including five community councils representing geographic or ethnic segments of the community. The sheer number of potential interagency contacts is staggering. If each agency had only one contact yearly with one other agency in this community, there would be more than 6500 contacts.

During the interviews a total of 39 specific organizations or agencies, not including the 7 hospitals in the community, were named as having some program or planning relationships with the respondents' agencies dealing with problems of the chronically ill. Additionally, for 6 out of the 7 hospitals named there was some specific type of organized relationship with one or more of the study group. To indicate the extent of the interagency relationships, 22 of the 39 agencies identified as particularly important for meeting the problems of the chronically ill were each named by administrators from 3 or more of the study agencies. Eight of these were named by all respondents: the 6 in the study and 2 additional ones (the school system and the welfare department). At the conclusion of each interview the respondent was asked to suggest names of other persons in the community who would be able to give information about community health services. Five of the respondents interviewed were named by all persons from agencies other than that of the named person. A high degree of interagency knowledgeability also was evident in that respondents from those agencies providing direct services to clients reliably specified the type of service provided, pertinent intake policies, and other relevant information about the service program of each agency cited.

Coordinative Efforts

Sixteen different interagency committees were specifically identified on which two or more of the study respondents were serving. Some were advisory committees organized to provide for interagency coordinated planning, while others related to specific project activities of the parent agency. Other coordinative activities were mentioned but not identified specifically enough for comparison. Six types of voluntary community groups, such as church organizations and service clubs, were mentioned as being involved in volunteer projects of the study agencies. These volunteer services included provision of clerical services, friendly visitor services, transportation aid and, occasionally, financial assistance.

No attempt was made to obtain a measure of time involved in these coordinating relationships, but even from this small number of interviews an extraordinary amount of time and energy was reported. The interviews presented an impression of a group of capable and cooperative health professionals, each giving generously of his own and his agency's time and energy to build and maintain coordinative relationships. But each respondent cited a long list of "unmet health needs" (20 or more were cited by each respondent), each was concerned about abortive attempts to meet these needs, and each seemed discouraged with movement toward solution to these problems.

With this reported amount of energy going into coordinative efforts, why did each administrator interviewed feel that the greatest problem in providing services for the chronically ill was lack of coordination?

PROBLEMS INHERENT IN COORDINATED PLANNING

Further analysis of the interview content indicated that, regardless of their interest in and their willingness to enter into cooperative relationships, coordinated planning for the agencies in this community seemed to be inhibited by three major barriers:

1. The specific mission of each agency, with the underlying differences in technical work requirements and differences in environmental constituencies from that of each other agency, resulted in differences in defining and identifying community health service needs.

2. Agencies view community needs and assess their effectiveness in meeting these needs in differing ways, leading to selective attention on the means by which each agency copes with problems in its particular

environment rather than on a critical analysis of the underlying problem.

3. The sheer volume and magnitude of required interactions within a complex administrative organization and between the agencies within a community reduce available energy for cooperative action.

Differences in Definitions of Health Needs

This first barrier is analogous to what March and Simon describe as subunit ideology within an organizational system.[10] The particular structure within which people work requires attention to the particular mission of the unit. A review of the history of these agencies showed that each one was formed initially to provide a particular kind of activity in response to a particular perceived need in the community. Once the organization came into being, a system was set into motion that was sustained in an exchange process with other systems in the environment. The output of each agency system, such as a particular service to certain clients, is part of the exchange process, and in return the organization receives from its environment skilled personnel, money, space, information, equipment, clients, legitimation, and support.[11] The administrator responsible for maintaining the environmental support relationships of his agency would be expected to perceive the agency's environment in relation to the mission of the agency. Therefore, since each respondent had been asked to identify needed community health services, it was possible to compare the type of needs most often mentioned with the stated mission of the agency. All needs mentioned were listed and classified into four categories, as follows:

Type 1—Client Needs. When a specific service needed by individual clients was identified, it was classified as a "client need." Examples are "Transportation is a big problem. People are house-bound and unable to get out." "Isolation and employment are the biggest problems." "No service in general counseling for the patient at home."

Type 2—Administrative Needs. When the orientation to the item was administrative or dealt with lack of manpower, the item was classified as an "administrative need." Examples are ". . . the utilization of nutritionists in working with community groups and in classes." ". . . additional staff to do case-finding and home-visiting in depth." "There should be more orientation for workers on services of other agencies."

Type 3—General Social and Economic Needs of the Community. When an item was mentioned that focused on a general community problem or an activity that related to community social planning or legislation, it was classified in this category. Examples are "The quality and quantity of medical services vary geographically." "There's a need for more hospital insurance and medical insurance programs." "I don't think priorities (in all services) are in the right place."

Type 4—Coordinative and Organizational Needs. Responses were classified in this category if they emphasized interagency activities. Examples are "There seems to be a lack of clear-cut control of nursing homes in the County." "More coordination of the type practiced at the county rehabilitation unit is needed" (a joint agency activity). "There are good services that need to be coordinated, and some need to be more strategically located."

Six of the nine respondents indicated needs in each of the four areas. Since more than one respondent was interviewed in each health department, and since the administrative positions of the respondents differed in some degree, only a general comparison of the total responses for each agency was possible. The percentage of responses by category was calculated for all respondents in each agency and for all respondents. Table 1 shows the proportionate emphasis placed on each category of need in relation to the particular agency's mission. It is interesting to note that the agencies that provide direct client services did not all emphasize client needs: The health department respondents as a group mentioned administrative needs most often, and the visiting nurse association, administrative and coordinative needs.

This differential in emphasis among agencies is not unexpected when the mission of the agency and the type and scope of activities performed are considered. The relatively large and diverse professional staff of a health department with its responsibility for a broad variety of community health services would account for a perspective on administrative problems. The visiting nurse association, with the next largest number of personnel but with a singular mission of providing professional nursing care to ill patients in the community, would be likely to have a great many administrative and coordinative problems. The voluntary agency and the social welfare council are similar in that their respective missions look to the stimulation of community-wide support for programs rather than to the delivery of direct services. The disease focus of the voluntary health agency, however, does create an interest in the patient with a particular type of problem, and this is reflected in the difference between the pattern of needs identified by the voluntary health agency as compared with the social

TABLE 1. *Respondent's Emphasis by Category of Community Health Need in Relation to Mission of the Agency*

Mission of Agency[1]	*Health Need Cited*[2] *Client*	*Administrative*	*General Social & Economic*	*Coordinative*
Health departments "The primary goal is to provide total health service to the community."	X	XXXX	XX	X
Visiting nurse association "Professional nursing care on a visit basis to acutely and chronically ill patients in their homes, stressing the rehabilitation nursing phase so that permanent disability can be prevented."	XX	XXX	—	XXX
Voluntary health association "Coordinates community services, public and private, that help meet the special needs of cardiac patients."	XX	XXX	XXXX	X
Social welfare Council "The purpose is the solution of health, welfare, and recreation problems through research, coordination, social planning, and citizen action."	—	XX	XXXX	XXX
Social service unit, county hospital "We see every patient who comes into the hospital. It is a generalized service. We deal with problems related to the illness."	XXXX	—	XXX	—
Emphasis in combined responses from all respondents	X	XXX	XXX	X

[1] As given in interview.
[2] Key: xxxx = more than 50% of needs cited.
xxx = less than 50%, more than 25% of needs cited.
xx = less than 25%, more than 10% of needs cited.
x = less than 10% of all needs cited.

welfare council. It also should be noted that the major responsibility of the respondent from the social service unit of the county hospital is the direct provision of a specific client service, and thus more attention may be placed on client needs than would have been found had the general administrator of the hospital been the respondent.

Selected Clientele

Each respondent was more attentive to the needs of the selected group of clients his agency was most likely to serve. For example, the social service unit of the county hospital and the social welfare council placed emphasis on low-income and minority groups, while the health departments and the visiting nurse association spoke for the most part of the low-income group and the aged. The voluntary health agency, on the other hand, emphasized the middle-income or the medically indigent group.

Thus, the frame of reference for defining a community service need reflected the respondent's and his agency's domain of influence. Although attention cannot be placed everywhere, there is a major problem inherent in these different viewpoints. If effective community action toward meeting gaps of service in a community is to come about, it will be necessary to delineate priorities beyond individual agency domains. When each agency pays attention to its particular domain, interagency planning tends to concentrate on areas of mutual concern and unless plans are made for incorporating the many community interests into the interagency planning process (as is hoped for by including consumer participation), the community health service needs will be dealt with segmentally and the inevitable gaps in services will continue to occur.

Differences in Definitions of Common Problems

It is apparent even from this limited number of agencies that community health service needs were identified in quite different ways that mirrored the respondent's currently defined domain of activities. Different goals and objectives lead to dissimilar definitions of problems, and this in turn can lead to unresolvable conflicts about means of bringing about problem solution. Levine and White have shown how different goals created conflict within the independent voluntary health agencies and the United Fund.[12] This type of conflict was seen among the agencies when a particular instance of cooperative activity was cited by representatives of the two agencies involved: The work that one person had put into the project was viewed as a voluntary contribution by one respondent and as doing someone else's work by the other. In another situation a proposed plan of action was reported by one respondent as minimally providing for a badly needed service, and the same plan of action was described by another respondent as believed to be too ambitious an undertaking.

Areas of need were often defined by respondents in terms of a predetermined solution rather than as a precisely defined problem. Perhaps the best illustration of this difference in ways of defining a problem is that of the community's basic transportation problem. Here are five ways in which it was discussed:

1. "A study was made of transportation services for the handicapped. Public transportation is poor, and volunteer transportation is not a feasible solution. A commercial organization is now investigating possibilities—agencies will be asked to finance the services. I don't think the agencies here will be able to provide the necessary funds."

2. "I would suspect transportation to medical services would be a problem. The county hospital services are not decentralized. That's the problem. Everyone has to come into the central area. Those people in greatest need of the services of the county hospital are the farthest away."

3. "Some services need to be more strategically located."

4. "Transportation is a big problem. The people are housebound and not able to get out. We use the Volunteer Bureau once in a while for transportation."

5. "Transportation is another problem that has not been solved."

In the first description three alternative solutions to transportation are mentioned; in the second and third the problem is defined on the basis of changing location of services rather than the development of new transportation facilities; in the fourth the definition is in terms of a particular type of client and a service for him; while in the fifth the problem is stated generally. There is general agreement about the difficulty of closing a geographic gap between clients and facilities, but quite different solutions are proposed in the description of this need. Any coordinated community action to solve this problem would require a more detailed definition of all aspects of the problem and agreement on the method of solution. These data suggest that the different ways of describing the general problem of transportation, with which each agency was attempting to cope, are formed in the image of the agency's coping response. This may have occurred because the problem of transportation is not considered to be in the "health" domain. Whether this phenomenon of problem definition in the image of coping response is more likely to occur when the underlying problem is out of the particular group's sphere of influence or whether this is a universal phenomenon is a question needing further study, but it is an important question for those concerned with planning.[13] Consensus among community groups about priorities in planning will be extremely difficult to obtain when problems are identified in terms of each agency's coping responses.

We have not made a distinction between cooperative planning or coordinative planning in this chapter because the semantic differences between cooperation and coordination appear to be irrelevant in the context of comprehensive health planning if it is assumed that either term implies concerted action on the part of two or more agencies. Every respondent indicated that one of the most pressing problems was a "need for coordination," but the form of coordination identified differed, depending upon the category of need described. Table 2 shows examples of cited needs for coordination by the category of need.

Responsibility for Action

Quite different levels of action are required to provide for the varied service needs identified in the interviews. For example, "The county hospital and welfare department should set the same standards for nursing homes" is a specifically defined suggestion of action, but it involves the domains of several agencies and extra-community action on the part of the state welfare department. A "centralized loan closet" involves an internal reallocation of agency resources already felt to be inadequate for other pressing needs. To carry out a "complete survey of health needs," activity outside any particular agency's sphere of influence is needed. To provide "more hospital and medical insurance" requires negotiation in a much broader part of the community than the usual health agency system.

In answer to the interviewer's question, "Who in the community could or should take responsibility for developing such activities [those identified as needed by the respondent]?" there was no pattern of expectation for implementation. Since needs were usually defined in terms of the things seen to be preventing the achievement of the agency's mission, it would be logical to expect that the respondent would not have a clear-cut idea about what could be done about it because otherwise some action would have been taken. Two kinds of answers

TABLE 2. *Examples of "Needs for Coordination" Cited*

Community Health Service Need	*Examples Cited*
Client-centered	"(Patients need follow-through)...there is no preplan discharge program from the hospitals...."
Administrative	"The employment bureau, those selecting persons for courses in nurses-aide training, should have more knowledge of the needs. More coordination between them and the nursing agencies could better the situation."
General economic and social	"Public transportation is poor and volunteer transportation is not a feasible solution. A commercial organization is now investigating possibilities. Agencies will be asked to finance the service. I don't think agencies here will be able to provide the necessary funds."
Coordinative	"There is a lack of clear-cut control for nursing homes. (There needs to be coordination) over the regulations for nursing homes for welfare patients between the county welfare and the county hospital."

were received from the question: "I don't know" or "I suppose any one of a number of agencies could." In cases where action had been unsuccessfully attempted, there was not a clear-cut diagnosis of why the action was abortive, e.g., "I guess I was working with the wrong committee" or "Money is necessary."

A large amount of agency personnel time was being spent in serving on a variety of committees organized for coordinative purposes. Most of these efforts consisted in information exchange. Whenever a particular cooperative program between two or more agencies developed, it appeared to have been initiated because of a particular problem one agency was attempting to solve. Areas of mutual program interest between two agencies probably evolved because of this highly developed network of information exchange, but among these agencies studied there was no clear-cut norm or expectation of assignment of responsibility for initiation of action. Although all agency personnel expressed a commitment to the general idea of coordinated action, the concrete examples reported involved only a minor adjustment agreement among several agencies.

The problems of initiating action in this community seem to be of two dimensions: First, the constraints of agency mission and method of operation restrict the development of common definitions of common problems, thus preventing consensual motivational forces to be brought to bear on the problem; second, methods of work also are related to the purpose and domain of the agency and there are very few areas in which there is a common mode of work among several agencies so that joint development of new activities or change of current action could be initiated.

The literature suggests that conflicts and difficulties come about in interagency cooperative efforts because an activity may be perceived to be threatening the domain of another agency. In these interviews there was little evidence of this threat aspect and, in fact, the problem seemed to be quite the reverse. For example, one health department acted with an expressed explicit policy of strengthening other agencies whenever possible, and this was recognized by personnel from the other agencies. In another situation an aggressive case-finding program on the part of one agency that involved actual review of another agency's records and attendance at staff case conferences was viewed as very helpful by the respondent from the second agency.

Coordinated planning will affect different levels of organizational work. At the immediate and specific program activity level, a high degree of cooperation can be obtained at the output interfaces or linkages between agencies, where the activity adjustment meets mutual organizational need. This is the type of coordination that the community had been able to achieve through strong efforts to provide informational exchange. Where solutions to problems may require policy changes but minor resource allocation change, it would seem that the major problem in planning will be that of finding a means of coming to consensual agreement about priorities for action. Where, however, solutions to community health problems will require a concerted redistribution of community resources, the threat to agency integrity becomes real and explicit.

Availability of Organizational Energy for Planning

As noted previously, a great deal of organizational energy in this community seemed to be going into coordinative and communicative efforts. Interviews were difficult to schedule not because of reluctance on the part of the respondent but because of their heavily committed schedules. Each respondent mentioned having numerous interagency committee responsibilities. These were felt to be extremely important yet time-consuming. Several respondents from the larger agencies indicated there was a problem of finding the time to share new information even within their own agencies. Data were not available to ascertain actual personnel ratios or to estimate the amount of time spent on interagency activities as compared with intra-agency activities, but the emphasis on administrative needs by all respondents suggests that these agency administrators are finding that the current energy expended is not effective. Although there was evidence of innovative program activities within each agency, the interorganizational emphasis was on information exchange rather than on implementation of new service areas. Planning requires a great deal of committee and staff time, but implementation of a plan requires an even greater commitment of personnel time and energy. In those agencies where direct services were provided, time had to be devoted to keeping staff informed about even minor changes in policies of the particular agency and of other relevant agencies that occurred over time. For example, where there are large staffs of public health nurses there is a continual orientation of new members of the staff to program policies of all agencies with which they may be expected to work. Additionally, as program policies shift and are adapted to varying needs, the staff must be kept abreast of these changes. Where specific coordinative programs had been developed between these study agencies, e.g., in the development of joint planning for hospital discharge of patients so they could be followed by the public health nurse, an increasing amount of time was required for information change. Each new interagency activity, therefore, reduced available personnel time for rendering services.

In the voluntary health agency and the social welfare council, where most work is accomplished through volunteer committee activities, time is needed for orientation of committee members. As one program administrator stated it, "The terms of office are for one year, making continuity of programs difficult. The staff barely has time to acquaint the leaders with the program before there is a change in the leadership."

From each agency's point of view, several particular problems were cited in the interviews as problems in implementing needed community health services. These were (1) The lack of staff time and money to initiate new activities. (2) The problems of maintaining continuity of current activities. (3) The amount of staff time required to maintain currency of needed and relevant information. (4) The lack of any community mechanism to develop continuity of support for demonstration programs or new program changes. (5) The lack of appropriate means for periodic priority-setting in agency activities and means for evaluating effectiveness of current activities.

All these problems are interrelated and perhaps can be summarized as a lack of plans for planning. Priority seemed to be given in each agency to the most pressing and immediate problems of the current work output. No agency has unlimited resources and, in general, Parkinson's law holds true: "Work expands to fill the time available."[14] Where there are highly trained, dedicated persons providing services in a rapidly expanding community, need is ever present and quantitatively increasing. The health professional expects and is expected to search continually for health needs and, therefore, needs will continually exceed the ability to meet them. Case loads of personnel may be heavy, but the health professional continues to be concerned about the "unmotivated client" and the "unmet need." Although needs were requested in the interviews, no respondent questioned the idea that there would be needs. This phenomenon of continual search around current problems means that work is never completed, and there is always a gap between available budget and manpower and the normative expectation of what ought to be done.

Attention to the problems of the immediate and current situation has certain dysfunctional consequences, because it reinforces traditional activities and prevents a search for alternative and creative ways to meet current or future needs. For example, in this study most respondents were concerned only with community health services needed by patients from public assistance, by the medically indigent, and by the aged. There seemed to be an implicit assumption that if only the patient's income were adequate he would be able to obtain needed services through private resources. In some areas, such as transportation or dietary services, this is probably a valid assumption. However, this emphasis on persons with inadequate income (certainly a major problem for organized community health services) suggests that the services of the health and welfare agencies are geared primarily to obtaining access for clients to currently available services. The gap between what is possible to obtain in the community and what large segments of the population are financially able to obtain is so large that little agency time and energy are available for developing new or innovative services that no person in the community, regardless of his income level, can now obtain.

Another factor that tends to reinforce the status quo is the way in which health programs have been categorized. Levine and White have indicated that agencies specialize in a particular functional area, such as a particular disease problem, a particular type of clientele, or a particular process.[15] For example, the "disease and organ" voluntary health agencies depend upon private donations for a particular area of interest, such as heart disease, and feel it is their public responsibility to use those funds for the intended purpose. Although every voluntary agency takes some part in promotion of certain general community functions that relate to their mission, they feel they are expected to spend the greatest amount of their effort in the particular categorical area for which the money was collected. For governmental agencies the widespread use of the expenditure or line item budget requires an accounting system by categorical activities. Evaluation then is concerned more with counting activities completed than with measuring the effectiveness of these activities. Innovative program change that requires reallocation of resources within an agency is also more likely to be questioned by legislative bodies than is repetition of previously accepted sets of activities.

IMPLICATIONS FOR COMMUNITY PLANNING

From these interviews with administrators of community health service agencies, several factors have been identified as potentially constraining influences on coordinative planning for comprehensive health services. These include differences in priority given to the type of community need identified; differences in the way commonly recognized needs were defined in terms of the agency's own coping responses to the problem; current pressures and demands for agency time and manpower; lack of clear-cut community norms for allocation of agency responsibility for initiation of new activities; and amount of organizational energy and time required for initiating and implementing changes in program activities.

One could describe this community of agencies as an interlocking web of activities and relationships that was in a static equilibrium or stable state. There was recognition that the traditional patterns of services were not adequate for the community's increasing needs for services; yet no one agency had the power, the money, the manpower, or the motivation to take on the responsibilities required for a major expansion or change in its or in the total pattern of provision of services. To take on such responsibility means eventual reallocation of current agency domains and disruption of present carefully nurtured, cooperative relationships and entails risking the present level of economic and public support of current activities.

In his model for analysis of the interorganizational field, Warren states the problem as follows:

> To summarize briefly, the people of a metropolitan community are not organized for making centralized rational choices among values which cannot be maximized simultaneously. Various values are

> allocated to specific CDO's (community decision organizations) for maximization. These CDO's, in turn, are the protagonists in a sort of sociodrama in which the "mix" gets worked out in some relation to respective resources and skill in their use, and within the framework of the range of acceptability of the composite decision to the large and important sectors of the community.[16]

He makes some tentative suggestions for restructuring the interactional field of the community decision organizations that might produce a more desirable mix for increasing the satisfying levels for each value sought. Five of his suggestions involve increasing the intensity of communication and feedback of information among the CDO's. The coordinative activities reported in this study indicate that, even with an intensive effort at information exchange among the agencies and with a strong commitment among the agency administrators for cooperative efforts, the complexity of the administrative problems involved in even small collaborative efforts prevented development of coordinated planning at any but the most immediate program level activity.

It is possible that under the impetus of current legislation truly comprehensive planning for community health services will become viable. However, the experience of this community with its history of cooperative effort suggests that effective planning will not be achieved unless some of these agency problems are met.

If community planning is to be a consciously organized, forward-moving process, it must take into account the dynamic needs of a continually changing future as well as correction of the deficiencies of the present. A viable planning structure not only should be flexible but should also enhance the opportunities for the many kinds of community decision-making that occur.* A few suggestions appear to us to be relevant. Kerr White has presented an excellent case for the development of equal but competitive health care systems to provide choice for the consumer.[17] The ultimate test for the effectiveness of each system would be its ability to gain and maintain its share of the market. Some of the regional medical programs under Public Law 89–239 have formed quasi-holding-company types of structures wherein the member agencies compete for the available resources.

* Paul Diesing has identified five kinds of rationality in societal decision-making: logical rationality that emphasizes the logic of cause and effect; economic rationality that searches for the most efficient allocation of resources, given an ordered set of objectives or values to be achieved; social rationality that seeks to maintain social integration; legal rationality that sets the ethical parameters of action; and political rationality that determines a structure within which the four other kinds of rationality can be served.[18]

Would it not be possible to develop within a community, for area-wide or regional planning purposes, types of coalition organizations in competition with each other for the community's support of their plans and in which each agency member holds a strong stake in the competitive position of its coalition organization? For example, such coalitions might be formed of competing *ad hoc* task forces charged with finding alternative solutions to the same problem or with establishing Kerr White's competitive systems. An adaptation might be developed of the competitive technique used by industry and by governmental agencies in letting competing contracts or in paying for preliminary work on competing bids. See chapter 10 for a further description. The current local agency battles for the role of the regional planning agency under comprehensive health planning could perhaps be channeled into a more fruitful competitiveness if there were less pressure for the formation of a single planning agency to service all planning functions. If a single agency is to be preferred, then provision should be made at least for the following:

1. A forum function where community planning issues can be debated openly and in the light of adequate study and information and where support or nonsupport of community agency programs can be communicated to the public.
2. A consensus-forming function where the present situation can be evaluated in terms of future needs rather than in relation to past standards and where interests can be bargained for and negotiated.
3. A competitive mechanism for assuring the development of alternative means of achieving solutions to the community's health problems involving the agencies expected to implement plans.
4. A continuous input of information from all segments of the community with constant feedback to all relevant decision centers, and appropriate use of technical expertise in the analysis of emerging health problems and their potential solutions.

To provide for all this within one planning structure is organizationally difficult, because in most attempts to coordinate activities a hierarchical structure seems to evolve. The formation of competing planning units within a directing and coordinating body might provide the impetus for the spontaneous development of more effective organizational forms to meet the comprehensive health needs of the community.

There is an increasing demand for services in every area of community health. In the absence of a centralized decision authority, and with the relatively weak market situation of the current organizational system, there is a diffusion of power and influence. Individual agencies seem to have become impotent in developing the qualitative changes needed for meeting community health service needs. There is evidence that the strategies of coordination used in the past have been increasingly ineffective in developing viable interorganizational action. The development of competitive planning structures should be worth consideration as a possible alternative.

References

1. Robert Morris, "New Concepts in Community Organization," in *The Social Welfare Forum*, New York: Columbia University Press, 1961, p. 128.
2. Martin Meyerson and Edward C. Banfield, *Politics, Planning and the Public Interest*, New York: The Free Press, 1955.
3. Sol Levine and Paul B. White, "The Community of Health Organizations," in Howard E. Freeman, Sol Levine, and Leo G. Reeder (eds.), *Handbook of Medical Sociology*, Englewood Cliffs, N.J.: Prentice-Hall, 1963, p. 341.
4. Lloyd E. Ohlin, "Prospects for Planning in American Social Welfare," in Robert Morris (ed.), *Centrally Planned Change: Prospects and Concepts*, New York: National Association of Social Workers, 1964.
5. Charles Press, *Main Street Politics: Policy Making at the Local Level (A Survey of the Periodical Literature Since 1950)*, East Lansing, Mich.: Institute for Community Development, Michigan State University, 1962.
6. Aaron Wildavsky, *Leadership in a Small Town*, Totowa, N.J.: Bedminster Press, 1964.
7. Robert C. Wood, *1400 Governments: The Political Economy of the New York Metropolitan Region*, Garden City, N.Y.: Doubleday, 1961.
8. Godfrey Hochbaum, "Health Agencies and the Tower of Babel," *Public Health Reports*, 80 (1965), 331.
9. D. L. Hink, and Mary F. Arnold, "A Study of the Adjustment Techniques of Patients and Their Families to the Non-medical Needs Resulting from Chronic Illness: Results of a Pilot Study," Mimeographed.
10. James G. March and Herbert A. Simon, *Organizations*, New York: Wiley, 1958.
11. The idea of exchange relationships among agencies can be found in many current references. See Sol Levine and Paul E. White, "The Community of Health Organizations"; Peter M. Blau, *Exchange and Power in Social Life*, New York: Wiley, 1964; James D. Thompson, *Organizations in Action*, New York, McGraw-Hill, 1967.
12. Sol Levine and Paul B. White, "The Community of Health Organizations," p. 334.

13. Feldman and Kanter discuss this phenomenon as a problem of search behavior. See "Organizational Decision-Making," in James G. March (ed.), *Handbook of Organizations*, Chicago: Rand McNally, 1965, p. 622.
14. C. Northcote Parkinson, *Parkinson's Law*, Cambridge, Mass.: Riverside Press, 1962.
15. Sol Levine and Paul B. White, "The Community of Health Organizations," p. 331.
16. Roland L. Warren, "The Interorganizational Field as a Focus for Investigation," *Administrative Science Quarterly*, 12:3 (December 1967), 414.
17. Kerr White, "Primary Medical Care for Families—Organization and Evaluation, *New England Journal of Medicine*, 227:16 (October 19, 1967), 847.
18. Paul Diesing, *Reason in Society; Five Types of Decisions and Their Social Conditions*, Urbana: The University of Illinois Press, 1962.

V

ORGANIZATIONAL PERSPECTIVES

THE ORGANIZATIONAL ARRANGEMENTS WHICH TAKEN TOgether constitute the health system are many and varied. This is a further reflection of the system's complexity. There are several different ways in which these arrangements can be characterized for purposes of understanding and comparing them. One is in terms of the nature of the organization–client (consumer) relationship. Certain types of organizations—for example, the private medical practitioner—have a *direct* relation to a "patient" and their major focus is on his level of health. The exchanges that take place in this situation, the laws, the traditions, and the normative expectations surrounding them are different than they are for organizational arrangements that are supposed to relate to the "community as a whole." Though the latter also deal directly with individuals who may be in need of information or care, their primary concern is said, somehow, to be with the level (distribution) of health in the *community*, and the exchange that occurs has a different meaning both to the participants and to those who might be evaluating them. Thus, in these types of organizations the criteria for judging efficiency and effectiveness, for example, will be different than in the case of the former. Using this same scheme, other types of organizational arrangements in the health system are more difficult to place, e.g., professional schools and associations, laboratories, voluntary associations, and certain federal and state agencies. The relation of their activities to the ultimate consumer is more indirect.

Another way to view the various organizational forms is implicit in the word *system* itself. We have been talking about health as a system, a patterned arrangement of activities and values loosely linked by virtue of their various contributions to a common output. In such a model, organizations are subsystems or constituent units of the over-all health system and they may be identified according to their contribution to this over-all system.

Open systems theory tells us that system maintenance and performance—the taking in of resources (input), the transformation of these resources into services or goods, and the exchange of these "products" (output) with the environment—requires that certain functions be fulfilled: production, support, maintenance, and adaptation.* Production, as the name implies, is activity involved in the direct transformation of resources—skills, knowledge, capital, and equipment—into services or goods for the ultimate consumer or client, i.e., the "patient" or the community. Here we might place such diverse organizational arrangements as private or group practice, hospitals, and at least portions of local health agencies, clinics, laboratories, etc. Other organizations such as professional associations, voluntary associations, and state and federal health bureaucracies provide more of a support function since they help relate the health system to the larger political–economic environment of the society and help generate resources as well as legitimacy for it. A portion of the maintenance function—the training, indoctrination, and socialization of "actors" in the system—is fulfilled by colleges, universities, and other educational institutions that are turning out skilled, motivated human resources. Another portion, that of controlling the over-all system and allocating rewards and sanctions within it, is the function of certain political and adminis-

* Daniel Katz and Robert L. Kahn, *The Social Psychology of Organization*, New York: Wiley, 1966, especially Chapter 3.

trative bodies as well as some professional associations. The adaptive function is clearly provided by the organizational subsystems involved primarily in planning or basic and applied research. Such organizations help the total system anticipate and adapt to social, scientific, and technical change.

It is clear that these distinctions are not watertight nor were they meant to be. Some organizations, for example, perform several functions. The hospital can be a teaching and research institution as well as a place for providing health care directly to patients. Professional associations are concerned not only with relating occupational segments of the health system to the larger society but also with exerting a certain degree of control over other organizations in the system. It is also clear that though these diverse structures can be said to be contributing to a central output—public health—in their actual day-to-day operations most do not consciously view their activities in the way we have been characterizing them here. In fact they concentrate on more discrete goals, suboptimizing in terms of them often to the disadvantage of the health system as a whole. The conception presented here provides a rough way of relating the variety of organizational arrangements to each other and to the notion of a health system.

Such a perspective is doubly necessary because the essential unity of the chapters in this part, which deal with several discrete conceptual schemes and apply them in a variety of organizational contexts, would be missed. These essays are about small parts of the total organizational complex constituting the health system. They have in common the fact that each deals with a problem at a fairly micro level. That is, the concern is with a single type of organization or even with only a very limited aspect of one type of organization rather than with the more macro problem of the health system as a whole. They differ in terms of the dimension on which they are focusing, e.g., decision-making, economies of scale, and cost–benefit analysis. They also differ in terms of the intentions of the individual authors. Some, such as those writing about decision-making or the life cycle of a health agency, are concerned with providing further theoretical and descriptive insights into more general organizational phenomenon. Others are more interested in marshaling empirical data for testing (in a loose sense of the word) some particular theory or model. Still others are seeking to provide rather pragmatic tools and analytic concepts that might have some immediate, if limited, use in administration. They should be read as individual essays but understood in this broader perspective.

18

The Life Cycle Dynamics of Health Service Organizations

David B. Starkweather & Arnold I. Kisch

Most descriptions of health service organizations presume that these agencies exist in a static state. In fact, however, they are in constant evolution. One of the leading students of formal organizations has stated: "The only permanence in bureaucratic structure is the permanence of change in predictable patterns, and even these are not unalterably fixed."[1]

What are these changes and how can they be described? Do they form a pattern which might be useful in predicting the future course of a specific organization? This chapter examines the "natural history" or "life cycle" of organizations in general and seeks to apply certain theories and findings of sociologists to health service institutions.

EFFECT OF THE EXTERNAL ENVIRONMENT

Life cycles of organizations are analogous to those of biological structures.[2] Organizations may be thought of as having strong wills to survive. Stages of development from birth to death are evident. Some organizations have normal development while others apparently have arrested development. All are influenced by and have an impact on their environment.

Studies of health service organizations often focus on the changes that can be wrought through manipulation of internal features. The sociologist's perspective, however, takes greater cognizance of the ecology of an enterprise—its relation to society at large and to the external forces which constantly exert pressure. These forces are often subtle and may go unrecognized. Yet the long-run success of an enterprise will depend more on its ability to adjust to changing values and demands of society than on administrative efficiency, particularly if this efficiency serves inappropriate or obsolete ends. The survival of an enterprise may become contingent on its readiness and ability to reorganize to adapt to changing conditions in society.

Some institutions appear to have greater control of their destiny than others. They more often take the initiative. Within the health services, those institutions that offer highly visible, dramatic, and valued services, such as the acute care general hospital, are in this category. They tend to endure despite their frequent low efficiency. Other health service organizations, such as public health departments, do not enjoy such well-articulated status. (For a discussion of organizations with intangible goals, see Warner and Havens.[3]) Their social worth is likely to be questioned even though they may be highly efficient in the sense that they seem able to make limited budgets go a long way. Public health programs additionally are very dependent on economic and political factors influencing their external environment. Treatment organizations, in contrast, are usually more self-contained and thus better able to direct their destinies from within.[4]

A BASIC DILEMMA

Service-oriented organizations are often caught between two sets of objectives: the organization's desire on the one hand to serve its clients and its need on the other hand to serve its sources of financial support. Only in a few organizations are these objectives compatible. For most organizations they pose a dilemma. In this chapter we present four phases of a typical health service organization's natural history and describe these phases in terms of the relative pressures brought to bear in each by the organization's commitment to these two sets of objectives.

In economic terms this is called the separation of consumption and control, and enterprises may be classified according to the degree of control exerted by the consumer. It is high in small businesses, lower in large businesses, weak in oligopolies or private monopolies, and nonexistent in public monopolies such as the post office.[5] One would think that medicine, particularly private practice, would rank high on the consumer-controlled list. No relationship would seem more personal and direct than the doctor–patient relationship. Yet it is the nature of a profession to say that the provider rather than the buyer "knows best" and, therefore, must control the relationship. Thus most medical and health-related institutions rank low in consumer control and rank close to public monopolies in the amount of true leverage possessed by the user.

Health service organizations are not fully described by traditional economic theories of the firm. Nevertheless, they too must respond to the relative pressures of client (patient) service versus financial support and allocate their resources accordingly.

Figure 1 presents in diagrammatic form the life cycle of a typical private medical or health agency.

There is of course the inherent danger of oversimplification in a diagram such as Figure 1 and in the interpretations that follow. Features attributed to one phase in the cycle are in fact part of a time continuum. And we do not imply that the sequence and relationships diagramed in Figure 1 always occur under every condition or that no other factors are involved. Yet a certain artificial sharpening of the boundaries in the evolutionary process may enhance appreciation of the manner in which organizations change. This typology should properly be viewed as a point of departure in a realm where virtually no systematic studies have been conducted.

PHASE I: THE SEARCH PHASE

In this phase of its life cycle an organization is of course young and small, having been created in response to the pressure of social forces. As described by Sheldon Messinger, the organization is in *ascendancy*, resulting from the concern of its leaders and members that something be done to transform social discontent into effective action.[6] The rate of innovation is high, permitting policies or procedures to be quickly modified as personnel seek the proper approach to problems that first generated the organization's formation. Patients or their representatives are formally or informally included in the decision-making process of the organization, and their suggestions and criticisms are sought with genuine interest.

At this stage there is much jostling, bargaining, and latent competition between the new agency and better established enterprises within

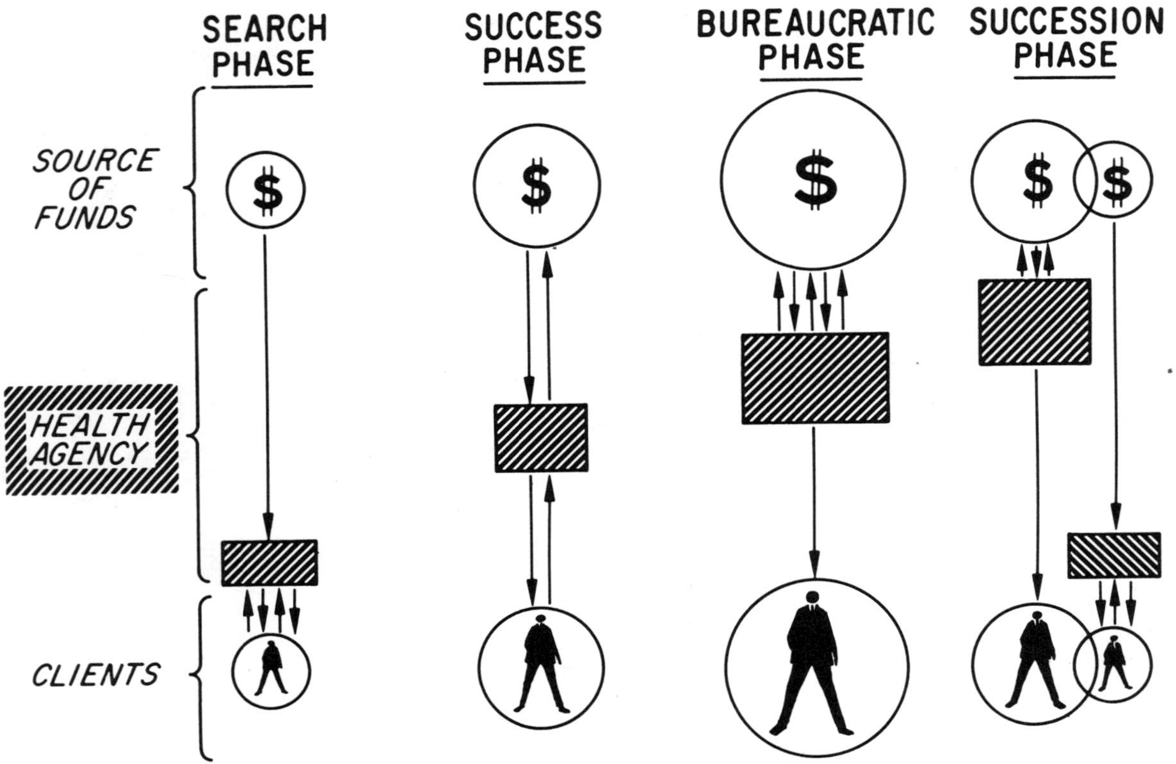

FIGURE 1. *Stages in the Life Cycle of Health Service Organizations*

the community, with each organization seeking its most favorable posture relative to the others. The new agency examines its own capacity and the world around it to discover where its services can most effectively augment the existing pattern, where financial resources are to be found, and upon whom these financial resources are dependent. At this early stage a maximum proportion of the agency's resources are devoted to service, since it is through this mechanism that the agency seeks to secure a firm position in its environment. Organizational decisions made at this point will have an important influence on the entire future course of the institution since important commitments have to made during these formative times. The role developed for the organization in the end actually may be forced from the outside rather than acquired by deliberate design from within.[7] If however a role acceptable to society cannot be developed at this stage, the agency will likely die.

The administrative structure of an agency at this phase is informal and open. The staff is growing, and there must be an opportunity for new members to be fully integrated. There is an egalitarian feeling between staff members, and policies are developed by sharing and pooling the perspectives and judgments of many. In this phase the leadership element is crucial, but here again there is a built-in dilemma. The leader in this stage must set a tone of flexibility and permissiveness if the organization is to make essential adjustments to its new environment. However, the agency also badly needs a charisma, since public recognition can best be achieved at this early time by the personal visibility of the agency's chief official. Unfortunately the qualities of charisma and the qualities of participative leadership are not often found in the same individual. This dilemma is never overcome by some organizations. The leadership requirements remain in conflict or the organization finds itself unable to make the subsequent crucial transition from personality control to institutional control—the "routination of charisma" (Max Weber).[8]

Another characteristic of the leadership element in this phase is that its competence is usually more in subject-matter rather than in administration. The small organization demands relatively little by way of management, and its resources flow in large measure toward its professional and patient service work.

There are other obstacles that must be surmounted before an organization can pass into the second, or "success," phase. James March and Herbert Simon define stress as the discrepancy between aspiration and achievement, and there may be either too much or too little stress in an organization. If achievement comes so early that stress is low, the result is organizational apathy. Under these circumstances the agency will not collapse but its innovation and expansion will be slow. If aspiration remains well above achievement, stress will be too high and may result in frustration or desperation. March and Simon define optimal stress as a condition when the "carrot is just a little way ahead of the donkey."[9]

Whether an organization thrives depends largely on the welcome or hostility accorded it by the community at large, and in the search phase this is dependent in large part on the quality and appropriateness of the services rendered to patients. If the community permits the organization to succeed in its initial purposes its staff will likely advocate expansion in order to extend the organization's benefits to more persons. The enterprise will then have survived the most critical time of its life and will begin to assume the qualities of the success phase. Ironically it is at the first phase in its life cycle, when an organization's zeal and motivation to achieve its objectives are highest, that it runs the greatest risk of failure. A small organization may be destroyed by circumstances that a larger organization would overcome. The leaders of young enterprises seem intuitively to recognize this fact. As the search for the proper type and mode of service is completed and the essential elements of an effective agency are assembled the usual progression is to broaden the base of operations in order to secure initial gains.

An example of a health service agency in the search phase is the neighborhood health center. It was created in response to social forces arising from the urban ghetto. Out of the genuine desire of civic and government leaders to transform this discontent into effective action, the notation of "maximum feasible participation" of urban ghetto consumers was formed. From medical care planners came the idea of the neighborhood health center as an important extension of the existing system of medical care delivery. Imagination and innovation have characterized the establishment and early operation of neighborhood health centers, as evidenced by the considerable variety among centers in different cities. There has been much jostling and bargaining between the new centers and the established institutions that deliver medical care—nearby hospitals, public health departments, etc. Even the relationship of the centers to their "parent" body, OEO, is unsettled. Within the organization of most centers there is a sense of high expectation, group esprit, and widespread sharing of problems and decisions.

The personal qualities of center directors seems critically important, with some centers on the brink of failure for lack of appropriate leadership. Certainly there is evidence in some centers of incongruity between aspiration and achievement. A few centers seem to have "arrived" so quickly that they have foreclosed on opportunities for future program development and financial support from other agencies and institutions. For some, these foreclosures may be the prelude to organizational demise. For other agencies (more numerous) the aspiration–achievement relationship is reversed: Lack of success has led to frustration, apathy, and dissension. There centers that have experienced these reactions also may be unable to sustain themselves as permanently viable organizations.

Five to ten years would be a reasonable time estimate of the search phase of neighborhood health centers. As indicated in the general typology, the role of the centers that survive this initial period will depend as much or more on forces outside the centers as from their internal dynamics. A number of these forces have yet to be fully registered: the impact of established political and government structures, the degree to which centers are embraced by hospitals and "mainstream" organized medicine, and the appropriation of funds from national legislation. These forces represent "input constituencies" of neighborhood health centers. Like all constituencies, in some way they must be served.

PHASE II: THE SUCCESS PHASE

Sol Levine has advanced the notion that there is initial and periodic competition between health agencies for three scarce commodities—patients, staff personnel, and financial resources.[10] This competition continues until there is a rough consensus between new and established agencies as to the proper allocation of manpower, money, and clientele to each. An organization will have worked its way into a favorable position in this distribution by the time it reaches the success phase. In order to obtain that favorable position, the organization will have had to alter both its objectives and its structural means for achieving those objectives. Initial radical objectives are mitigated in favor of strengthening and preserving the organization. Yet in this process a dilemma is presented: Organizational strength leads to survival, but it also generally leads to a surrender of some of the agency's initial motivating ideals.[11]

"Formalization" is the term used to describe the internal structural changes that occur during this phase. There is reduced dependence on the personal attributes of the founding leaders and an increase in more routinized control.[12] Jobs become specialized, and a hierarchy of authority is developed. A central administration develops, strengthening management. Organizational rewards of money and status are extended to staff personnel who previously obtained their satisfaction more from client service. The staff's attention becomes divided between immediate patient needs on the one hand and future-oriented requirements of securing the enterprise's financial base on the other. By and large a satisfactory balance is achieved, with enough administrative focus to avoid the risks to survival inherent in the search phase and still enough client focus to foster the provision of needed services at adequate levels of quality. These composite features are listed by Peter Blau as the prerequisites of "adjustive development." They include a professional orientation to job and patients, staff employment security, establishment of a working group that commands allegiance of the staff, and the absence of basic conflict between professional staff and management.[13]

The success phase is not without its serious problems. Organized and centralized planning and control are obtained at the expense of individual initiative. Both are needed for continued success, but few organizations seem able to achieve a sustained balance between the two.[14]

What drives an enterprise beyond this success phase? Why could evolution not stop at this point—to the satisfaction of clients and staff and for the best over-all social good? One reason is that the enterprise finds it difficult to assess its true successes and failures. As more attention is devoted to the mechanics of day-to-day operations the indices of over-all performance become obscured. Only in retrospect is the shift away from pursuit of primary goals observed. At the time there is an illusion of steady progress, and the agency moves on, seemingly advancing but in reality quite possibly retreating.

With good fortune an organization will in time sense that social conditions are changing, perhaps to the point where wholly new purposes are indicated. Economic and psychological interests of officials may then promote a displacement or proliferation of the agency's aims.

The history of voluntary agencies outside the health field contains many examples of such modifications.[15] The YMCA gradually recast its goals from religious and spiritual to recreational and social in response to a general secularization of society. Following its popularity as a quasi-political force the Townsend Movement was transformed into a social organization for the elderly.[16] An example allied to the health field is the assumption of active blood donor programs and civil emergency services by the American Red Cross when the nation no longer demanded all of its capacity as a relief agency for fighting men. Perhaps the best-known example of deflected goals in an actual health agency is the change that took place in the National Foundation after the successful accomplishment of its original target, the control of infantile paralysis through development of the Salk vaccine. Sociologist David Sills attributes this remarkable perseverance to a wide acceptance of the foundation by the public and to its being "an organization as committed to a means as to an end."[17]

Additional evidence of decline of the success phase is a shift in the balance of the professional–administrative relationship in favor of increased administrative control. The desired personality specifications for the agency's leadership undergo change, and subject-matter specialists who led the organization in its early development are replaced by executives with strong managerial skills. This change in the type of control seems inevitable even though one might wish that leadership patterns that encouraged both innovation and effective implementation could be preserved.

The timing of the leadership transition is very important. It can come prematurely through overemphasis of the agency's need for effective communication and command, thereby denying an organization innovative leadership at a time when it is still badly needed.[18] On the other hand its occurrence can be excessively delayed, leaving the organization unprepared for the time when charismatic leadership eventually departs.

A dramatic example from the business world is that of the Montgomery Ward Company in the late 1940s and 1950s. The company was managed almost single-handedly by its domineering and dramatic chief executive, Sewell Avery. However, he refused to reconsider an economic prediction that envisioned a catastrophic national depression following World War II (as had occurred following previous wars). Because of this he held most of his company's assets in liquid form and failed to invest in corporate growth and expansion.[19] Signs began to appear that the much-feared depression would not materialize. Yet Avery held to his position during a time when rapid and important expansions were being undertaken by other merchandising companies. Sears Roebuck captured most of the enormous retail business that was available to whichever mail-order company was prepared to respond to the new market.

The change in character of leadership, sometimes arranged by design but frequently occurring ad hoc, largely dictates the future course of an organization and the rate of its advance into the much less productive phase that often follows the success phase. Few boards and councils that make executive selections clearly see these implications. As a result the leadership in health service organizations frequently oscillates for a time between exclusively professional and strictly managerial types, with neither providing the combination of qualities the agency could ideally use.

Still, such difficulties are seldom sufficient to destroy an enterprise. A degree of autonomy has been established by this time that permits the organization to survive. What does occur due to the shifting and reshifting of directions resulting from changes in leadership is a wasteful expenditure of organizational energy. In this a certain momentum and social force is lost that seldom is regained. In the ultimate it leads to institutional stagnation.

One final factor important to the success phase in the life cycle of organizations is the almost universal drive toward bigness. Our achievement-oriented American culture equates growth and bigness with success. There is a certain preoccupation with size for its own sake rather than for what it might accomplish. In many ways this interest is warranted, since the present technical and economic structure of society gives advantage to larger institutions that are denied to smaller ones. These advantages include the most fundamental one—a greater chance of long-run survival.

Yet there is a special anachronism when the features of large institutionalism are applied to the health services. With the exception of environmental sanitation almost all of these services center on the relationship between a patient and his doctor. Many of the traditions of American medicine flow from this dominant theme. This highly personal type of relationship, however, is the antithesis of the kinds of relationships that characterize large institutions. As advances in medical diagnosis and therapy require more and more institutional support for the physician, this dilemma grows in importance. Milton Roemer and Ray Elling have stated that "the problem is to take advantage of modern technology through a rationally organized division of labor while at the same time meeting the varied needs of each individual patient.[20] It is precisely this problem that besets a health service organization as it struggles to avoid drifting toward an ineffective and stifling state of bureaucracy.

An example of a health service agency that is experiencing success, with some indications of drift toward the bureaucratic phase, is Kaiser Medical Entities. In the late 1940s Kaiser displayed features of the search phase. It attracted national attention and respect for its innovations in prepayment, group practice, and hospital service. The

Kaiser Plan offered satisfaction for patients in comprehensive care, access to specialists, supervision of medical practice, and low cost. In its early years the Plan struggled financially, requiring support from client organizations (unions) and its parent enterprise (Kaiser Industries), in addition to its premium income.

In twenty years Kaiser expanded into the imaginative complex of interlocking organizations implied by the word "entities." It is heralded as a successful and well-run system for financing and delivering medical care, even by most of its early, vocal, and determined critics.

We will not detail this success story here, as it has been well-chronicled elsewhere. Yet lest success run to Kaiser's organizational head, some indications of advancement through this second phase should be identified.

The Entities have no real assessment of client satisfaction, since the number of patients who use non-Kaiser physicians for diagnosis or treatment has not been determined. As for clinical services, Kaiser's position of leadership in comprehensive care has been challenged. One union that originally provided financial sponsorship for Kaiser has been unable to obtain psychiatric services from Permanente physicians, and as an alternate has established its own psychiatry program. Separate dental services and drug purchase benefits have likewise been established.

Kaiser seems less able than in prior years to influence its environment; to a greater degree it is influenced by circumstances beyond its control. For instance, Kaiser would like to open its membership to new enrollees but is frustrated in doing so by the increasing demands upon its staff and facilities from "ingrowth" of membership groups already under contract.

The executives of Kaiser's several regional organizations admit to spending much of the time in internal coordination of the component parts—the Health Plan, the Permanente Medical Group, the Kaiser Foundation hospitals, and the administrative services. Kaiser headquarters, where many decisions are made. is at a point considerably removed both geographically and in number of hierarchic layers from patients in clinics and hospital beds—patients who sometime view Kaiser as an unwieldy bureaucracy.

This is a somewhat critical appraisal of an enterprise that has come to be regarded as a model health service organization. Yet we should underscore what in the long run (fifty years) may become an important and worthwhile countervailing force within the organization. Unlike most medical and hospital enterprises, the Permanente Medical Group and Kaiser Foundation hospitals are heavily dependent on the

Health (Insurance) Plan. And the Plan, though not controlled by policyholders, must ultimately satisfy premium-paying patients. This arrangement may check what would otherwise become creeping bureaucracy, providing Kaiser with periodic pressure from consumers to revitalize and innovate services.

PHASE III: THE BUREAUCRATIC* PHASE

In general, as an organization becomes more complex in its internal workings it also becomes increasingly differentiated from the larger social system.[21] Its gains in autonomy are made at the sacrifice of sensitive communication with social reality. While the public may seem to suffer most by this development, the agency itself is the ultimate loser. Changes in social forces that are not met by responsive adaptations on the agency's part lead to a lack of public interest in the agency's mission. Reduced public concern in turn eventually causes a diminution in the flow of public resources to the agency. This phenomenon can be seen in the historical flow and ebb of the public health movement.

One reason for social detachment is that an agency may come to depend on certain groups of clients, patrons, or special-interest parties for primary support. These parties themselves may be out of touch with society's mainstream. Each "special" group demands of an agency its share of attention, thereby lessening the agency's capacity to respond to unmet public needs. Of such nature is the attention of public schools to PTA's and of welfare departments to political councils.

One activity that can counter this tendency is innovation. A widely held sociological theory is that a change in social structure will produce some form of conflict and that conflict will generate innovation. But if innovation is stifled by an elaborate organizational structure, new ideas usually will not see the light of day. A common practice of bureaucracies faced with this problem is to establish official innovation departments called "research and development," "systems division," "patient relations," etc. While institutionalized invention is better than none at all, it is a poor substitute for a more natural and spontaneous

* The word "bureaucratic" has several different meanings. Sociologists frequently use the definition of Max Weber: An organization guided by official rules, a systematized division of functions, an official hierarchy, a technically competent administrative staff, separation of management and ownership, etc.[22] A second and common use of the word suggests organizational rigidity, overemphasis on procedural detail, and "red tape."[23] This chapter attributes both meanings to the word, implying that Weber's preferred form of authority, as manifest in many organizations, has undesirable side effects.

type of creativity. Further, such departments often produce additional complexity and conflict within an organization. This is particularly true when the departments are staffed by persons who lack operational experience. Another difficulty lies in the fact that once an official innovation department is created within an organization, the rest of the personnel tend to assume that innovative thinking is no longer required of them.

In the bureaucratic phase a fairly rigid conformity to procedure develops. There is an overemphasis on discipline and control to the point that they become values in themselves, leading to decreased ability to adjust to changing reality. Means tend to become ends and to displace original organizational goals.[24]

As the organization grows its internal structure changes through the addition of staff necessary to assure adequate communication and coordination. Activities previously done informally are now done by a rising proportion of the total personnel complement given over to staff control functions.* Such organizational maintenance work naturally bleeds energy from the enterprise's productive capacity.

It is at this point that the more imaginative people begin to leave the organization. They are usually replaced by less enthusiastic functionaries who can live with the large quantity of daily ritualism and who tend to settle down to minimum levels of performance.[26] This unfortunate circumstance is outlined by March and Simon as the last of a three-stage decline in which the organization first loses the ability to adjust to new demands, second loses its ability to alter external circumstances to suit its operation, and finally resorts to adjusting its "aspiration level" downward to an "achievement level." (The reverse, of course, is the case in the search and success phases.)[27]

What happens to patient care in health service organizations that are at this stage of their life cycle? Few officials of the organization really know. Informal communications concerning patient needs no longer can reach the higher levels, and no one lower in the organization is empowered to alter policy. Furthermore, there may be a clear disadvantage to employees in displaying sensitivity to unusual patient needs. When confronted with a nonroutine situation an employee of an organization in this phase of development is likely to fare better if he sticks to the prescribed rules than if he attempts to bend the rules in

* There is conflicting evidence as to whether this "administrative component" continues to increase in greater proportion than the growth of an organization (a phenomenon popularized as Parkinson's law). However the evidence is fairly clear that during the *early* stages of an organization's growth the proportion of administrative personnel increases.[25]

order to serve the patient. It is often better not to bother one's superiors with problems if one is interested in promotion. In short, it is usually better to be organization-minded than client-minded.[28]

Faced with a block in upward communication, high-level officials may attempt a top-down form of communication in which patients or their representatives (at this stage often called "public representatives") are invited to participate in organizational decision-making. This co-optation often becomes a mere semblance of communication. In its fictitious and manipulative form it not only fails to capture the clients but blocks any real expression of problems and requests.[29]

When an organization is unable to bridge the world of management and the world of patients the job of communicating from one to the other may fall to an outsider, quite possibly a journalist.[30] Reporters bypass the internal communication system by publicly transmitting client complaints directly to the top bureaucrats. Thus board rooms and council chambers sometimes echo with the accusation: "I didn't know a thing about it until I read it in the newspapers!"

Examples of the bureaucratic phase in a health agency is the Los Angeles County Department of Charities. The department is an unwieldy combination of hospital and welfare services. It is massive, employing more personnel as a unit of government than do five states. It is totally dependent on the County Board of Supervisors for allocations of operating funds. The department's organizational inflexibility was publicly dramatized in 1966 when efforts were made to reorganize the department into separate agencies of welfare, adoptions, and hospitals.[31] Obsolete administrative mechanisms were revealed in a strike of the department's social workers. These employees, in close proximity to clients, struck not only for higher wages but in protest of working conditions. It soon became apparent that important personnel policies could be resolved only by the County Board of Supervisors. The department was devoid of the normal executive authority necessary to make adjustments.

What was true in respect to employees also seemed to hold in respect to at least some clients. This was revealed by the McCone Commission investigation into causes underlying the Watts riots of August 1965.[32] The 3000-bed County Hospital, locally known as the "Big House," was found to be eight miles distant and one hour of public transportation away from Watts residents. Yet it was in effect the only hospital available to most of these low-income people. More than distance, Watts residents complained bitterly of long waits, lack of coordination, and an atmosphere of indifference at the hospital. Plans for a new hospital to provide more immediate service to Watts residents received mixed support from the Board of Supervisors and failed to obtain the requisite two-thirds approval of the county voters in a referendum election. Plans were then developed to build the hospital with private funds through a complex financial arrangement that would retain ultimate public ownership of the hospital even though it was established under separate and private corporate identity[33] (in the terms of our typology, a form of organizational succession).

SUCCESSION PHASE

What is it that triggers a large, stagnant organization to metamorphose —to spawn a new unit—and thus start again the full organizational life cycle? To a degree this process is a mystery, particularly as to time and detail. Yet in one form or another it seems to be inevitable. One set of forces in the process is clearly external to the organization. The flow of resources to a unit that is serving society poorly or inefficiently is eventually reduced. The enterprise, possessing a will to survive no less than that found in living organisms, thereupon may develop an entirely new form that is better suited to the temper of the times. More commonly, however, a new unit will be established within the old organization to compete successfully for clients. Such a phenomenon occurred in the auto industry some years ago. One auto maker prospered for several years by producing compact economy cars exclusively. This firm was quickly matched by new sideline offerings of small cars by established big car manufacturers.

Within health service organizations the transition appears to be caused more often than not by severe conflict arising between professional ideals and bureaucratic discipline. The need of the professionals within the organization to exercise more individual responsibility and their identification of new ways to serve patients often result in the elaboration of a new unit. Perhaps at first the new unit is intended only as a planning activity, but often it blossoms into a full and quite independent existence. The evolution of mental health departments from public health departments is an example.

Thus a valuable ingredient is buried within a large bureaucracy—the ability to generate new organizational forms. From the point of view of service the offspring may be a great improvement on the parent; yet credit for its survival and success belongs in part to the older organization from which it sprang.

A final example concerns the labor–management health and welfare movement. It illustrates not so much the current position of a specific agency relative to one stage of organizational change but rather the long-term process of organizational evolution.

In the late Middle Ages of European civilization there was no separation of skilled labor and management. This was the era of craft guilds, when health and welfare services were arranged through organized guild associations and societies. The Industrial Revolution, first in Europe and then in America, witnessed a separation of labor and management. The disregard by factory owners of workers' health prompted both protective-labor legislation and strong unions. Many unions developed benevolent societies which, at the turn of the twentieth century in the United States, were important mechanisms for providing medical care to workers and their families. These labor, ethnic, and fraternal welfare societies were succeeded by the more efficient and dependable prepayment plans sponsored by doctors and hospitals. But as bureaucratic forms these in turn became unresponsive to labor's needs. We are currently witnessing the amazing growth of union–management health and welfare funds. These trust funds are at present searching for the best combinaton of continued pressure for maximum performance from established health services and union-designed "direct" programs. As a result of trust fund practices the concept of "dual" or "multiple choice" has evolved to offer labor and consumer groups more responsive and varied health service packages.

History suggests that trust funds will not remain the final organizational form to serve laborers. There will be subsequent transformations as agencies continue to alternate between attention to client needs (laborers as union members) and recognition of external sources of financial support (negotiated employer contributions, which constitute reductions of corporate profits).

SUMMARY AND DISCUSSION

The features characteristic of each phase of the organization life cycle are summarized in Table 1.

The model presented in this chapter is not intended to describe accurately the life cycle of public in contrast to private medical or health agencies. This is so for a number of reasons. First, in public agencies it is often government rather than the agency itself that responds to the client's (voter's) needs. Government thereupon will dictate change within an institution, even though that institution may not be responsive to its clients' wishes. In this way the relationship between client and government becomes the arbiter of change, rather than the relationship between client and institution. Second, public agencies tend to bypass the search and success phases and to begin life near the bureaucratic phase, proceeding thence immediately to the succession phase. Only in the succession phase do they give rise to second-generation organizations that then go through early phases of the organizational life cycle. Also, in public agencies there is more chance for an institution to continue over time in the bureaucratic phase despite the fact that it has lost much client support and displays excessive organizational rigidity. This survival often relates to political considerations important to government but totally external to the organization and its immediate clientele. This again reflects the fact that government and not the client ultimately decides the course of public, as opposed to private, agencies. In this regard it might be well to point out that the government of course is ultimately controlled by the people. However, this control body is a large amorphous mass, quite different in nature from the smaller well-defined "public" that makes up the patients or clients of a particular health agency.

Beneath the progression of organizations through the different life cycle phases there are some basic principles that perhaps set the limits or indirectly influence the course of events. One is the necessarily recurrent process of reappraising goals—of defining the desired relation between an organization and its environment.[34] A change in either the organization or its environment demands reappraisal and probable alteration of organizational policies and goals. Some enterprises do this job better than others, and a given organization may have greater success in doing so at some times than at others. This is a particular problem for health service agencies where the technical and social environment is constantly changing.

A second underlying principle is that decisions often are not determined by an organization's officials but seem to emerge as circumstances compel. We have noted that health service organizations actually may be rated on a continuum ranging from organizational control over environment to environmental control over organization.

Another principle brought into focus by dividing the organizational life cycle into stages is that leadership personnel well-suited to one stage are often ill-fitted to another. Militant picket bosses are needed to organize unions, while more subtle negotiators are needed to refine and advance the initial victories.[35] The innovator–entrepreneur Henry Ford would be out of place in Ford's present-day board rooms filled with consensus conscious executives. It is hard for the controlling

TABLE 1. *Characteristics of Life Cycle*

CHARACTERISTICS	
GENERAL FEATURES	
Age	young
Size	small
ECOLOGICAL FEATURES	
Relationship to environment	influences environment
Adaptability	adaptable
Relationship with other agencies	conflict and adjustment
Public visability	low
image	clear
Pressure groups	few (client oriented)
Risk of failure	high
CLIENT FEATURES	
Client satisfaction	high
Numbers served	few
Responsiveness to clients	high
ECONOMIC FEATURES	
Financial stability	unstable
Productivity	increasing
SERVICE FEATURES	
Range of services	narrow
Manner of rendering services	direct
Operating methods	changing
ORGANIZATIONAL FEATURES	
Goals	frequent redefinition
Progress toward goals	accelerating
Aspiration-Achievement gap	movement toward aspiration
Time perspective	future
Administrative flexibility	high
Innovation	dispersed, individual
Influence of sub-units on decision making	many influential sub-units
Communications	informal
Focus of leadership	outward
Leadership expertise	subject-matter oriented
Authority of leader	charismatic
Type of staff organization	equalitarian
Maintenance of system	little effort expended
Scope of individual tasks	enlarging

STAGES			
→search →success →bureaucratic →succession (↺)			
→	→	→	old
→	→	→	large
→	→	→	influenced by environment
→	→	→	inflexible
→	→	→	accommodation
→	→	→	high
→	→	→	clouded
→	→	→	many (politico-economically oriented)
→	→	→	low
→	→	→	low
→	→	→	many
→	→	→	low
→	→	→	stable
→	→	→	declining
→	→	→	broad
→	→	→	direct and indirect
→	→	→	traditional
→	→	→	assumed fixed
→	→	→	decelerating
→	→	→	movement toward achievement
→	→	→	present
→	→	→	low
→	→	→	centralized, organized
→	→	→	one or few influential sub-units
→	→	→	formal
→	→	→	inward
→	→	→	management-oriented
→	→	→	bureaucratic
→	→	→	hierarchial
→	→	→	great effort expended
→	→	→	shrinking

members of organizations to see clearly what personality best matches the organization's needs of the moment, and it is hard for the individual who may be mismatched to accept this fact without personal affront.

This exposition has emphasized the inevitability of change: "What is a satisfactory adjustment for one group or circumstance is unsatisfactory for another."[36] While change seems inevitable, clearly there are instances when the precise stages described above are not followed by an organization—or not followed in the same sequence. Timing varies considerably. What seems to be needed is a set of indicators—clues that reveal whether an organization was moving away from its orientation to clients or patients and toward the latter stages of its evolutionary cycle. A good deal of research needs to be done before such indicators can be applied with reliability. In the absence of this research (and perhaps as a guide to research that any organization could undertake with its own staff) the following questions might be pursued:

1. How are mistakes corrected in the organization? Patients have questions and complaints, some legitimate and some not. A sampling could be made of these complaints to determine the percentage resolved to patients' satisfaction.

2. To what extent does communication take place on the problems of individual patients? At a certain level in an organization these become "translated" into general sets or stereotypes. Is this level of generalization near or distant from the level at which decisions are made that could correct the individual problems?

3. How much does the staff of an organization know about its patients—their social background as well as their health condition? This knowledge could be tested of persons at different levels of an organization, and variations could be noted between levels and between agencies.

4. Conversely, how much is the patient informed of the results of his contact with the organization?

5. Janowitz and Delaney have devised a test of "functional knowledge" of clients versus "substantive knowledge" of community persons and resources important to an agency's survival.[37] As part of this test questions are asked of clients. Then officials at various levels in the organization are asked to estimate the clients' responses. The degree of correlation between the two is a reasonable measure of the organization's ability to serve clients.

6. When communications exist, how representative are they of patients' actual feelings and needs?

7. How many contacts are there between top administration and patients being served?

8. Are solutions to client problems delayed until relevant information is passed up and down the organization hierarchy for decision? Or are persons in direct contact with patients sufficiently empowered to make the appropriate adjustments?

9. Is there consensus within the organization on what is to be done for patients and on how to do it? Is there agreement on who makes decisions concerning patients or where to go for decisions? This could be tested by posing real or hypothetical cases to various persons to determine the degree to which they agree on a course of action.

10. Is innovation in the method of rendering services allowed? If so, at what levels and with what mechanism for accepting or rejecting the ideas proposed? This could be tested by identifying suggested innovations and tracing the action taken upon them.

11. Can patients "negotiate" with organization rules?[38] A degree of flexibility is an essential of organizational effectiveness.

12. Finally, we should not overlook well-designed attitude surveys. Such information in itself would be revealing, but particularly so if correlated with the other measures suggested above.

One problem with the "inevitable change" theory is that it implies that organizations are in a state of helplessness—that they can do nothing but passively await whatever destiny is theirs by way of social evolution. To be contrary, seeking answers to the questions posed above would represent positive action on the part of an organization—purposeful effort to keep its conduct sensitive to society's problems. Mechanisms of review and self-criticism are essential. Viable organizations must undertake such appraisals periodically if not continually. It is in this process of rejection, renewal, or revision of programs and policies that organized action is—as it must be—perpetually reconstituted.

References

1. Peter M. Blau, "The Dynamics of Organization," in Amitai Etzioni (ed.), *Complex Organizations: A Sociological Reader*, New York: Holt, Rinehart & Winston, 1961, p. 343.
2. Mason Haire, "Biological Models and Empirical Histories of the Growth of Organizations," *Modern Organization Theory*, New York: Wiley, 1959.
3. Keith Warner and Eugene Havens, "Goal Displacement and the Intangibility

of Organizational Goals," *Administrative Science Quarterly*, 12:4 (March 1958), 539–555.

4. S. N. Eisenstadt, "Bureaucracy, Bureaucratization, and Debureaucratization," in Amitai Etzioni (ed.), *Complex Organizations*, p. 276.
5. Amitai Etzioni, *Modern Organizations*, Englewood Cliffs, N.J.: Prentice-Hall, 1964, p. 95.
6. Sheldon L. Messinger, "Organization Transformation," *American Sociological Review*, 20:1 (February 1955), 3–10.
7. Philip Selznick, "Critical Decisions in Organizational Development," in Amitai Etzioni (ed.), *Complex Organizations*, p. 356.
8. Max Weber, *The Theory of Social and Economic Organizations*, A. M. Henderson and Talcott Parsons (trans.) and Talcott Parsons (ed.), New York: The Free Press, 1947, pp. 324–386.
9. James March and Herbert Simon, *Organizations*, New York: Wiley, 1958, pp. 183–184.
10. Sol Levine *et al.*, "Community Interorganizational Problems in Providing Medical Care and Social Services," *American Journal of Public Health*, 58:8 (August 1963), 1183.
11. Peter M. Blau and Richard W. Scott, *Formal Organizations*, San Francisco: Chandler Publishing Co., 1962, p. 228.
12. Selznick, "Critical Decisions in Organizational Development," p. 358.
13. Blau, "The Dynamics of Organization," p. 350.
14. Blau and Scott, *Formal Organizations*, p. 247.
15. David L. Sills, "The Succession of Goals," in Amitai Etzioni (ed.), *Complex Organizations*, pp. 146–159.
16. Messinger, "Organization Transformation," pp. 4–8.
17. David L. Sills, *The Volunteers*, New York: The Free Press, 1957, p. 159.
18. Selznick, "Critical Decisions in Organizational Development," p. 358.
19. *Time*, October 6, 1952, p. 89.
20. Milton I. Roemer and Ray H. Elling, "Sociological Research in Medical Care," *Journal of Health and Human Behavior* (Spring 1963), p. 67.
21. Blau and Scott, *Formal Organizations*, p. 225.
22. Weber, *The Theory of Social and Economic Organizations*, pp. 329–330.
23. *Webster's New Collegiate Dictionary*, Springfield, Mass.: Merriam Co., 1949, p. 111.
24. March and Simon, *Organizations*, pp. 141–142.
25. Haire, "Biological Models...," pp. 292–293.
26. Bernard Levenson, "Bureaucratic Succession," in Amitai Etzioni (ed.), *Complex Organizations*, pp. 370–375.
27. March and Simon, *Organizations*, p. 182.
28. Etzioni, *Modern Organizations*, p. 99.
29. Blau and Scott, *Formal Organizations*, p. 101.
30. Etzioni, *Modern Organizations*, p. 99.

31. "Social Workers Return to Work After 17-Day Strike," *New York Times*, June 19, 1966, p. 26.
32. *Governor's Commission on the Los Angeles Riots*, December 1965, vol. 18.
33. Arthur Viseltear, Arnold Kisch, and Milton Roemer, *The Watts Hospital: A Health Facility Is Planned for a Metropolitan Slum Area*, Arlington, Va.: Division of Medical Care Administration, Public Health Service, U.S. Department of Health, Education and Welfare, December 1967, pp. 41–48.
34. James D. Thompson and William J. McEwan, "Organizational Goals and Environment," in Amitai Etzioni (ed.), *Complex Organizations*, p. 177.
35. Clinton S. Golden and Harold J. Ruttenberg, *Dynamics of Industrial Democracy*, New York: Harper & Row, 1942, p. 59.
36. Blau and Scott, *Formal Organizations*, pp. 250–252.
37. Morris Janowitz and William Delaney, "The Bureaucrat and the Public, A Study of Informational Perspectives," *Administrative Science Quarterly*, 2 (September 1957), 141–162.
38. Anselm Strauss *et al.*, "The Hospital and Its Negotiated Order," in Eliot Freidson (ed.), *The Hospital in Modern Society*, New York: The Free Press, 1963, pp. 147–169.

19

Organizational Decision-Making

L. Vaughn Blankenship

In the last decade or so, decision-making as an activity has become the focus for the development of some new theories, some new ways of thinking about administration and human behavior in organizations. These theories represent somewhat of a departure from other ways of viewing organizational phenomenon in that they are generally dynamic, they usually assume that man wants to be rational to the best of his ability, and they are clearly most appropriate for understanding or describing those administrative acts requiring most in the way of cognitive rather than overt behavioral activities—for example, planning, budgeting, staffing, policy-making, and resource allocation. In short, they place the emphasis on *thinking* as opposed to *doing*. How do men think when they problem solve? How should they think given certain ends or goals?

Theories about decision-making can be broadly (and imprecisely) divided into two types: those which are primarily normative and those which are primarily descriptive in character. These distinctions reflect something about the substance of the theories, the way they are written, the terms they use to describe administrative behavior, and the methodologies they imply. The real roots of the distinction, however, lie in the *purpose* of the theorist and the specialization and division of labor that has occurred within those occupational groups concerned with decision theory.

Normative theories of decision-making, as the name implies, are concerned with how individuals and organizations *should* make decisions or *can* make decisions most efficiently and rationally, given a certain set of objectives. Among other things their aim is to provide the intellectual basis for developing techniques for clarifying goals and alternatives and making "optimal" decisions. They have grown up in the traditions of industrial engineering, applied economics, statistics, and rationalistic psychology, and their proponents are usually housed in professional schools where there is a close and self-conscious link between the world (and problems) of the practitioner and the world of the academic researcher and teacher.

In such an environment, understandably enough, the utility of theory to the decision-maker becomes a major rationale for its development, a test of its value, and the main criterion for choosing which theory is best. While many may be interested in more "basic" problems or in simply "understanding" decision-making, the ultimate justification for the activity is the utilitarian one, and the products of such an environment are skilled administrative technicians prepared to put their theories and methodologies at the disposal of the decision-maker:

> The theory of administration is concerned with how an organization should be constructed and operated in order to accomplish its work efficiently... [The] "principle" of efficiency should be considered as a definition rather than a principle: it is a definition of what is meant by "good" or "correct" administrative behavior. It does not tell *how* accomplishments are to be maximized, but merely states that this maximization is the aim of administrative activity, and that *administrative theory must disclose under what conditions the maximization takes place.*[1]

Descriptive theories are more concerned with how people *do* make decisions and the way in which certain things—personality, hierarchy, technology, status systems, politics, and environmental factors—influence these choices. To the extent that the question of values or goals intrude into such theories, they are merely one more piece of objective datum to be measured and analyzed in terms of their behavioral consequences. The major justification for this activity (and here is the *real* difference) is intellectual and altruistic: knowledge and understanding are worthwhile ends in themselves. The ultimate test of a good theory is whether it advances understanding, and this is a test to be administered by one's professional colleagues rather than by a decision-maker in the hierarchy of some organization.[2]

Such theories and the empirical findings they produce obviously may lead to a concern for design and application (and it is here that the rather neat sounding distinction between normative and descriptive theories begins rapidly to break down). If, for example, we know something about group prestige distinctions and communication patterns and innovative behavior such as the adoption of new drugs by doctors, it is clearly possible to take the next step and suggest a new strategy for advertising or marketing drugs. In the past, however, individuals developing or using these descriptive theories have, ideally, been unconcerned about taking this next step and making a policy recommendation. If they did, they were, or *should* have been according to the traditions of "value-free" social science, very self-conscious about what they were doing so as to avoid confusing their role as a social scientist and their role as an adviser or social engineer:

> Now this is not to say that a social scientist who temporarily becomes a social engineer cannot exploit his data-gathering position to do a little pure science on the side. A man who consults with industry or labor and applies what little knowledge there is to a practical problem can indeed play simultaneously the role of social scientist. But this involves more than changing the language and sending his report to a different journal. It means he has to be clear about the different purposes of his effort and about the standards of success appropriate to each.[3]

In this chapter, then, the decision-making approach to the analysis of organization is generally outlined. It is done in the tradition of the descriptive rather than the normative orientation in that it presents some ideas on how individuals (probably) make decisions rather than on how they should make them. The emphasis is placed on some of the conceptual and methodological problems involved in looking at administrative behavior in this fashion. The perceptive reader will discover for himself how illusive the line between normative and descriptive becomes when one begins to analyze decision-making.

GOALS, POLICY, AND DECISION-MAKING

Those at the top of an organization—the chief executives: the boards of directors or trustees or supervisors—in a sense "make policy," they set objectives and goals. That is, they issue statements or write words on paper that express what they think *ought to be done* by other members of the organization. So far, however, such statements are merely utopian in the sense that they outline a set of ideals that are hoped for sometime in the future.

Over-all objectives or policies of the type we are discussing here for the moment are frequently stated very broadly—so broadly, in fact, that everybody agrees with them and they are of little value in making concrete, day-to-day decisions. Who really can disagree, for example, with the statements that the goal of a public health agency is to provide for the highest level of health care for the most people at a minimum cost? The operational problem with such statements becomes immediately apparent when an administrator has to decide whether to use some money in his budget to hire another public health nurse, raise salaries, or purchase some badly needed equipment. Which alternative will give the highest level of health care? Which will help the most people?

Such broad directives or general aspirations must be translated into more specific subgoals and, as such, they become the special concern of different parts of the organization: the marketing department, the personnel department, the accounting department, the maternal and child welfare department, the out-patient clinic, and so on. In other words, a group of people, organized as a subunit, are assigned certain formal responsibilities that presumably are related in some fashion to these over-all goals. The criteria for making decisions has become more explicit and limited, and organizational subgoals have now been embedded in the social structure of a group or department within the larger organization.

This factoring out of goals[4] does not stop at the departmental level. Departmental goals must be translated into still more specific objectives and assigned to divisions and sections and finally, at the very bottom, specific individuals—workers, salesmen, investigators, nurses, and secretaries. At that point, if every individual meets his assigned goal, by a process of addition the unit, department, and finally the organization meet theirs. Objectives become an important way of coordinating the individual efforts of the hundreds of people who make up the organization. No one individual below the top of the organization has to consider more than a few goals in making decisions since he can assume that others are paying attention to other objectives. He can specialize and become an expert in making a few selected decisions. The formal structure of the organization—the division into offices, units, bureaus, etc.—parallels the means–ends relationships between broad and more proximate objectives.

Implicit in this picture of objectives and organizations are several explicit things. At the top of an organization we have individuals whose role is to establish goals or levels of performance for the organization as a whole. At the bottom of the organization, far removed from them physically and socially, are those who actually implement these goals through their activities. What an organization *finally accomplishes*, the goals it finally realizes, ultimately depends upon the concrete actions and decisions of operatives—those tens, hundreds, or thousands of individuals who, on a day-to-day basis, make the product or provide a service to a client or customer through their joint efforts.[5] Those at the top can only influence these decisions very indirectly. Thus the superstructure of organization, the division of labor and specialization, may be viewed as a network of power and communication whose ultimate justification is its ability to influence the decisions of operatives when the critical moment arrives to decide.

This picture also assumes a great deal of rationality and power on the part of policy-makers, the people at the top. It assumes, first, that they see clearly where they want to go, the numerous ways of getting there, and which of these ways is best. It also assumes that they or their subordinates have the time and wisdom to translate policy into more and more concrete terms without altering, substantially, the original intent. It assumes, finally, that the people in the organization are malleable, that they are neutral instruments whose activities and attention can be modified without regard to their interests, training, or previous experience and that the consequences of change, in terms of policy implementation, can be perfectly predicted.

Just to state such assumptions is to point out the limitations of this model as a description of what, in fact, organizations actually do. Even with the aid of the most advanced computers and sophisticated analytical devices, policy-makers have neither the resources nor the mental capacity to make such demanding calculations. Furthermore, the search for information upon which to base judgment and the attempt logically to clarify goals represent costs in several forms: time, communication, lost opportunities, and often resistance to policy. Clarifying mutually incompatible goals can result in loss of support for a program since it makes it crystal clear to diverse groups in the environment or even to members of the policy-making body just what they stand to gain or lose.[6] Thus goal ambiguity or sequential attention to goals—focusing on one at one time and place and another at a different time and place—can be effective strategies for neutralizing or avoiding opposition to policy. In addition, since all the exigencies of the actual operating environment in which goals must be implemented hardly can be anticipated ahead of time, some discretion to modify practice in response to the environment must, of necessity, be allowed lower level officials. This, in turn, may result in a substantial change in goals or at least a shift in priorities among them.[7]

Finally, policy-makers usually *begin* with an already ongoing set of programs, skills, and commitments. There are numerous "sunk costs" in the form of investments in technology, training, and experience that can be forgone only at a substantial loss to the organization. Controls from the environment in the form of laws, contractual obligations, professional standards, fiscal requirements, reporting procedures, and organized public opinion extend into the organization. The *esprit de corps* and special "point of view" that most organizations build, only partly consciously, as a prerequisite to and consequence of coherent, consistent action on the part of its members is a potent force. These represent very real constraints on the policy choices realistically available and the extent to which they can be implemented from the top. Only at substantial cost and effort can policy-makers do much more than modify and adjust past orientations and behavior. The sense of what is feasible and what is acceptable and possible will usually win out over what is ideally desirable.

THE DECISION-MAKING ENVIRONMENT

We often tend to think of decisions in terms of *final choices*, as discrete events with a definite beginning and a clear end: The board of trustees is presented with a recommendation to purchase a computer or to add a wing onto a hospital, and they vote "yes" or "no"; a supervisor interviews three job applicants and decides to hire one—or maybe none, but instead sends a routine order to the personnel department asking it to send around more applicants: or a manager looks at cost estimates, considers the possible responses of competitors, and picks one of several possible prices at which to sell a new product. Certainly these are decisions, but this hardly exhausts the reality of decision-making.

Often, for example, by the time the final choice is made it is largely a *pro forma* matter. Take the decision of building a new hospital wing. By the time the board of trustees meets to consider this possibility, a number of other people and other decisions already have shaped the proposal on which they will vote. Normally the board does not review all the information considered by others before it decides, but it commits the hospital and the community in one way or another on the basis of recommendations it receives. In fact, Professor Parkinson has suggested, half facetiously, that there is an inverse relationship between the amount of time a board will spend considering an issue and the amount of money involved![8]

These recommendations, in turn, are the result of a number of decisions that subordinates or outside consultants have made about what the board needs or wants to see. Frequently they will be structured in such a way as to minimize the likelihood of negative consequences to those making the recommendations, especially if they know they are to be evaluated on the basis of them. To be sure, these expectations may be based on certain reality factors: understandings of what the board's formal powers are, previous experiences including how members have reacted to similar proposals and the kinds of questions they have asked, and informal communications with various board members. But they are filtered through the perceptual apparatus of subordinates or consultants and the interests they have in the outcome.

Even such hard data as figures on costs and savings or benefits involve numerous subjective decisions about which numbers or which time span is relevant, what the real costs are and how they are to be measured, and who benefits in what fashion. Much of the professional training of the accountant, for example, is given over to considerations of the many ways in which costs can be calculated, overhead distributed, and true value determined. As one consultant to a business firm said, "In the final analysis, if anybody brings up an item of cost we haven't thought of, we can balance it by making another source of savings tangible."[9] Under such circumstances, then, the board's final choice may be little more than a ratification of such previous decisions.

Sometimes, too, the choice is to do nothing—to make no decisions. In such instances there may be no overt indication that conscious choice has, in fact, been made. Occasionally the failure to decide is the result of conscious intent; sometimes it is the result of ignorance. This latter situation arises when we are unaware that the occasion for a decision exists or that there are alternatives open for us from which choice is possible.

Much advertising, for example, is intended to make the consumer aware of alternatives so that he can make a choice. It also is intended to call his attention to the need for making a decision by stimulating a desire for the product or service. A major concern of the salesman is to get himself into an organization and to make it aware of alternatives it did not know existed before. Efforts to tell the community about health and welfare services are, at least in part, attempts to let potential clients know that alternatives are available. Thus, not only does the client, customer, community, or organization go around looking for alternatives, but alternatives go around looking for customers or people with problems.

In short, then, the study of decisions is much more than the analysis of a *single choice point*. Instead we must look at all the activity and the considerations that preceded the final choice in time if we are to understand the nature of the decision and if we are to find out which objectives have been advanced by a decision or will be advanced by one. Also, by looking at the entire process surrounding a decision, we see that there are *many points* at which influence can be brought to bear to shape the outcome. In fact, the moment of final choice may offer the *least* opportunity to influence a decision except in an "all or nothing" sense. By that time lines of action have been clarified, compromises have been reached, thinking has been crystallized around certain solutions, and emotional (if not political) commitments have already been made by many involved in the decision process. Our attention, then, must be focused on the entire process of decision and on the environment in which it occurs.

Influence and the Decision-Making Model

Decision-making may be thought of as a series of interrelated experiences or events, some of which occur solely in the mind of the individual decision-makers and some of which involve his interaction with his environment. There are numerous "models" of the decision process that specify these various experiences as a decision evolves from initiation to final choice point. Some models have three or four phases; others have more. There is no one model that seems best, so we are free to pick that one we like. This being the case, we will describe decisions in terms of

1. Recognizing the occasions for decisions.
2. Analyzing the existing situation.
3. Identifying alternative courses of action and assessing the consequences of each alternative.
4. Choosing from among alternatives.

Let us look at each of the above in some detail and consider, in particular, the ways in which the organization can influence them.

THE OCCASION FOR DECISION

Recognition of the "occasion" for a decision means that the individual decision-maker scans his environment for cues that will cause him to realize that an event has occurred requiring some response on his part. He becomes aware that there is a discrepancy between what *is* and what *ought to be*, and this in turn triggers the subsequent set of actions. The cues may come from a number of different sources—e.g., clients, friends, professional colleagues in or outside the organization, superiors, subordinates, or the mass media. The available evidence suggests that individuals tend to be most sensitive to cues from superiors or, where close-knit and informal relationships exist, from peers, and considerably less attuned to cues from other parts of the environment.[10] They may also come in a more or less structured form—for example, a monthly balance sheet, an inquiry from a client, an application blank or a written directive as opposed to reports in the newspaper of a flood or a layoff at a local plant, a series of decisions by officials in a federal agency, or experiences in a series of conferences or professional training programs.

When we say that a cue is more or less structured we imply something about both the individual decision-maker and his organizational environment. Built into the individual's memory cells, on the basis of past experience and training, is the realization that certain events or the symbols of them are important to his job. They call attention to the fact that something has happened and that he is expected to make some sort of response, even if the response is to do nothing. When we talk about structured cues we also mean that there is a close relationship between the cue and the *possible responses*. It triggers off a definite set of thoughts and a range of imagined, correct actions.

A structured cue also indicates that search is built into the information system of the organization. It has an "intelligence" network, a set of standardized information-gathering and reporting procedures and certain ways of displaying and routing this data to appropriate people. In this fashion it influences profoundly what people will see. A relatively unstructured cue is generally the opposite of these things: it is unexpected and often nonrepetitive; there is not a routine way of picking it up in the sense that people specialize in searching for it. Often it is picked up by chance or by luck; often it may be overlooked. Finally, the relevance for the organization, its meaning in terms of goals or strategy, is not immediately clear.

The importance of the conception that the individual has of organizational objectives in this phase of the decision process is clear. Perceptions of reality, the cues seen and the responses made, to a large extent are determined by beliefs about departmental goals and responsibilities. In this sense the organization chart is a plan of action, a priority system for action. In a business, for example, those in a marketing department ignore many things that happen in their environment; they do not "see" them because they are not relevant to the goals of that department as they are understood. Even though things happen in their environment that would be of great interest to the people in production, the people in the production department never hear about it because the marketing people failed to see it or see it in a light that does not suggest it is of importance to production.

THE EXISTING SITUATION

The cue for decision-making is given meaning within the context of the present situation of the individual. This present is partly a function of the individual's location within the organization, his role in it, and the expectations he believes others have of him. It also is a result of his past experiences in interpreting similar cues. For both reasons the situational context in which cues are received is a powerful source of stability and conservatism within an organization. Past success in responding to a certain cue increases the likelihood that it will be interpreted and responded to in a similar fashion in the present. The danger, of course, is that the present situation is different. Thus we find the all-too-familar phenomenon of the decision-maker who is brilliantly prepared to "fight the last war," a phenomenon that at least in part lies behind the comments of the German sociologist Karl Mannheim on the nature of "bureaucratic conservatism":

> Every bureaucracy... in accord with the peculiar emphasis on its own position, tends to generalize its own experience and to overlook the fact that the realm of administration and of smoothly functioning order represents only a part of the total political reality. Bureaucratic thought does not deny the possibility of a science of politics, but regards it as identical with the science of administration.... Thus irrational factors are overlooked, and when [they] nevertheless force themselves to the fore, they are treated as "routine matters...."[11]

If the context gives meaning to the cue, the reverse also is true. The cue helps shape the situational context in which it will be perceived. If, for example, the decision-maker believes that the cue indicates a personnel problem, such as a secretary coming into his office in tears or an irate telephone call from a client, his attention will turn immediately toward those areas of his activities to the exclusion of other things. This may be the case even though it may turn out that there is no direct connection between the cue and the situation it led him to perceive.

A recent case study of decision-making in a business firm illustrates this process nicely.[12] A large manufacturing company had gradually been replacing some of its heavy equipment as money became available. One reason was that the old equipment was potentially unsafe for those working with it. Though concern for employee safety was a stated objective of top management, it was largely a latent concern. However, an accident resulted in the death of an employee on the job. Though there was no objective evidence that the event was in *any way* directly attributable to the existence of the older equipment, it nevertheless was interpreted in this fashion and management decided almost immediately to replace all the equipment at a speeded up and considerably costly pace. Thus a cue, in this instance a dramatic one, lead to a focus on one aspect of a situation—an aspect that hitherto had been latent, in spite of the fact that there was no overt causal relationship between the perceived situation and the event. The cue was objectively incidental to the decision that resulted, although it clearly triggered that decision.

While the analysis of the existing situation—surveying hiring practices or policies in dealing with clients, examining the present organization of the office, looking at current budget levels, questioning figures on utilization or patient load, etc.—is a major and definable step in the decision-making process, it is linked closely with the initial perception of a cue. The direction it will take and the conclusions it will lead to may well be embedded in the event that gave rise to the analysis in the first place: We find what we started out looking for.

IDENTIFYING AND ASSESSING ALTERNATIVES

Identifying a possible course of action and assessing the consequences are the next phases in the decision-making process. We would like to believe that the search for alternative solutions to a problem continues until a best one is found. Perhaps this belief in the ability of man to order his thoughts and to treat them as objects apart from himself—objects fit to be made public, dissected, and analyzed—is a pecular feature of the rationalistic, secular bias of our scientific–industrial culture. There are a number of factors, however, that quickly constrain this "ideal" model of (rational) human behavior and give it a rather different bent, as we shall see.

To begin, there is the very real fact that what is best is relative—relative to who (what system) is answering the question and when it is being asked. It is bound by both system reference and time. For example. from the respective viewpoints of a visiting nurse, a relief investigator, and a probation officer, what may appear to be the best way to deal with a family on ADC because there is a delinquent child and a father with a heart condition, from the perspective of the family or the community at large may appear to be the height of irrationality and a very bad choice of alternatives:

> The relief investigator, in pursuance of agency policy, urges the father to seek work; the visiting nurse counsels rest on doctor's orders. The assistance agency hunts a part-time job for mother; the probation officer bids her stay home to keep Johnny out of mischief. The truant officer warns Johnny against any more absences from school; the probation officer admonishes him not to miss his school-hours appointment at the court.[13]

Such a situation exists not merely because each decision-maker is located in a particular department or agency with a particular set of goals—the result, in part, of the factoring out process described earlier—but because there is still no good way of determining what is best from some more comprehensive, system point of view. In fact, it is not even certain how the relevant system (the who factor) and its goals may be identified. If we then add the time dimension and attempt to extend our conception of a relevant system in that direction (the when factor), the problem of defining what is best becomes almost insurmountable.[14] To paraphrase the old adage, what is one generation's meat (cheap way of sewage disposal) is another generation's poison (polluted rivers)!

Even if we could succeed in identifying the relevant system in time and place, it would usually be found to have multiple objectives. Take the apparently mundane problem of organizing secretarial–clerical skills within a department. We want to have high quality work—carefully typed letters and a convenient filing system so that letters can be found without too much difficulty—a reasonable level of morale among the secretaries (few things can be so disastrous for the usual office filing system, for example, than high turnover, and we do not want high-priced executives or professionals waiting for their work. Neither do we want clients or customers to be kept waiting for responses. Given these various ends, what is the best way to organize? Should we put all secretaries in a secretarial pool? Should each executive have his own secretary? Should some secretaries type, some wait on clients, some do filing, and some take dictation or run the mimeograph machine? How many typewriters do we need and what kind? Which organizational alternative, in short, will give us the neatest and most accurate correspondence, the least lost time, the best morale, the most satisfied clients or executives, and at the least cost? At this point our ability to pose such a complex problem exceeds our ability to solve it in any optimal sense.

This brings us, finally, to another set of difficulties, those associated with identifying and assessing alternatives in a systematic, comprehensive fashion. Anyone who plays a game of ticktacktoe for a period of time quickly learns that there are a limited number of ways to win the game and that two equally knowledgeable players will always end up in a stalemate. This occurs because the rules, structure, and outcome of the game are simple and bounded. In more complicated games with a much wider range of moves (alternatives) such as chess, it becomes computationally impossible for the individual player to relate each move he must make to all the possible countermoves of a knowledgeable opponent and these, in turn, to his own next move and so on to an imagined winning move.[15]

From a computational point of view, the decision-maker in an organization who would consider and trace all possible alternatives to some desirable end point, especially given the fact (as we have seen already) that end points are both difficult to identify and multiple in nature, is in a situation more analogous to the chess player than to the ticktacktoe expert. In fact, he may be even worse off since he, unlike the chess player, is identifying and weighing alternatives in an open as opposed to a closed (bounded) system of decision-making. It is still theoretically possible for the chess player to discover all possible moves and to trace through the consequences of each. This is beyond the realm of even theoretical possibility for our decision-maker in an organizational context. Even if he should undertake such a search, the costs involved would quickly outweigh any possible benefits.

What we discover, then, in looking at this phase of the decision-making process, is that it always and inevitably falls far short of the ideal model of search behavior. Instead, just as the environmental context in which a cue is received shapes the meaning of that cue, cue and environment also shape and direct the search for alternatives and the way they are evaluated. As we have already pointed out, in discussing the concept of the "structured cue," for example, the stimulus explicitly carries with it the suggested range of responses, e.g., when inventory falls below *X*, reorder using a blue sheet if it is a *Y* item and a pink sheet if it is a *Z* item. Even where possible responses are not quite so explicit, search is limited in other ways.

Take the example given above involving the problem of organizing secretarial skills. Seldom would it arise in a context where there had been no secretarial activities performed in the past. Someone had been performing them in some fashion. Thus the problem (as is most often the case in organizations) is not one of designing something in the abstract but of deciding how to adjust or change an ongoing arrangement.

A number of alternatives come readily to mind because it is a fairly conventional situation—one encountered frequently and thus a situation for which there are a limited number of conventional right answers embedded in the folklore of organizational and occupational subcultures. There are certain ways of organizing secretaries just as there are certain ways of organizing outpatient clinics, fire departments, or mass immunization drives that generally are recognized as making sense in terms of past experiences, legal or contractual requirements, and what is acceptable to the norms of the occupational groups involved. In the absence of prior knowledge of these ways, search consists of uncovering the conventional wisdom of organization, sometimes with the help of an outside management consultant, sometimes by seeing how others have done it, sometimes by examining one's own past experiences, and sometimes by reading a manual on (or taking a course in) management theory and techniques.

The problem multiple goals represent in evaluating alternatives is handled in different ways. Sometimes it is resolved by what has been called "sequential attention" to goals.[16] Continuing with our example of organizing secretaries, instead of looking at all objectives simultaneously—e.g., efficiency, speed, quality, quantity, and reduced cost or waiting time—and going through the onerous task of comparing alternatives on each of these dimensions, one alone, cost, is singled out as the focus of attention. The comparisons are made on this value, and the others are ignored or used to produce marginal adjustments in the alternative selected on the basis of cost. The particular objective that becomes the center of attention seems to depend on the initial cue that was received to initiate the decision, e.g., high turnover, a reduction in the budget, theft of a typewriter, complaints from an influential client, and the environment in which it was received.

Sometimes the problem of multiple goals is resolved through the process of comparing the imagined alternatives with the present situation.[17] Thus the question of objectives per se is ignored and the focus is put on comparing the present state with one or two possible future states in terms that seem relevant to the context in which the decision has arisen. Will alternative A or B reduce costs, improve quality, or raise morale over what we now have? What marginal adjustments can we make in the present setup to decrease the amount of time lost between when a letter is dictated and when it is sent out? The problem of finding some objectively "best" alternative becomes translated into finding one that is feasible under the present circumstances, makes good sense, improves the situation over what it has been, etc.

In recent years a number of significant and sophisticated techniques have been developed for improving the rationality with which decisions can be made. These include methods for identifying objectives and for assigning quantitative values to them on some systematic basis, arranging alternatives and calculating the best one in terms of such objectives, and displaying these processes or their results in such a way that the decision-maker can select an optimal mode of action.[18] The range of situations in which these methods have been applied to date has been limited, partly because of their inappropriateness to certain important classes of decisions, partly because they are costly for an organization to develop, and partly because they are difficult for the nonexpert to understand and accept. As they become better known and better developed, however, it seems quite clear that they will be adopted in some fashion by more and more organizations, especially for decision areas that are relatively bounded. That they will improve on the quality of decisions within such areas seems quite likely. That they will increase the over-all goodness of the system seems more doubtful. That men will continue to search for better ways of identifying needs and allocating resources to them seems certain.

CHOOSING FROM AMONG ALTERNATIVES

The series of events that has preceded this phase of the decision-making process have served to structure and shape it. Thus the final choice emerges gradually and almost unconsciously from the continual stream of events and thoughts that have preceded it in time. In fact, as discussed earlier in the section on the environment of decision-making, it often is difficult if not impossible for the individual (or group) decision-maker to recall just when he made a final choice among alternatives. The solution to the problem of reducing the distance between what is and what ought to be simply presents itself to the decision-maker as the natural and obvious thing to do.

In some situations, of course, it may appear to the outsider that the decision-maker at a moment in time has been presented with (or listed for himself) a selection of alternatives from which, by the exercise of conscious choice, he selects a winner. We have already seen, however, that there is much that is illusion in this image. The board of trustees votes "yes" or "no" on a bond issue. Was that the moment of final choice? Was it when the idea of a bond issue was first raised or when a consultant was hired and told to make recommendations on how to finance a new hospital? Was it when board members discussed the matter informally with the administrative staff or the consultants? Was it when the mayor gave his backing to the idea? Was it when a hurried caucus was held prior to the meeting so that some last-minute differences could be ironed out and the subsequent vote could be made unanimous? From a formal point of view we may be able, and in fact have, to pinpoint some moment and place of final choice since this is a prerequisite for fixing legal or political responsibility for a decision and maintaining the myth of authority. From the point of view of the decision process itself it has no such separate and distinct existence.

CONCLUSION

Theories of organization or administration are almost as numerous as the number of people writing textbooks about or doing research on the subject and are only slightly less numerous than the attempts to classify and codify them according to various schemes. At best they represent not rigorously formulated and interrelated sets of axioms and postulates from which hypotheses may be deduced or on which practice may be based but diverse mental sets—orientations, approaches, and frameworks—that serve to sensitize their adherents to certain kinds of questions or phenomenon to the exclusion of others. This certainly applies to the decision-making approach to the analysis of administration described in this chapter. It is not so much a theory as a set of constructs for organizing the "buzzing, blooming confusion" that is reality.

Ideally it would be nice if we did not have to depend upon others to do some of our work for us; if we could, by ourselves, conceive, design, and carry out the many activities involved in producing something we value—health, education, automobiles, butter—life would be much easier. Unfortunately, the things we could do would be necessarily limited as we would have neither the time, wit, nor resources to do very much in one lifetime. Since we must, of necessity, involve others in our schemes, the next best thing would be to arrange matters in such a way that they would do the same things and make the same decisions that we would if we were in their place. Unfortunately that is an extremely difficult task for reasons we are all intuitively familiar with: people have different experiences, they see the future in different ways, and they have different values. Because of this they tend to "see" different facts or to look at the same set of facts and draw quite different conclusions about what ought to be done. Thus, in this approach the study of administration becomes the study of the social psychology of individual and group problem-solving and of the conditions under which values or goals are best realized. The practice of administration becomes a problem in designing organizations and influencing decision-makers in such a way that the best possible decisions under the circumstances are forthcoming.

References

1. Herbert A. Simon, *Administrative Behavior*, New York: Macmillan, 1958, pp. 38–39 (italics added).
2. This brief description of the decision-making system of science is idealized. In fact, we know very little about the criteria used by scientists in evaluating their theories and findings. See, e.g., C. West Churchman, *Prediction and Optimal Decision Making*, New York: Wiley, 1961, especially Chapter 3.
3. Harold L. Wilensky, "Human Relations in the Workplace: An Appraisal of Some Recent Research," in Conrad M. Arensberg *et al.* (eds.), *Research in Industrial Human Relations*, New York: Harper & Row, 1957, p. 36 (italics added).
4. Victor A. Thompson, *Modern Organization*, New York: Knopf, 1961, especially Chapters 2 and 3.
5. Herbert A. Simon, *Administrative Behavior*, especially Chapter 2.
6. Wilbert E. Moore and Melvin M. Tumin, "Some Social Functions of Ignorance," *American Sociological Review*, 14 (December 1949), 787–795. For an example of how this can affect policy-making, see Martin Meyerson and Edward C. Banfield, *Politics, Planning and the Public Interest*, New York: The Free Press, 1955, especially Chapter 8.
7. Peter M. Blau, *Dynamics of Bureaucracy*, Chicago: The University of Chicago Press, 1955, Chapter 2.
8. C. Northcote Parkinson, "High Finance, or the Point of Vanishing Interest," in *Parkinson's Law*, Boston: Houghton Mifflin, 1957, pp. 24–32.
9. Quoted in R. M. Cyert, W. R. Dill, and J. G. March, "The Role of Expecta-

tions in Business Decision Making," *Administrative Science Quarterly*, 3 (December 1958), 340.

10. Robert V. Presthus, "Toward a Theory of Organizational Behavior," *Administrative Science Quarterly*, 3 (1958), 48–72, and Rensis Likert, *New Patterns of Management*, New York: McGraw-Hill, 1961, Chapter 4.
11. Karl Mannheim, *Ideology and Utopia*, New York: Harcourt, Brace & World, 1936, p. 119.
12. R. M. Cyert, W. R. Dill, and J. G. March, "The Role of Expectations in Business Decision Making."
13. Harold L. Wilensky and Charles N. Lebeaux, *Industrial Society and Social Welfare*, New York: The Free Press, 1965, p. 253.
14. For a suggestive exploration of this problem of time see C. West Churchman, *Prediction and Optimal Decision Making*, especially Chapter 2. See also C. West Churchman, "On Large Models of Systems," *Internal Working Paper No. 39*, University of California, Berkeley: Space Sciences Laboratory, June 1966, for a discussion of the general point presented here.
15. "While there are only about 30 possible moves in an average chess situation, a consideration of all possible replies, and so on, leads to a number on the order of 10^{120} paths from the initial state to terminal states in chess." Julian Feldman and Herschel E. Kanter, "Organization Decision Making," in James G. March (ed.), *Handbook of Organizations*, Chicago: Rand McNally, 1964, p. 615.
16. Richard Cyert and James March, *A Behavioral Theory of the Firm*, New York: Wiley, 1964.
17. For a case example see R. M. Cyert, W. R. Dill, and J. G. March, "The Role of Expectations in Business Decision Making."
18. Roland N. McKean, *Efficiency in Government Through Systems Analysis*, New York: Wiley, 1964, and Russell Ackoff, *Scientific Method: Optimizing Applied Research Decisions*, New York: Wiley, 1958.

~20~

Economies of Scale in Outpatient Medical Practice

Richard M. Bailey

Almost every recent major speech or article by persons interested in the organization and delivery of health services has referred to the term "economies of scale." Careful analysis of these uses of the concept quickly reveals that the meaning either is not well understood or that differing interpretations are used to support disparate positions or philosophies. Clearly the concept needs concise definition if it is to function usefully. This chapter attempts to define the concept "economies of scale" as it is conceived in the literature of economics, to discuss the uses (or misuses) of the concept in the field of health care, to consider proper applications of the concept to the production of health services, and finally to relate the concept to some empirical data recently collected by the author as part of a research project designed to measure scale economies in the practice of internal medicine.

The concept of economies of scale derives from that area of economics concerned with understanding the activities and operations of productive enterprises—microeconomics. The concept is a significant component of microeconomics because it attempts to explain how various resources may be combined within any given firm in the most efficient manner. It is apparent from observation of the economy in general that the number and size of the firms that constitute different industries vary widely: the automobile and steel industries have few firms of giant size; the retail food industry has many firms of relatively modest size; the television repair industry has many firms of small size. A fundamental postulate is that each firm within the industry seeks to find the optimal size to maximize long-run profits—the objective of the business enterprise. Optimal size differs among the various industries, however, because of many factors such as the relative price of the goods and services used in the production process, the size and location of markets, and so on. But for the individual firm it should be emphasized that profit alone motivates finding the "correct" combination of inputs—land, labor, and capital—to produce the desired product at the lowest unit cost. Obviously the different combinations of inputs available to the firm to yield the desired product are many, but only the optimal combination yields the maximum profits. This, then, is what is generally referred to as economies of scale—the search for that size of productive enterprise that uses the optimal combination of inputs to obtain highest rate of return.

Economists believe that initially most industries are subject to increasing returns to scale (as size increases, efficiency increases: so unit costs decrease and profits rise). Beyond some point, constant returns to scale set in (i.e., there are no further economies of scale—when output is increased in any proportion, there is also a proportionate need to increase all inputs). Finally, decreasing returns to scale occur beyond a certain size of firm where centralization of authority causes inflexibility and rigidity; here the costs of producing additional output rise and diseconomies become apparent.

Usual attempts to measure economies of scale empirically center around two types of data: rates of return on invested capital (profitability) and physical volume of output resulting from a given quantity of one or more inputs (productivity). Profitability is the measure most frequently used to analyze economies of scale among firms in an industry because of the availability of financial data collected and published in numerous reports to stockholders, trade associations, and governmental statistical agencies. The profits of firms, moreover, can be viewed as a measure of collective efficiency. That is, even though certain activities of the firm may be inefficient and unprofitable, the final profit data are cumulative evidence of over-all efficiency in all production and marketing operations.

One prominent economist, George Stigler, has argued that a good measure of scale economies in a given industry can be found by observing the changes that occur in the size groupings of firms over time.[1] In effect, Stigler's survivorship principle explains that as changes in technology, resources, and markets arise, the effects are felt by individual firms though changes in production costs and profits. Firms that adapt to the new conditions become more profitable vis-à-vis their competitors—often through altering their production methods and scale of activities. Firms that are slow to adopt new production techniques eventually fail or are merged into other firms as a means of retaining a favorable competitive position. Thus over time the goal of profits forces firms to change their scale of operations and the most efficient size of firm becomes evident by observing industry trends.

Efforts to analyze the efficiency of firms in an industry by focusing upon productivity rather than profits are fraught with many problems. First, most firms in an industry do not produce the same mix of products. Many product lines may overlap, but except in rare cases each firm emphasizes one or more groups of products in which it possesses certain competitive advantages. A chemical company is not a chemical company is not a chemical company (with all due apologies to Gertrude Stein), though each may be classified as a member of the chemical industry. Second, even though similar products are produced, it may be extremely difficult to assign production costs to a given process and make cross-firm comparisons; e.g., how are overhead costs allocated? Finally, there is the issue of what is needed to produce the final product: The important objective, after all, is the product the customer buys. Each firm has resources different from its competitors—more capable managers in Department A, less skilled machinists in Department B, and so forth. The efficiency of individual activities is of real interest to the corporate executives who have production line responsibilities *within* the firm. But measures of efficiency that are important *between* firms are directed to final products or a mix of products, not to steps in the production process. Since these measures of efficiency are combinations of a conglomerate mix of activities that literally are impossible to measure empirically by counting detailed units of inputs and comparing them with units of output, one is almost forced to fall back upon the all-inclusive measure, profitability. In summary, economies of scale that exist between firms in a given industry generally can be examined more readily through financial data than by focusing upon specific inputs and outputs in the production process.

In the field of health care, the concept of economies of scale is frequently used to mean something quite different from that described above. Some people—notably physicians—are primarily interested in increasing income by achieving economies of scale in the microeconomic sense; others are more interested in the greater possibilities for increasing physician productivity. The physicians, as producers of medical services, are attuned quite legitimately to costs of production and level of income.* Taking a Stiglerian view of outpatient medical practice as an industry, it is evident that the long-run trend is toward practice organizations of larger scale. Coupling this trend with data frequently reported showing that physicians in groups earn higher incomes than those in solo practice,[2] an economist may readily conclude that his understanding of the effect of the profit motive on individuals and organizations has again proven itself: Economies of scale must exist in outpatient medical practice because over time more physicians are practicing in larger organizations; the higher incomes of group physicians not only explain the motivation for changing the scale of practice but are reflections of the changing technology and methods of producing medical services that are responsible for generating the higher physician incomes.

When considering economies of scale in medical practice, a significant but often overlooked point is that of changes in the number of services that may be offered as practice size increases. The typical solo practice is limited in the number of services that can be produced. Most services connected with patient care require the direct involvement of the physician in the production process. All services that require special equipment or technically trained personnel must be obtained outside of the practice. In essence, one might say that diseconomies of scale appear to exist in solo practice in that many inputs, mainly laboratory or x-ray services, cannot be economically incorporated into the production process of the practice.

As practice size increases, one of the first noticeable changes in most medical groups is the inclusion of a laboratory. Reasons for adding a laboratory as part of the practice are many and varied, but the crucial point is that it enlarges the variety of services to be produced and sold by the practice. In the process of adding a laboratory, some substitution of paramedical personnel time for physician time doubtless occurs. Multispecialty clinics almost always add x-ray facilities also. The x-ray unit, like the laboratory, adds to the variety of inputs that the individual physician has at his disposal to use in producing medical services and again offers the possibility for substitution of paramedical personnel time and capital equipment usage for physician input. The difficult question at issue, though, is how much do these

* It should not be interpreted that this argument hinges upon physicians being profit maximizers in the normal meaning of the phrase. But, it is contended that after a physician has decided how he may like to practice medicine (solo, group, hospital-based specialist, etc.), he will behave like other professionals — attorneys, university professors, and others — in attempting to maximize his income. Income may not be a primary objective, but it is a strong secondary one.

changes in production possibilities (substituting other personnel and equipment for physician time) really increase efficiency in physician productivity? Although an initial response might be that physician productivity would inevitably increase, at least two other alternatives should be considered: One, given the extreme difficulties in measuring productivity using the physical inputs and outputs technique mentioned above, the only other option is to use income data. But income data in larger groups reflect a composite of the entire medical practice activities. Thus, to the extent that the laboratory and x-ray functions are profitable to the medical practice, income differences among various scales of practice may be influenced more by the profits earned by these adjuncts than by increased physician productivity. Second, the difficult and largely unresolved problem of quality differences must be considered. If the greater variety of inputs available in the larger scale practices is used primarily to improve the quality of medical services produced, the productivity of physicians may not be increased—at least as far as the economist can measure and define productivity. Several open-ended questions thus remain that are not easily answered at this point but are reconsidered later.

Consumer representatives, governmental agencies, and most socially motivated people concerned with the field of health care generally use the term economies of scale to include a broader set of ideas than a mere lowering of the costs of producing medical services. Because these individuals are more consumer-oriented, their concern over physicians' proper organization to realize the advantages of economies of scale does not stop at the point of lower production costs but extends to an even higher objective—that these scale economies be passed along to the consumer. These interest groups are concerned with promoting economic efficiency within outpatient medical practices as a means to an end, not as an end in itself. More specifically, their focus is upon economic efficiency as it affects the pattern of resource allocation in the economy as a whole, not just within the medical practice. This concept falls within the purview of welfare economies where the criterion of efficiency applied is not profits but whether a particular pattern of resource allocation is preferable to another as it affects consumer well-being. The notion of economic efficiency as used in this context would declare that a particular distribution of resources (e.g., 90 % of all physicians practicing solo and 10 % in groups) would be efficient if and only if it is not possible to make one person better off without making anyone else worse off by altering the production process. An increase in the efficiency with which medical services are produced through grouping of physicians in a clinic in this example could result in more total services being provided to patients—without increasing the burden upon physicians or their assistants—and, hence, yield an increase in the total satisfaction of consumers. An emphasis upon reallocation of physician resources into larger practice organizations appears to be sought by the above-mentioned groups with this specific objective in mind: to improve the well-being of the patient–consumers at no extra cost to the physician–producers.

It is obvious from this discussion that producers and consumers interpret the term—economies of scale—quite differently. As long as these separate views are obscured by a common term imperfectly understood or defined, there is a danger that the actions of the various parties may lead to eventual open conflict. At that time the separate interpretations of economies of scale will be made clear. But by that time it may be too late to reconcile opposing views on a sensible basis—hence the plea for better understanding and communication now.

The rationale used repeatedly by medical spokesmen to preclude further governmental involvement in the practice of medicine is that such interference with the free market process is unnecessary because of the high degree of competition that exists in this service industry.[3] By assuming a high degree of competition, a tight economic argument can be developed to show that the activities of the physician–producers will be harmonious with the best interests of the patient–consumers. This is so because it is a basic tenet of economic theory that the necessary conditions for an efficient pattern of resource allocation (the welfare economics view) are satisfied in a perfectly competitive economy.[4] The key properties of a perfectly competitive economy (or industry) as summarized in a leading economics textbook are:

> 1. All factors and commodities are sold at fixed prices which are the same for every buyer and which no individual buyer or seller can change.
> 2. In the long run there is an equality of quantity supplied and quantity demanded for all products, with the prices at which this occurs being the minimum possible prices at which the producers would be willing indefinitely to supply these products.[5]

Anyone reading this quotation necessarily will be hard put to cite a number of industries to which these properties can be applied. There are few. The quotation must be viewed as a theoretical proposition that is only more or less approximated in real life. At the other theoretical end of the spectrum we have those industries in which the seller is so large and powerful that he dominates the market, fixes all prices rigidly, and produces what he wants to when he wants to—the true monopolist. In such cases economic efficiency and consumer well-being are adversely affected. Most firms and industries lie somewhere along the spectrum between these two extremes of perfect competition and monopoly. The point that needs making here, though, is that by any reasonable economic criteria one can gather, outpatient medical practice in the United States today can hardly be called a sharply competitive industry.

Most economists who have written on the topic regard medical practice as a highly monopolistic industry,[6] but in fairness it should be said that most of these men have taken a sweeping overview of the entire profession. A more correct interpretation of the outpatient medical practice industry is that it embodies many elements of monopolistic competition—i.e., each seller (physician) is in competition with a limited group of other sellers with regard to some services and with different sellers for different aspects. This then implies that a considerable amount of market power is held by the physician–producers although a high degree of competitiveness exists in some areas. The significance of this statement should not be overlooked. If outpatient medical practice is made up of many organizations engaged in monopolistic competition, then the statements of medical spokesmen are misleading; e.g., consumer well-being cannot be maximized by producers acting with the belief that what is best for them is best for their patients.

Proceeding one step further, those persons interested in promoting the growth of large-scale outpatient medical practices to achieve scale economies—with the expectation (or hope) that efficiencies so gained will result in lower prices for medical services—are likely to be disappointed. If scale economies are present, but physicians act like competitive entrepreneurs and take essentially what the market will bear, gains from improved efficiency will be absorbed by the physician–producers and not passed back to the consumers. If the market in which outpatient medical services are sold is really competitive, the physician–producers will not be able to benefit personally from scale economies except in the short run as one or more physicians develops a production-increasing or cost-reducing lead over his competitors. On the other hand, if the market in which outpatient medical services are sold is of the monopolistic competition type, changes in medical practice organization that yield scale economies will redound primarily to the benefit of the physician–producers. These benefits, of course, can be of several types: more (or fewer) patients may be treated, incomes may rise, prices may not be lowered, more leisure time may be taken by the physicians, or some combination of these alternatives may occur.

At this point it may be valuable to introduce some data gathered by the author during April 1967. The data were collected as part of an ongoing research project concerned with empirical measurement of economies of scale in the practice of internal medicine.* Approximately 90 internists engaging in fee-for-service practice in the San Francisco Bay Area are cooperating in the study. The size and distribution of the outpatient practices ranges from several solo practices up through four multispecialty clinics in which as many as 30 or more physicians are employed. Although the primary focus of the study is on the activities of internists, there are so many areas of similarity and overlap between the medical and surgical specialties that generalizing from the data on internists to include other physicians can be justified easily.

It is the intent in this section of the chapter to test a number of hypotheses that flow from the observations and theories discussed above against data from the study. Before evaluating data, though, it may be worthwhile to summarize a few of the foregoing statements and hypotheses.

First, it is asserted that outpatient medical practice is not highly competitive—it contains many elements of monopoly that give the producers considerable power to decide what medical services will be produced, what prices will be charged, and what inputs will be used in the production process. Second, it is recognized that there is a great range in the size of outpatient medical practice organizations with a notable tendency for practices to become larger. Especially notable is the trend away from solo practices. Third, as practice size increases, physician incomes rise on average and physician income is deemed an appropriate criterion for measuring the effects of economics of scale. Fourth, the higher incomes of group physicians may be due partly to economics of scale and partly to the enlarged opportunity to sell other services as integral inputs of the production process, i.e., a bundle of services (notably laboratory and x-ray) rather than physician services alone. Finally, in light of the market power of physicians noted in the first argument above, one should not expect to find that economics of scale achieved by physicians in the larger practice organizations will necessarily be passed on to the patient. The suboptimizing objectives of a higher income or shorter work week for the physicians may well take precedent over the optimal societal objective of increased consumer satisfaction.

* This research is supported by the USPHS, Division of Medical Care Administration, Health Economics Branch, Grant No. CH–00232.

TABLE 1. *Revenues, Income, and Working Hours of San Francisco Bay Area Internists, April 1967*

I	II[1]	III[2]	IV[3]	V[4]
Practice Size	*Average Revenue per Internist*	*Average Profit per Internist*	*Average No. Hours Worked per Internist*	*Average Profit per Hours Worked*
Solo	$4777	$3090	225	$13.73
2-man	5842	3644	223	16.34
3-man	6107	3389	208	16.29
4-man[5]	4973[5]	2971[5]	207[5]	14.35[5]
5-man	6441	3900	195	20.00
6–10-man clinic	6750	3742	187	20.01
11–15-man clinic	6676	3221	203	15.87

Data from 70 internists:

[1] Revenue data are based upon the total productive effort of the physicians during April as reflected in dollar billings for services rendered, not cash payments received.

[2] These figures may not reflect the exact distribution of income to each internist because of the unit of measure noted in footnote 1 and also because the income-sharing arrangements in multiphysician groups are based upon partnership agreements that may divide income on grounds other than straight production.

[3] The hours worked data were obtained from special diaries maintained by each internist for each day of the month and include time spent on research, study, hospital staff meetings, practice-connected travel, etc., as well as on direct patient contact activities.

[4] This is computed by dividing Column III by Column IV.

[5] For purposes of analysis, the 4-man practice data are excluded from consideration. The reason for such exclusion is that in all of these practices at least one of the four physicians was substantially underemployed during April 1967. Each of these practices had been 3-man partnerships until Summer 1966, when a new, young man joined as an employee–prospective partner. The expectation was that in a short time these physicians would have a practice load comparable to that of the senior partners. This was not the case by April 1967. Thus, even though the hours worked per internist were comparable to other size practices, the patient load and revenue data were distorted by the underemployment of the junior men.

Table 1 presents completed data on income and length of working hours during April 1967 for 70 of the 90 internists participating in the study. Rejecting the data on revenues and profits of internists in the 4-men practices as abnormal (see footnote 5 in Table 1), the revenue data in Column II seem to indicate that economies of scale exist among the various sizes of practices. Although average dollar production and practice size increase concomitantly, profit increase is not as steady. This discrepancy between dollar production and profit growth rates results from the higher overhead expenses that accompany increases in size of practice. Thus, dividing income by the average number of hours worked per internist generates these observations:

1. Using income per hour worked as a criterion of the most efficient scale of medical practice, it appears that there is no one optimum size of firm.

2. The significant breaks in income per hour between the solo and 2-man practices and the 6–10- and 11–15-man clinics may indicate the presence of diseconomies of small and large size, respectively. Neither observation is surprising. In most industries a large variety of different-size firms can be found coexisting with one another at any one time. As Stigler notes, "This persistence can only be explained by the fact that there is more than one optimum size."[7] Since each firm has a somewhat unique set of resources and product mix, efficiency as measured by profits may reflect many different patterns of production that may be optimum, each in its own right. Caution, of course, also must be exercised when interpreting the significance of the breaks in income, particularly among the larger practices, because the data cover only one practice each in the 5-man and 6–10- and 11–15-man clinic groupings. At the lower end of the size spectrum, though, the extent of diseconomies in solo practices is quite clear-cut.

Table 2 contains a disaggregation of sources of revenue earned by the internists in the study and focuses attention upon the various

TABLE 2. *Sources of Internists' Revenue by Per Cent, April 1967*

	Revenue from Personal Services						
I	II	III	IV	V	VI	VII[1]	VIII
Practice Size	*O.V.*	*A.E and C.H.P.E.*	*H.V.*	*H.C.*	*Revenue from Lab & X-ray*	*Other Revenue*	*Total*
Solo	33.5	13.7	34.6	3.1	4.8	10.3	100.0
2-man	26.2	12.5	23.1	3.1	18.5	16.6	100.0
3-man	27.1	16.2	20.2	2.7	20.4	13.4	100.0
4-man	28.0	11.5	19.9	3.5	26.0	11.1	100.0
5-man	25.8	12.9	18.7	3.6	28.3	10.7	100.0
6–10-man clinic	26.8	14.1	9.9	0.5	36.5	12.2	100.0
11–15-man clinic	26.7	12.7	10.6	1.6	38.9	9.5	100.0

Abbreviations: O.V. — office visit; A.E. and C.H.P.E. — annual examination and complete history and physical examination; H.V. — hospital visit; and H.C. — house call.
Data from 70 internists:
[1] Includes revenues from injections, EKG, and miscellaneous.

methods by which physicians in different scales of practice use the productive resources available to them.* For example, in this study it was found that every practice of three or more internists either had a laboratory within the offices or a financial interest in a laboratory in the immediate vicinity to which patients were referred. In the 2-man practices, about 60% had such an arrangement. Since the use of the income criterion as a measure of economies of scale includes all activities of the practices, the larger practices were found to use a greater mix of inputs in the production process. Accordingly, Table 2, Column VI, shows that a significant factor contributing to physician incomes in all practices of two or more internists is revenue from laboratory services. Solo practices too small to support a laboratory profitably show very little revenue earned from this activity. The contrast between solo internists and others also shows up markedly in the measures of revenues received from office visits and hospital visits (Columns II and IV, respectively). The solo internist has essentially one thing to sell—his personal services. Internists in the larger practices, by internalizing laboratory and x-ray facilities within the firm, are selling a bundle of services of which many are provided by other personnel.

Linking the data from Table 2 with those from Table 1, we are able to explain the greater profit per hour of work in the multiphysician practices as due in large part to profits from laboratory and x-ray facilities. The greater number of inputs sold by the internist increases the total price of a patient visit in the larger practices. The solo physician, on the other hand, loses this revenue because he must refer his patients elsewhere to obtain these input services. As size of the physician organization increases, the bundle of services that can be profitably sold likewise increases.

On the other side of the coin, the much larger share of revenue earned by solo internists from hospital visits—especially when contrasted with the largest clinics—exhibits another interesting point. The solo internist may find it necessary to hospitalize patients more frequently

* In the production of medical services the physician's role is that of an agent for the patient. He combines his own skill and knowledge with inputs of other services that he deems needed to produce an effective diagnosis or treatment—the patient does not purchase these services independently. Output of medical practice is defined here as those units of physician-patient contact (office visits, for example) that result in the use of various inputs (physician time, laboratory tests, injections, etc.). Thus laboratory and x-ray services produced in the practice are viewed as inputs to the production process. The inclusion of such inputs by the internist in his treatment of patients amounts to a sale of additional services and adds to the internists' contribution of revenue in the practice. The costs of such service inputs are charged against the internists as part of overhead.

than other physicians do to obtain detailed diagnostic information. Also, he may have more elderly patients, on the average, which would increase the incidence of hospitalization. As a result, his volume of hospital visits and share of income accruing therefrom is high. In the clinics many diagnostic procedures frequently can be done on an outpatient basis using the extensive laboratory and x-ray facilities that are available. Thus there are two kinds of trade-offs that seem to occur among the small- and large-scale practices: on the producer side, income from hospital visits vs. income from the sale of laboratory and x-ray services; on the consumer side, diagnostic workups done in the hospital as an inpatient vs. in the clinic as an outpatient. The implications of these kinds of trade-off in terms of the most efficient allocation of resources are interesting to speculate upon but are beyond the scope of this chapter.

One of the primary factors stimulating interest in economies of scale is the quantity of medical services that can be produced. More specifically, there is great interest in increasing physician productivity so that the total volume of medical services produced per physician can be enlarged. In this context, physician services are viewed as a vital component of medical services—obviously they are not the only component. Table 3 measures the units of service that the internists produced during April 1967. Essentially these are output units that involve physician–patient contact; other units of service that can be viewed as inputs to the production process are not considered. No attempts have been made to assign weights to these output units, although it is recognized that the average time spent per physician is greater for some services than for others.

It is clear from Table 3 that the average number of patient contact services produced by solo physicians was above that of internists in any other practice size classification. Even if weights were assigned giving due credit to the longer periods of physician time used in producing examinations, the solo internists would still lead. In the classifications of hospital visits and house calls, the pattern of the physician-produced service units is most marked. Here it is most evident that internists in the two largest multispecialty clinics produce a relatively small number of hospital visits and house calls. Physicians in the 2–5-man groups have similar production patterns in the hospital visit and house call categories.

The data can be explained in several ways, depending upon one's point of view: (1) The solos and small practice physicians are "patient-oriented" while the larger practice physicians are "technically or science-oriented"; (2) there is not a direct correlation between the

TABLE 3. *Physician–Patient Contact Services, San Francisco Bay Area Internists, April 1967*

Practice Size	*Average Physical Units of Services Produced*[1]				
	O.V.	*A.E.*	*C.H.P.E.*	*H.V.*	*H.C.*
I	II	III	IV	V	VI
Solo	215	10	15	142	11
2-man	165	14	12	77	16
3-man	176	15	18	97	12
4-man[2]	154	10	10	81	13
5-man	201	—— 32[3] ——		86	15
6–10-man clinic	207	11	27	30	3
11–15-man clinic	173	20	9	28	5

Abbreviations: O.V. — office visit; A.E. and C.H.P.E. — annual examination and complete history and physical examination; H.V. — hospital visit; and H.C. — house call.

Data from 70 internists:

[1] Although the solo internists represented in the study scored higher than internists in other size practices in terms of "averages," the range of physical units of services produced was much wider than in any other practice size. Comparisons of practices using the median rather than the mean narrows the differences between the solo internists and the other group physicians.

[2] For purposes of analysis, the 4-man practices data should be discounted for the reasons cited in Table 1, footnote 5.

[3] All examinations were merged under one classification.

number of patient visits and the quality of care provided—it may be inverse; (3) the solo and small group physicians have a different type of patient load than do the clinics; and (4) the clinic physicians get the "tougher" cases. When additional data are analyzed, some explanations can be offered that hopefully will be more than pure speculation. Any explanation at this point would have to be subjective. But the point that we need to return to is this: How do the data at hand confirm or reject the hypotheses raised earlier in the paper? Specifically, do economies of scale exist in outpatient medical practice and, if so, are the benefits so gained passed on to the patient?

From the data presented in Tables 1, 2, and 3, the following points seem clear: (1) Economies of scale—as measured by the profit criterion—are present in outpatient medical practices. Since the profit criterion is the one most used by producers with maximizing profits, we may conclude that a definite incentive exists for physicians to practice in medical organizations larger than the solo form. Because the scale economies appear to extend over quite a range, however, it is not clear just what size of practice is optimum in terms of profitability.

(2) In terms of total hours worked per month, physicians in solo and 2-man practices work approximately 15–30 hours longer than those in the larger practices. If a physician desires to maximize income and minimize the length of his work month, a practice size larger than 2 men seems to be in order. (3) The source of economies of scale in outpatient medical practices—again using profits as the measurement criterion—may lie more in the internalized laboratory or x-ray facility than in the production of more units of physician–patient contact services. Whereas solo internists in the study relied upon the sale of their own personal services to generate almost 85% of total revenue, internists in the two largest multispecialty clinics earned only 51% of revenue from such physician–patient contact services. Almost 39% of revenue generated in the largest clinics came specifically from laboratory and x-ray services ordered by the internists and produced by clinic personnel—at a profit, obviously. The ability to sell a complete package of medical services in the clinics can be contrasted with the limited package of solo physician services. The result is higher incomes for those physicians who are in the larger practices. (4) A review of the average total number of unweighted units of physician–patient contact services produced by internists in practices of different size indicates that the solo physician produces the greatest personal proportion of such services. This may or may not represent "good" medical care. But for those who are interested in economies of scale as a means to producing more medical services, it cannot be concluded from these data that the larger practices are accomplishing this end. Rather, physicians in these practices appear to be working fewer hours, having fewer physician–patient contacts, and enjoying more leisure time. In the process they are making higher incomes.

In his excellent book *Ferment in Medicine*, Dr. Magraw summarized a number of views on group practice that should be repeated here. "In theory group practice should lessen overhead expenses by increasing efficiency, should cost the patient less as these savings are passed along to him, and should provide a greater range of service to the patient than would be otherwise available. Actually not all these theoretical advantages hold true consistently, although the last one usually does.

"As in any other element of medical care, group practice can be organized either from the standpoint of the convenience or needs of the doctor or the needs of the patient. When it is organized according to the doctor's needs, it is primarily a scheme for the division of labor... when it is organized from the standpoint of the patient, group practice offers a synthesis of care, and some one physician covers the whole field, drawing on the others as necessary."[8]

In this chapter it has not been possible to discuss the advantages and disadvantages of group practice organizations. Working from a base of economic theory, attention has focused upon the predominant type of outpatient medical practice organization—the fee-for-service practice. Data gathered exclusively from fee-for-service practices in the San Francisco Bay Area have been matched against an economist's interpretation of the incentive and competitive structure of these medical practice organizations with the objective of finding (1) whether economies of scale exist in larger practices, (2) the sources of these economies, and (3) the way in which these economies benefit the physician–producers and the patient–consumers. There is great similarity between these findings and Dr. Magraw's statements.

In deference to the physicians' practicing in fee-for-service groups—both single and multispecialty—the author does not find their behavior to be in any way capricious. Like the producers of most kinds of services—be they professionals or businessmen—there is a strong element of self-interest in the way each organizes its work activities. Many physicians have worked excessively long hours in the past (some still do). Many have had too little time for leisure and study and travel. No one can be condemned in our society for seeking "the good life." However, the hard facts of life in this country today reveal that there is a shortage of physicians. The response to this shortage that is sought by consumer-oriented individuals is to encourage physicians to increase their productivity—to make more medical services available in a given period of time. The data presented in this paper indicate that fee-for-service group practice physicians, especially those in the large groups, may be responding not as the consumers would like but in a contrary manner. This response is made possible by many factors, the most important of which appears to be the ability to maintain (or improve) one's income in the groups by selling a larger bundle of services than is possible in small-scale practice. As a result of making profits upon the scale of these tie-in services, the physician may be able to work fewer hours or see fewer patients.

If consumer-oriented individuals are to achieve their objectives of making more medical care services available through the group practice of medicine, careful attention must be given to the structure of the industry. What types of group organizations are required? How may new incentives be devised to encourage physicians in fee-for-service group practice to produce more patient visit services, not just more services per patient? These groups must make a strong case that they are providing medical care of improved quality or that by having all services immediately available they can save the patient's time or that the number and quantity of laboratory and x-ray services produced along with the visit to the physician are less costly over-all than if purchased elsewhere. Not until such a case is built on these grounds and with considerable supporting evidence will it be clear that economies of scale as they presently exist in medical practice do not shower more benefits upon the physician–producer than upon the patient–consumer. An often and unfairly criticized comment made by my colleague, Joseph Garbarino, merits careful consideration:

"There are undoubtedly increases in efficiency that result from group practice, but there are some offsetting considerations. Supporters of this form of medical organization often point out the advantages that accrue to participating physicians as compared to those in solo practice. These include regular working hours, reduced off-duty hour demands, regular and often lengthy vacations, and participation in formal retirement programs. Note that, considered by itself, each of these acts to reduce the weekly, annual, or lifetime output per physician. Substantial increases in operating efficiency would be needed simply to offset these factors."[9]

If we carefully think through what these statements of the benefits of scale economies mean for consumers, not producers—considering the market imperfections inherent in medical practice and the sub-optimizing profit goals of the physician–producers—how else can we approach the question of who presently benefits most in fee-for-service group practice? The time has come to put on the hat of a cynic from Missouri and demand: "Show me!"

References

1. G. J. Stigler, "The Economies of Scale," *Journal of Law and Economics*, 1 (October 1958), 54.
2. For example, see W. N. Jeffers, "A Financial Look at Internal Medicine," *Medical Economics* (September 4, 1967), 109; A. Owens, "Physicians' Economic Health: Holding Up," *Medical Economics* (December 12, 1966), 80; S. D. Pomrinse and M. S. Goldstein, "The Growth and Development of Medical Group Practice," *Journal of the American Medical Association*, 177 (September 16, 1961), 765; and W. Weinfield, "Income of Physicians," *Survey of Current Business* (July 1951), 9.
3. The position recently expressed by the president of the AMA on the "com-

petitive enterprise" nature of medical practice is one of many examples of organized medicine's belief that the market will resolve all problems. See M. O. Rouse, "Organizing and Delivering Health Care," *Journal of the American Medical Association*, 201, 378.

4. K. J. Cohen and R. M. Cyert, *Theory of the Firm: Resource Allocation in a Market Economy*, Englewood Cliffs, N.J.: Prentice-Hall, 1965, p. 294.
5. *Ibid.*
6. For example, read M. Friedman, *Capital and Freedom*, Chicago: The University of Chicago Press, 1962, p. 137; or R. A. Kessel, "Price Discrimination in Medicine," *Journal of Law and Economics*, 1 (October 1958), 20.
7. G. J. Stigler, *The Theory of Price*, 3rd ed., New York: The Macmillan Company, 1966, p. 158.
8. R. M. Magraw, *Ferment in Medicine*, Philadelphia: W. B. Saunders Co., 1966, p. 246
9. J. W. Garbarino, "Price Behavior and Productivity in the Medical Market," *Industrial and Labor Relations Review*, 13:1 (October 1959), 14.

21

Estimating Costs of Laboratory Error to the Patient

Edward L. Cavenaugh

Economic analysis can aid the manager in his decisions about allocation of resources within a given program, but such decisions depend upon his having adequate data. This chapter is a report of the development of a method for obtaining information on one type of cost that along with other data can be used in determining priorities in the allocation of resources in a laboratory improvement program.

THE LABORATORY IMPROVEMENT PROGRAM

The clinical laboratory is an essential component of the health care system because the physican uses laboratory information about the patient in his diagnosis, treatment, and management of illness. Although standard laboratory procedures are expected to be used, the maintenance of quality control is dependent upon a number of factors—for example, skill, training, and knowledge of the personnel carrying out the tests; handling of the sample from the patient to the laboratory; and variability in the testing materials. Thus one of the management problems of the laboratory is to increase the reliability and accuracy of test results. Because of this variety in the range of factors that can affect the final reliability of information about the patient provided to the physician, broad-gauge efforts are being made by laboratories and by governmental agencies responsible for laboratory control to reduce the probability of error.[1] Error is a relative concept in that the variations found in dealing with biological phenomena must be considered as well as the variation in the reliability of the testing procedures.

Laboratory improvement programs are designed to raise the level of laboratory performance by increasing the accuracy of laboratory-derived information about the patient. The major method by which this mission is operationalized is by using one or more of the following approaches:

1. *Training.* Teaching laboratory workers how properly to perform various test procedures.
2. *Consultation.* Providing expert assistance in solving specific scientific problems encountered in performing laboratory tests.
3. *Licensure.* Requiring each laboratory to be licensed before it can accept and test specimens, or each employee to be licensed before he can perform any test procedure on specimens used in the diagnosis and treatment of patients.
4. *Proficiency testing.* Using "unknown standard samples" to evaluate any laboratory or employee's capability to produce an accurate test result.
5. *Research and development.* Improving test procedures, reagents, processes, and methods for use in routine laboratory operations.
6. *Standardization activities.* Standardizing test procedures, reagents, and methods used in routine diagnostic, clinical laboratory work.
7. *Quality control.* Designing procedures to assure accurate test results or to recognize that a test procedure is "out of control" in time to keep the report from reaching the physician using the information.

The Problems of Resource Allocation

The problem of resource allocation with a laboratory improvement program is difficult in that, in addition to the several program approaches which can be used to improve performance levels of laboratories, there are more than 200 laboratory tests performed in clinical laboratories. Thus there is not only the need to choose the most appropriate program approach from among the several alternatives—i.e., that which will result in improvement in laboratory proficiency—but also the problem of selecting from among the many tests carried out in laboratories in a way in which an optimal return on investment can be realized. For example, for any one test it may require extensive research and development to achieve a minimal change in performance level, while for another test the performance level may be increased greatly by less costly means.

In the laboratory improvement program no data are available to determine costs resulting from problems that remain unabated. Little if anything is known about the "at risk" groups, age differentials, or disease entities most likely to occur or about other losses that will result if program efforts are not effective.

Thus a measure of performance is needed to determine the most productive approach or mixture of approaches that can be applied to some limited number of tests. Systems concepts as described by Churchman[2] provide a basis for viewing each component of the health care system in its relation to its objective. In determining the measure of performance for a laboratory improvement program, the "system" may be defined in several ways: the laboratory itself, the laboratory–physician system, or the laboratory–physician–patient system. If the broader system is used, then the data on the costs of laboratory error to the patient and the society must be determined in order to provide a way of quantifying progress in the laboratory improvement program.

DEVELOPING A MEASURE OF PERFORMANCE

If the laboratory improvement program objective is to make available adequate and accurate laboratory services for all citizens regardless of where they reside in this country, a measure of performance is needed to aid in measuring progress toward this goal. Since the ultimate purpose of the program is to benefit the patient and the society, this can be stated as "minimizing" economic losses suffered by the patient because of laboratory error."[3] Patients' losses, stated in economic terms, can be used to measure each component part of the total system's contribution toward achieving the health care objective. Subsequently, decisions about resource allocations can be made in such a way as to reduce those errors most costly to the patient.

Data Needs

In this study, before an economic measure of patient loss per laboratory error could be determined, the following information was needed: (1) a list of possible consequences of laboratory error; (2) the cost of each such consequence stated in dollar values; and (3) the number of times each such consequence could occur when a laboratory test result was in error.

Consequences of Laboratory Error

A list of consequences was prepared that was believed to be exhaustive but not mutually exclusive. These appear in the appendix to this chapter. A dollar cost was determined for each consequence using various data.[4] For purposes of this study, laboratory error was defined as "any test result which is different enough from true value to cause the medical management of the patient to be different from what it would have been had the true value been known."[5] This broad definition was required in order for each consequence to be judged from a common base.

The number of times a given consequence could occur presented a difficult problem. There are no data available that can be used to make such a determination. It was learned that when a laboratory error occurs, none, one, two, three, or more of the listed consequences could occur. The most logical approach to the problem appeared to be through the use of probability statistics. In other words, information on the likelihood that each consequence would occur given 100 laboratory errors was necessary if any cost data were to be developed. From the data needs as identified, a crude equation was developed for use in solving the problem. The equation is

$$MPC = Pe_1 \cdot Ce_1 + Pe_2 \cdot Ce_2 + \dots Pe_n \cdot Ce_n$$

where:

MPC = most probable cost per laboratory error
Pe = probability that a given consequence will occur
Ce = cost of the consequence stated in dollar values

Data are not available on the consequences of laboratory error, since the error is not generally recognized. However, in their experiences with patients physicians have had to deal with the problems of laboratory error and would be the most likely source of data on the consequences of error. Therefore, a decision was made to use an expert panel of physician–judges to obtain a subjective estimate of the probability of occurrence of each consequence.

To test the feasibility of using such a method in obtaining costs of laboratory error to patients, it was not practical to work with all 200 laboratory tests. A decision was made to use three tests that were believed to be different in their probable cost to the patient, given an error of equal magnitude in each. An expert panel of laboratory directors (seven pathologists, and three M.D.–Ph.D.'s) ranked a series of laboratory tests according to three characteristics: probable impact on the patient if the test results were in error, number of times the test was ordered in relation to all other tests, and the medical specialty most likely to order the test. Three clinical tests were selected that were judged to have a high to low impact on the patient if error occurs. Prothrombin time was judged to have a probable high impact on the patient; blood urea nitrogen, a medium impact; and cholesterol, a low impact. All three were ordered frequently and were familiar to internists, the physician group used to estimate probability of occurrence of consequences of laboratory error.

After the three tests had been selected, a panel of 40 internists was selected and each was asked to give his opinion of how often he thought each of the 11 consequences would occur for each test if there were an error in the laboratory result. The panel was not chosen as representative of all physicians but as experts in the relevant field of knowledge as judged by their certification in internal medicine. Staff members from three different hospitals were included.

It was learned during pretests of the methodology that laboratory error can be either low or high relative to "true" value and that the consequences will differ depending upon whether it is to one side of true value or the other—that is, whether it is a "false positive" or a "false negative" error. For this reason a decision was made to evaluate each test for both kinds of errors.

The physician–judges were asked to give two kinds of information for each test and for each type of error. First they were asked to indicate what they would do if a report came in from a laboratory that was presumed to be correct but was actually of a certain magnitude of error. For example, if the test result had been significantly different from what they had expected, they might order more tests or they might not recognize that there was something unusual about the information and they might do nothing. Each of the seven consequences was not independent of any other but represented what would have occurred as a result of the first decision about the laboratory test. From this information an estimate was made of the number of times a particular consequence was likely to occur given a single laboratory error. An arithmetic mean was derived from the responses of the 40 physicians (Table 1, Column 1). Then the physicians were asked to estimate how often those events would occur per 100 laboratory errors. This provided a probability estimate of the likelihood of occurrence of each event (Table 1, Column 4).

TABLE 1. *Most Probable Cost of a Laboratory Error by Event, and Total Cost per Error for Each Laboratory Test Evaluated*

Prothrombin Time — Erroneously High

Event	(1)[a] *Number of Events per Error*	(2)[b] *Cost per Event*	(3)[c] *Total Cost of Event*	(4)[d] *Probability Event Will Occur*	(5) *Cost per Error*
1. Nothing	—	—	—	—	—
2. Repeat test ordered	1.35	5.34	7.21	78.4	5.65
3. Battery of tests ordered	1.28	7.80	9.98	15.5	1.55
4. Extra appointments	0.95	7.50	7.12	42.3	3.00
5. Unnecessary drugs	0.50	1.34	0.67	23.9	0.16
6. Unnecessary procedures	0.18	20.67	3.72	3.1	0.11
7. Unnecessary hospitalization	1.60	52.67	84.27	39.0	32.86
8. Temporary disability	1.58	22.56	35.64	36.4	12.90
9. Partial permanent disability	2.60	67,428.00	175,300.00	—	1,753.00
10. Total disability					
Income loss	1.00	67,428.00	67,428.00	—	674.00
Extended care	1.00	45,000.00	45,000.00	—	450.00
11. Death — income loss	1.50	67,428.00	101,442.00	—	1,011.00
				Total cost	3,944.00

[a] Compiled from completed interview forms and divided by the number (40) of judges to obtain an average number of events per error.
[b] Obtained from the three hospitals serving in the study. The cost shown here is an average cost for the three hospitals surveyed.
[c] As is.
[d] Represents the arithmetic mean as determined for the 40 judges.

Data Tabulation

The formula $MPC = Pe_1 \cdot Ce_1 + Pe_2 \cdot Ce_2 + \cdots Pe_n \cdot Ce_n$ was used as the basis for arriving at a cost per error for each of the tests evaluated. The procedure used is best described by an example. For Event 2, "repeat test ordered. (original test result is questioned because of history and physical findings),"* the total number of times a repeat

* See the appendix to this chapter.

test would be ordered was divided by the number of judges (40) to arrive at an average number of repeat tests per error—in this case 1.35 (Table 1, Column 1). The average cost per laboratory test being repeated ($5.34) was multiplied by the number of tests per error (1.35) to obtain a total cost ($7.21) for repeat tests per error (Table 1, Column 3). This total cost of the event was then multiplied by the probability that a repeat test would be ordered to obtain the probable cost per error for that particular event (Table 1, Column 5).

FINDINGS AND IMPLICATIONS

When costs per error for each test had been stated in economic terms, errors in prothrombin time tests were found to be much more costly to the patient than errors in either blood urea nitrogen or cholesterol (Table 2). Thus subjective probability can be used to provide an approximate base for assigning an economic value to the probable costs of laboratory error. This, in turn, provides a measure of performance for allocation decisions within a laboratory improvement program.

The 40 interviews conducted in this study indicated to the investigator that the private sector of medicine is aware of the difficulties in rationalizing the patient care system and, although they recognize that their individual responses are educated guesses, they are willing and able to provide information that will aid in developing needed data. The development of a method for obtaining cost data used in setting priorities and allocating resources that is stated in terms of the cost to the patient and the society provides a base for making decisions with the larger system in mind.

Cost per error depends upon what is included in the system studied. For example, to determine the costs of laboratory error to the laboratory subsystem, one cost figure is used. If, however, the system is expanded to include hospital, drugs, physicians, and patient, the result is a much higher figure and a clearer picture of the true cost of laboratory error. In prothrombin time, when the total system is included (the patient plus all of the other costs), the average cost per error reaches a staggering total of approximately $7500. Table 2 shows the probable cost per laboratory test error according to the unit of analysis.

Cost per error when the total system is included demonstrates what would otherwise be lost when program-planners fail to attach a monetary value to all measurable effects of error. The difference between an average cost per error of $5.75 in Table 2A and $7557 in

TABLE 2. *Probable Cost per Laboratory Error for Three Tests by Direction of Error and Unit of Analysis*

Test	*High*	*Low*	*Average*	*Priority Rank*[a]
A. Repeat Tests and Battery of Tests[b]				
Prothrombin time	7.00	4.50	5.75	3
Blood urea nitrogen	20.00	11.00	15.50	1
Cholesterol	13.50	4.00	8.75	2
B. Repeat Tests, Battery of Tests, Physician Visits, Drugs, Medical–Surgical Procedures, Hospitalization, and Extended Care[c]				
Prothrombin time	493.00	1,729.00	1,111.00	1
Blood urea nitrogen	290.00	1,589.00	939.50	2
Cholesterol	76.00	598.00	337.00	3
C. Repeat Tests, Battery of Tests, Physician Visits, Drugs, Medical–Surgical Procedures, Disability, and Death[d]				
Prothrombin time	3,944.00	11,170.00	7,557.00	1
Blood urea nitrogen	1,056.00	9,007.00	5,032.00	2
Cholesterol	420.00	3,421.00	1,921.00	3

[a] Priority rank is based on average cost per error to the patient.
[b] Includes costs for Events 2 and 3 (see the Appendix to this chapter).
[c] Includes costs for Events 2–7 plus extended care costs for Event 10 (see the appendix to this chapter). These are all "direct" costs by definition.
[d] Includes costs for Events 2–11 (see the Appendix to this chapter). These are direct and indirect costs of laboratory error.

Table 2C reflects the difference in perspective that the legislative bodies and the public would never be aware of if an economic value were not assigned to "life and limb." Of course, any monetary value ascribed to life is an arbitrary one at best. Nevertheless, if the same value is used throughout the analysis of a given program, it will indicate where to allocate resources for the greatest chance of an optimal return. Without this measure, only a part—and usually a very small one—of the magnitude of a given problem is recognized.

Values and Decisions

The problem of values must be recognized and handled in the use of economic data as a basis for decision-making, especially in the health field. If only economic values were used in laboratory improvement programs, for example, the decision might be reached to put Test A in the lowest possible priority ranking because it is almost exclusively for the diagnosis and medical management of senior citizens. When measured in purely economic terms, the older person's value is small compared to the value ascribed to a person in the 15–24-year age group. Therefore, economic values must be regarded only as a useful tool when allocating resources. In instances involving social values, such as our belief that all of life is valuable and should be maintained to the limit of our resources, the program director can use economic data to see where his resources are going and what is being lost in order to maximize these social values.

Many other considerations are involved in allocation decisions in laboratory improvement: for example, the probability of the error occurring and the causes of such errors and estimation of by how much this probability of error could be reduced. However, without some estimate of measurable benefit, in this case reduction of loss to the patient due to laboratory error, there is no way to compare alternative actions.

SUMMARY

Subjective probability offers one approach to the use of economic analysis in the health field. It lacks the objectivity of other statistical techniques but provides a much more useful approximation of economic costs of illness than any other method available. Knowing the costs associated with illness or "poor health" is the first step toward use of cost–benefit analysis in program justification and optimal allocation of resources within program areas. Data developed in this study showing a cost per laboratory error demonstrated that the use of probability estimates provided a technique sharp enough to show clearly a marked difference in cost per laboratory error. With this technique information can be obtained that will be useful in setting priorities and allocating resources for optimal returns to the system under study.

APPENDIX:

Possible Consequences of Laboratory Error

Event	*Description of Event*
1. Nothing	Medical management of the patient is not changed, test result is disregarded, and no repeat test is ordered.
2. Repeat test is ordered	Original test result is questioned because of history and physical findings.
3. Battery of tests	A more detailed series of tests is ordered to determine validity of the original test. This could also occur if original test result indicated a disease condition not suspected from history and physical findings.
4. Extra appointments with physician	This includes hospital rounds and private office visits required for additional laboratory tests, therapy, and a more detailed diagnostic study.
5. Unnecessary drug therapy	Patient receives medication because of the original laboratory error.
6. Unnecessary medical or surgical procedures	It may or may not involve hospitalization. Examples include transfusions, biopsies, X-ray studies, and appendectomies.

7. Unnecessary hospitalization	Patient is kept in the hospital or admitted because of the erroneous laboratory result. Examples include time required for additional laboratory tests, time required to initiate or stabilize therapy, special facilities needed for diagnostic study, and perform surgical or medical procedures judged necessary.
8. Temporary disability	Impairment to the extent that the person is unable to carry out his usual activity.
9. Permanent partial disability	Impairment of body function to the extent that the person cannot earn a livelihood but can care for himself. Examples would include partial paralysis and mental impairment.
10. Permanent total disability	Impairment of body function to the extent that the individual is unable to earn a livelihood and is unable to perform routine personal care such as eating, bathing, using the bathroom, and dressing himself.
11. Death	When death is attributable to the laboratory error. Examples include transfusion reactions, hemorrhage, and reactions to drug therapy.

References

1. Two major laws have been enacted that put pressure on state and federal governments to become more active in assuring accurate laboratory test results: (1) P.L. 89–97, 89th Congress, July 30, 1965, "Social Security Amendments of 1965." This law requires that any laboratory providing services to recipients of medical care under provisions of this law must meet specified requirements. And (2) P.L. 90–174, 90th Congress, December 5, 1967, "The Clinical Laboratories Improvement Act of 1967." This law gives the federal government jurisdiction over all clinical laboratories engaged in interstate commerce.
2. C. W. Churchman, *Systems Approach*, New York: Delacorte Press, 1968.
3. E. L. Cavenaugh, *The Use of Systems Concepts in Designing a Laboratory Program*, unpublished doctoral thesis, Berkeley: The University of California, 1968.
4. Cost data used were adapted from D. P. Rice, "Estimating the Cost of Illness," *American Journal of Public Health*, 57:3 (March 1967), 424–440; D. P. Rice and B. S. Cooper, "The Economic Value of Human Life," *American Journal of Public Health*, 57:11 (November 1967), 1954–1966; and H. E. Klarman, "Syphilis Control Programs," in Robert Dorfman (ed.), *Measuring Benefits of Government Investments*, Washington, D.C.: The Brookings Institution, 1963, pp. 367–414. Cost data provided from three hospitals representing their charges for hospital stay, drugs, procedures, and laboratory tests. Dr. R. M. Bailey, personal communication on cost per office visit to internists in the Bay Area of California.
5. E. L. Cavenaugh, *The Use of Systems Concepts in Designing a Laboratory Program*.

22

Health Officer Decision-Making: A Case Study

Mary F. Arnold

With our current interest in the rationalization of societal and organizational decisions, it becomes important that we understand more fully the process by which decisions come about. The following case study is a report of the way in which decision-making occurred in a project undertaken by a health officer in a small county health department. Essentially it was a planned exploration by the administrator of the organization's informational resources to assess the feasibility of undertaking a new set of organizational activities.

Although as an administrator the health officer makes decisions for his organization. these decisions are made by an individual problem-solver. Students of decision-making who start with the organization as the unit of study have difficulties in reconciling organizational outputs with individual decision-making models; while those who start with the individual as the unity of study tend to view the organization as a constraint on the individual, thus bypassing the task or mission problem of the organization in which the individual is a member. The former, in defining organizational goals, either takes the administrator's (or those of the top administrative hierarchy) expressed goals as the surrogate for the collectivity's goals or accepts the actual output as representing a consensual goal. Those whose concern is with the individual do not address themselves to the problem of rational behavior for the collectivity, except as they may assume that stability is an organizational goal.

From the point of view of the student of the administrative organization, the problem of compatibility of individual decision-making with organizational decision-making is still an unsolved problem.

INDIVIDUAL DECISION-MAKING BEHAVIOR

Students of individual decision-making have usually concerned themselves with problems of motivation and with the processes of human problem-solving and learning. Newell, Shaw, and Simon's model of human problem-solving is a theory of information-processing behavior, when the system is presented with an actuating stimulus:

> In its simplest aspect, the problem-solving process is a search for a solution in a very large space of possible solutions.... We postulate an information-processing system with a large storage capacity that holds, among other things, complex strategies (programs) that may be evoked by stimuli. The stimulus determines what strategy or strategies will be evoked; the content of these strategies is already largely determined by the previous experience of the system. The ability of the system to respond in complex and highly selective ways to relatively simple stimuli is a consequence of this storage of programs and this "active" response to stimuli.[1]

This theory, however, is concerned only with how information is used to solve a problem. It does not concern itself with the motivational aspects of selective attention to stimuli, nor does it consider the problem of competing stimuli over time. It does not tell us why the problem is defined as a problem to be solved.

MODELS OF DECISION-MAKING

There are two basic models of decision-making, and most discussions of problem-solving and decision-making behavior are based on variations of one or the other position. The first is the rational model, which assumes that the goals or the problem is given and that the organism or system solves this problem by seeking out and selecting an optimal solution to the problem on the basis of rational decision rules. This rational model is compatible with the assumption of the logical positivists that goals are given in the sense that they are ethical in character and cannot be assessed or evaluated in terms of their rationality.

The second model is a heuristic or learning model, in which the problem or goal is diffuse and undefined and the system is seeking a new aspiration level at the same time it is selecting the means of achieving this new state. This model involves two processes: the continual redefinition of preferred goal states, and adaptation of programs of action as new states are determined from the assessment of previous decisions and as new information from the environment is obtained.

These two models are not incompatible with each other, because the rational model can be included as a subprocess of the learning model. Cyert and March, for example, suggest that the firm is an "adaptively rational" system rather than an omnisciently rational system.[2] Gore also discusses these two models and their relationship:

> decision-making is not a smooth-flowing process dispensing choices when and where they are required. Rather it is a twisted, unshapely, halting flow of interactions between people, interactions that shift constantly from a rational to a heuristic mode and back again. Sometimes tortuous, sometimes effortless, these interactions face in two directions at once. First, they must maintain a viable ideology as the basis for energizing the undertaking.... Second, they must maintain an elaborate system of action embodying the requirements of a logical consistency.[3]

In the case study reported here, the project of the health officer could be categorized as planned "intelligence activity" as opposed to "design" or "choice" activity, although all three kinds of decisions are involved in the process.[4]

The health officer's project was stimulated by a contact from a representative of the state health department who indicated that his unit had some money to use in ascertaining what information a local health officer could collect and use in developing a cardiovascular disease control program for the community served by a local health department. Because of the nature and size of the jurisdiction served by this health officer's department,* it had been felt that this might be a feasible place to make such a study, if the health officer were interested.

To fulfill this project, the health officer had two major problems to solve: the generation, selection, and choice of the means by which

* A county health department is generally an administrative unit under the county government; the health officer is usually appointed by the governing body, but there may be requirements as to his qualifications imposed by state (or local) statute. In some counties, such as the one in this study, there may be a professional administrative officer who serves a coordinating and liaison function between the governing body and its various administrative departments.

the desired end could be achieved and the selection of a feasible objective that could be achieved by available means. It can be seen, over the period of the study, that the strategies evoked by the stimuli of new information shifted between means and ends problems.

METHOD OF STUDY

The case study was conducted over a year's time. The investigator became aware of the health officer's plans to undertake the project in its formative stage and obtained permission to study the decision processes in the project after the preliminary ideas had been developed. Data were collected on a periodic basis through 15 taped interviews with the health officer over the period of the project. Interviews were generally two to three hours in length and, during the peak activity of the project, were obtained weekly. Because of heavy pressures on the health officer's time, these interviews often provided the only block of "thinking time" that the health officer could set aside. Since the presence of the interviewer, as well as the recording of the interview, obviously introduced new elements into the process, the interviewer must be considered as part of the interactional setting. However, since the interviewer's comments also were recorded, it was possible to trace certain effects of the interview interaction. Probably the major influence was the time it afforded the health officer to think aloud. Because of this verbalization, fleeting ideas may have become more explicit and fixed and may have been influential in the health officer's decision to defer action at the end of this project. However, since very few health officers have any major changes in agency activities in this particular health area, the writer believes that the interview situation was not a major factor in the final decisions on the project.

The general form of the interview was first to consider what had happened since the previous interview, following which the health officer was asked to project future plans. Occasionally the interviewer asked specific questions about the outcome of previous plans, as a deliberate stimulus; but most often the health officer was not reminded of previous statements nor was the transcript shown to the health officer. The content of the interview sometimes digressed widely from the immediate project activities, but much of this digression provided clues as to how and why decisions of the health officer had been made. All materials produced by the health officer for the project were provided to the interviewer. On two occasions recordings were made of conferences the subject had with outside consultants. This made it possible to have information on the expectations the health officer had of the consultation session before it occurred, on the actual interaction, and on what results followed from the consultation situation.

DECISION PROCESSES OVER THE STUDY PERIOD

Preliminary Developmental Stage

During the first conference with the state health department representative the idea developed that the health officer might personally undertake the project rather than hire another person to do it under direction. The health officer reported:

> I said that it ought to be the health officer, and he said, "Why?" Well, if we got some other physician to do it, it would be somebody coming into the county cold who would first have to learn the county and make contacts with members of the medical society and the hospital administrators and all the voluntary agency executive directors, etc. I thought probably I could do the work more efficiently and faster for a given amount of time and per dollar than anyone that we would hire from the outside who would have to learn the community, its problems, its resources, etc., and make the personal contacts. I saw this as something that would depend a great deal on interpersonal and interprofessional or intraprofessional relationships in the community, because some of the things that we would probably be getting our noses into are rather sensitive areas; for example, looking at hospital records, autopsy records, maybe even looking at the records in some private physician's office.... I felt it had to be somebody whom the medical profession knew and had a certain amount of respect for and trust in.... I pointed out we already had a precedent for an administrative arrangement for lending personnel to some community effort... if I played my cards right, I would probably get the county to let me do something like this, but we would have to have funds under the research contract to allow for hiring another physican in the department half-time... to do some of the routine stuff that requires a physician but not necessarily the health officer. [Tape 1.]

After the preliminary discussions with the state health department representative in March, the health officer talked over the idea of doing such a project with some key professional friends in the community, including several physicians and a voluntary agency executive. But it was not until June that further details were discussed with the state health department representative. Following this second conference the health officer at a routine meeting with the county administrative officer first broached the subject of doing the project within the administrative organization of the county. In the preliminary discussions the health officer sought assurances of support of the project ideas and suggestions as to feasible means of carrying it out. Finally, in August (about five months after the first contact), the health officer prepared the first draft of a grant request needed by the state health department if the project was to be funded:

> Summer was busy as summers always are... so I didn't have very much time, and I'd make a start here and there on writing up a protocol but didn't get very far. But finally I decided time was passing—I've got to take the bull by the horns and get moving on this. I didn't do a thing but, oh, I guess over a couple of weeks... I had been jotting down ideas on paper and thinking a lot. I recall now that I'd been thinking about this protocol a number of times as I stood in front of the mirror in the bathroom in the morning.... Anyway, I finally decided that this had to get done if the project was going to get done, so I just took a Sunday one day when I was not on call and went to the office... I think I spent about seven hours there.... This was just flowing from my fingertip onto the typewriter.... I did very little rewriting, and I had it all ready to be typed up and sent to the State Health Department the next day. [Tape 1.]

After minor suggestions were made by the contracting agency, a second draft of the contract was submitted in September. Once the contract request was submitted, the next problem was recruitment of staff:

> In the meantime one of the things I had to be working on after I got the second draft submitted was to start beating the bushes for personnel. We knew we were going to have to have a clerk on a half-time basis and a half-time physician in the health department. The statistical consultation we weren't too concerned about, because I knew we could get some free from the state health department and we had the money in the budget for other fee-for-consultation basis. [Tape 1.]

However, almost another month went by before the contract from the state health department was received. The next problem that was anticipated was getting approval from the county board of supervisors. Advice was sought from several sources in the community before a formal request was made:

> Well, for better or worse my letter about this contract came up as the very last item on their agenda at 5 o'clock in the afternoon. The letter

> was read; they approved it; it was passed. We couldn't decide whether it was that I had answered all the questions that they possibly could have thought of or they had done all their homework so that they knew what it was all about, or at 5 o'clock they weren't interested in arguing. ...Anyway, it went through very smoothly and without any trouble whatsoever....The contract finally came to us on the 29th of October, dated October 1st, and the board approved the contract and approved its signature by the chairman on the 9th of November. It was only last Friday (December 2) we finally got the four copies of the contract back from the board of supervisors so that we could forward them to the state health department again....I didn't want to proceed spending too much money or hiring people until I was sure we had that contract back signed by the board. [Tape 1.]

The preliminary development of the project and implementation of the contract took about nine months. During that period a specific plan of action had evolved from the original general idea. Once the health officer's interest was stimulated, thought began to develop on how the project might be done. The stimulus had occurred at a time when the health officer was bored with "paper shuffling," and this project offered an opportunity for intellectual stimulation that was congruent with the mission of the organization administered by the health officer. The first major decision that was made was that the health officer would undertake the project personally rather than direct someone else. This decision shaped the specific plan of action since all decisions on the project became those of the health officer, an individual decision-maker, rather than the alternative possibility of having to develop consensual decisions between the person guiding the project and the one executing it.

The strategies called up from the previous experience of the health officer first involved the problem of assuring support from significant persons within the community since the image of the goal of the project called to mind information collection from relatively sensitive sources (i.e., patient records). Exactly what might be involved in a cardiovascular disease control seemed to be implicitly assumed at this stage of the project. Information collection may have been the point of reference at this stage, because of the interaction with the state health department representative, and therefore it was assumed that information about data was what would be funded. The objectives stated in the contract represent a mixture of means and ends:

> 1. To determine what data related to morbidity and mortality from cardiovascular diseases are already being routinely collected in the County.

2. To determine what data are needed by a local health officer for planning programs for the prevention and control of cardiovascular diseases.

3. To identify sources of these needed data in the County.

4. To evaluate these data from the standpoint of: (a) fesasibility of collecting them; (b) their accuracy and completeness; (c) their usefulness for: (1) Immediate program planning, (2) Continuing surveillance, (3) Establishing a baseline profile of the community with respect to cardiovascular disease, (4) Forecasting future needs, or long-range planning.

5. To identify gaps in data needed for effective planning of programs for the prevention and control of cardiovascular diseases.

6. To develop within the Health Department a community-wide cardiovascular disease data index. [Grant Contract of Project.]

The state health department had emphasized the development of an analysis of the community's information system and was willing to contract for such. All parties to the transactions seemed to assume that there was a clear-cut general model for a cardiovascular disease control program; in other words, if information were adequate a program of action would be available. (Later in the project, this assumption was questioned.)

Contact Phase

The first step in the search of the problem space had actually taken place during the preliminary stages of developing the project, when the health officer had thought about where data might be available and had made a preliminary list of potentially available sources of data. These strategies for search came from the intrinsic knowledge the health officer had of the county, of laws and regulations regarding the collection of vital data, and of the patterns of medical care in the community. Once the contract was made final the next major problem was to obtain access to the potential data. Death certificates were immediately available in the health department itself, and these were the first source of data to be used. However, access to other data required permission from other gate-keepers. At a suggestion from the contracting agency, an abstract of the protocol was prepared and mailed with personal letters to key persons:

I have numbered in order of writing and mailing the letters that I have written trying to open doors of access to data. [Tape 1.]

The first group of letters went to the coroner and to the head of a group of pathologists who work with the coroner's office; the next to the medical director of a home care program in the county and to a key hospital administrator. In each case the initial persons to whom letters were sent were well known to the health officer and considered to be "friends of the health department":

> Again I started with the one I knew best.... I have known him for a long time; he has always been most cooperative with the health department. He is a brilliant administrator.... I wrote him that X and Y, two people whom he knows very well, already had a general familiarity with the project. [Tape 1.]

The strategy in gaining access to data was therefore one of expanding upon a trust relationship between professional colleagues:

> All this I said in an attempt to reassure them that only a medical person will be sticking a nose into these records and that no patient-identifying information will be broadcast, more than anything. I am going to have to know patients' names when looking at patient records because if I want to compare, for example, information on a given patient on a death certificate, and there might be a hospital record on that patient, an autopsy report on that patient, and a private physician's office chart on the patient. I will obviously have to know the names or I can't correlate the data. [Tape 1.]

The professional relationship of the physician to his patient is a highly salient value with problems of confidentiality of records and of professional cooperation. It was this particular area of trust that was of greatest concern to the health officer. Much of the health department's activities depend upon having the trust of the medical community. Thus anything that would diminish that trust relationship because of the project had potential consequences for the future activities of the health department. Even the earlier decision that the health officer should be the individual to undertake the project was made with this risk in mind: "I felt it had to be someone whom the medical profession knew and had a certain amount of respect for and trust in." This feeling had been continually reinforced by informal discussions held with consultants during the early, formative stage of the project.

During this initial contact phase the fact that the health officer was interested in problems of cardiovascular disease began to spread within and outside the community. There had been a meeting in October with the physician in charge of a heart unit at the nearby hospital and members of the state health department to which the health officer had been invited and at which some mention had been made of the project. The early informational discussions with various key members of the professional community had paved the way for the more formal contacts by letter. However, the health officer still expressed a great deal of uncertainty about how the medical society should be approached to gain its support:

> I was mainly concerned about whether they would have any objections about letting the health officer stick a nose into medical records in the community.... So far I have only talked about autopsy reports, just private autopsy reports, and patient records in hospital record rooms. I said nothing in this letter to them about maybe wanting to get into records in private physician's offices. This, of course, will be a matter of consent of the individual physician. But I still wanted them to know that only a medical person was going to be looking at these patient records. It wasn't going to be a nurse; it wasn't going to be a social worker, clerk, statistician, or anybody else; just one of their medical colleagues.... Just sort of a reassurance in letting them know really what is going on. [Tape 2.]

A second strategy of maintaining the trust relationships of key groups in the community was the use of the device of an advisory committee. Key individuals were asked to serve, and key groups were asked to name a representative. The advisory committee at this stage was used as a device for maintaining communication and trust with persons felt to be keys of access to information. Later the advisory committee, which actually never met together, was used as a kind of subjective reference group for thinking about what the key members of the community would support in the way of a disease control program:

> It goes without saying that first they should be people officially representing the medical society. Then I wanted people who would have contact with patients with cardiovascular disease...a pathologist because I wanted access to autopsy records and a medical social worker from the welfare department because at the time there was the MAA program. [Tape 2.]

First Learning Phase: Attention to Means

Some three years prior to this project the health officer had been very much interested in the use of computers for medical resords. An image seemed to have been formed by the health officer of a system of strategies for obtaining an ongoing community profile of disease:

> We are just now trying to see where are the data, what are the data, how good are they, can you get to them, or do people object to having you get them, etc. So the basic evaluation of the data or description of the data and then the analysis of the data has to be done to get the community background of the burden of cardiovascular disease in the community.... In other words, the community profile of cardiovascular disease. Okay, you bring that up to date; you bring that up to point A in time. Now, do you then stop and go back to all your old ways of letting data accumulate randomly and scattered here and there if nobody went looking at it and go through this again in five or ten years? Or once you've brought your data up to date at a given point in time, then do you, from that point in time, develop a new method of collecting, filing, storing, analyzing, and retrieving data?... I can't see why it would be such a chore if a physician has a supply of cards or sheets with places to fill in the following: patient's name, age, sex, race, birthplace, occupation, number of years in that occupation, place of residence, number of years in that residence; then presenting complaint, final diagnosis, and have the secretary mail it into a centralized data-processing center in the county once a week. At the end of a month the health officer can get a report: How many cases of this, that, or the other type of cardiovascular disease have we in the County? Where are they? Who are they? etc. [Tape 2.]

This image of a dynamic computerized profile of particular problems in the community was a sort of generalized criterion against which the more specific problems of assessing the availability and validity of the data were evaluated. At a later stage in the project this image changed, but initially it provided the direction for the first part of the learning phase.

The first set of data to be reviewed was that immediately available, the death certificates in the health department. This review revealed several decision problems not explicitly faced before: the decision as to a definition of cardiovascular disease and the problem of assessing the validity of the information, as well as the question of what additional information, not available on death certificates, would be useful in obtaining the hoped for "community profile."

The first problem of definition was solved on a medical–technical basis, but it continued to be a source of uncertainty throughout the project since the condition of the cardiovascular system often was not revealed in autopsy reports; and later attempts to obtain data on morbidity revealed discrepancies between the pathological conditions listed in autopsy reports and the diagnoses entered on the death certificates. The first criterion for validity was a logical validity, particularly following comparison of death certificate information with the autopsy report. But the problem of determining what information would be useful for a "community profile" was not faced in this first review of death certificates:

> So, if we are looking just at death certificates, we want to have some idea of what the duration of cardiovascular disease or cancer was in this individual; the length of time of having the disease presents a burden of morbidity from the disease to the community. You can't get it from the average death certificate. [Tape 4.]

Upon learning how poor the data were on legally required documents, the health officer generalized this learning to other potential sources of data. Informal contacts also acted as reinforcements to this learning. It was at this point in the project that the image of a community profile began to deteriorate. The health officer began to question the validity of nursing home records, as well as of hospital records, except as the information might be collected directly from the patient's attending physician:

> Because I have to feel that somewhere before this project is over we have got to get some sample reporting from physicians, I feel this is the only way we will get an idea of the total load of cardiovascular disease in the community. Death certificates, you have the end; hospitals, you have the late stage; and how are you going to get at the physician's records currently? Now if we ever want to get the load of cardiovascular disease in the community up to a given point in time (which would involve the physician's going back and going through their records to see what they have at this point), this is something else. And I shudder to think about how we would get this information. ... This we will have to work on; we have got to face it if we are trying to find out what a local health officer needs to turn the cardiovascular disease burden in the community and what sort of services this community needs; we have to have this information. So I will have to face this a little later in the project. [Tape 4.]

There was also a great deal of uncertainty in considering strategies for obtaining reports from physicians:

> I haven't quite decided yet whether to ask them to report only on new patients who come to their attention, since I could hardly ask them to go back and pick up all their existing case load of patients with cardiovascular disease. This would be too much, so I will probably ask them if they will report to me on new patients with cardiovascular disease developing in any of their existing patients. I could provide data sheets; all they would have to do is check something or fill in blanks. Their office aides could *almost* fill in these and mail them back probably once a week. [Tape 4.]

Several weeks later the health officer reports on a conference with a consultant, and we find the ideas about sources of data are further narrowed:

> I pointed out that it had occurred to me that every bit of medical information on a patient in a community originates with the physician, and so why go through all this other rigamarole if you can just get physician reporting? [Tape 6.]

As the difficulty of obtaining useful data from existent records became clearer, this gradual shift in strategy became more pronounced. By February 11, in answer to a question of the interviewer—"In retrospect if you had to do the protocol over again for this at this point in time, would you change it any, or not?"—this shift is quite obvious:

> Up to this point I am fairly well satisfied with the protocol. We have presented ideas about all sorts of sources and data that we may not even look at in the end, but at least they come to mind. Better to have everything and then throw out what doesn't seem useful rather than to list just a few things.... Sources of data? Vocational rehabilitation records? Hospital emergency room records? I think I told you last week one internist said not to even bother to look at them... there is nothing in them... medical records in the welfare department related to categorical recipients who need medical care?... I am reserving judgment about those, they may be worthwhile... vocational rehab...? Again that is getting pretty late in the disease.... There's a lot of prior information that's gone before anybody ever gets to vocational rehabilitation.... This vocational rehabilitation record is very superficial, skimpy knowledge, very late in the course of the individual's life history, and of no real value. This is why I say, "it is all going to come back to the physician." [Tape 6.]

However, at this time also the problems of obtaining data began to be balanced against an estimated payoff and cost:

> spot checks, though, are a nuisance to do unless you do this with a lot of different diseases.... The alternative for that would be to simply have ongoing household interviewing the way New York City is doing... so we plan programs on the basis of this information that it takes us a year to gather and summarize, and maybe the facts that the information indicates took place a year before that, so we are now two years behind.... And if you had to put the salary of a statistician into only getting at physicians to report, I think it would be a bad investment. [Tape 7.]

However, payoff implies that there are effects to action, and this becomes a problem of cause and effect. A decision for action is said to depend upon resolution of two kinds of beliefs: that of incidence, or one might call it salience, and that of causality. Throughout this health officer's project these two major aspects of problem-solving entered into the picture. The two images that appeared seemed to be general conceptual frameworks for these two problems within the problem-solving process. As it became more and more uncertain that information regarding incidence and the extent of the problem in the community could be obtained, the attention of the health officer began to focus on the problem of causation and the ends that logically could be achieved by action. The issue of the use of the information became important.

Second Search Phase: Attention to Goals

At about this time another activity in the project was started. A questionnaire was sent to health officers throughout the country to find out what other health departments were doing. Also the ideas of consultants were sought more vigorously, although the study of the death certificates and comparisons with autopsy reports continued.

The review of the death certificates had stimulated the formation of a new image—that of concentration on the etiology of the diseases in question. It became evident that the health officer had two general goals in mind for the health department: stimulating and coordinating community services (other than direct medical care) needed by the patients in the community and initiating preventive programs. For example:

> We will want to know the town of residence; that's basic epidemiology. We need to know where the patients live if we have to provide a service for them. We want to know their occupation and what is the relationship, if any, between occupation and cardiovascular disease. [Tape 3.]

Both these images reflect the health officer's beliefs about the mission of the health department, but up to this point in the project the community profile had been described for the most part in terms of services needed by the patients. Following the initial review of death certificates the epidemiologic interests in terms of etiology began to take primacy. By the middle of March this problem of the ultimate use of the data that might be collected became more salient:

> What will we accept as measures of success of a cardiovascular disease control program? In the first place, what types of cardiovascular disease will we single out for attention? Some of the advisory committee members have said individually, "Why don't we limit ourselves to coronary artery disease, strokes, and generalized arterial sclerosis?" Now this makes sense because it is the bulk of the deaths. Certainly, if we are interested in doing something about premature deaths from cardiovascular disease, the one area in which to work is coronary artery disease because a lot of others occur at the higher age level.... I think that it is totally unrealistic to say our goal should be to reduce premature deaths due to cardiovascular disease. Then we will have to set arbitrary standards of what we mean by premature deaths. [Tape 8.]

Second Learning Phase: Attention to Ends

Following this explication of a more definitive goal, emphasis in the search for information shifted more prominently to the epidemiology of cardiovascular disease. The health officer had begun to seek expert consultation and to search the literature regarding the etiology of cardiovascular disease. In one interview session the health officer gave a complete rundown of risk factors identified with the various diseases in the cardiovascular group, and each was assessed in terms of what could be done:

> Okay, if you find that the lipid factors in the blood led to the thromboses, find the people who have abnormal lipid factors in the blood and do something about them, if you can, if the patient will let you. Hum... obesity? Obvious. Diabetes? Treat it properly. Personality factors? Well, maybe you can and maybe you can't do something there. [Tape 8.]

Additionally, in continuing the review of autopsies and reports of those whose death certificates had no mention of cardiovascular disease, the health officer had found that in nine out of ten cases there was some mention in the autopsy report of at least moderate cardiovascular disease. This new information about the extent of the problem of cardiovascular disease, added to new information from the literature search, posed a new problem.

> It is a different kind of a program problem from setting up special clinics or special home care services for the people who already have advanced cardiovascular disease. So I think the health officer has to decide what kind of program he wants for his community. I think that probably one has to do with both at the same time because it is ridiculous to think about ignoring disease that is already there. These people are human beings; they are suffering; they have to have care and

> attention; we have to do something for them. But on the other hand there is no sense in doing something for these people while, at the other end, we are just continuing to feed into this group people with premature athrosclerotic disease because there is nothing on a preventive level being done earlier in life. So I think the health officer almost has a moral obligation, you might say, to attack both problems simultaneously and from the beginning even though he can only do a small bit in each. [Tape 8.]

The review of data sources continued during March, but the health officer's interest began to shift to how these data might be useful for evaluating the effectiveness of specific control measures that might be undertaken. There was still some concern expressed for the ill person; but the uncertainty of obtaining information about such persons was increasing. The health officer was also beginning to be quite dubious about ever being able to define a clear-cut goal for a preventive program.

> Your control program aimed at risk factors is going to look like heck, so I think that you have to know what you are dealing with anatomically. What is the pathological entity? And I think that this is going to be a difficult thing to do, especially for this county where the numbers are relatively small. It would have to go over a fairly long period of time over which you have to gather statistics; they are less valid because a lot of influences are entering into the picture that are confusing, so that one year is never the same as the year that preceded it. But I am convinced now you can't say that we will have a program to control cardiovascular disease and then we will evaluate it at the end of five years. [Tape 9.]

This period seemed to be the turning point in the project. The general problem space had been narrowed down to consideration of specific action possibilities:

> I am going to talk with A and B about the progress of the project and tell them some of the things that I have told you today, that I think we are all wet talking about a "cardiovascular disease control" program. There have got to be specific programs or specific types of cardiovascular diseases. And this isn't something that you whip through in a few months. [Tape 9.]

Completion Phase

Over a three-month period the process of learning had narrowed down the general problem into a somewhat new and specific image of focusing on particular preventive factors and on estimating payoff for working toward this. Discussions had been held with several of the key persons to whom the health officer had not previously spoken, but by this time the conversations reported were directed at what the health department could be expected to do about cardiovascular disease.

In the meantime changes in the health system itself began to be evident. Medicare had just been initiated, and the heart, cancer, and stroke legislation had been passed and regional medical programs were developing.

> So I feel just a little bit that this Phase I is going to have to slow down and wait until we see which way the medical care picture goes and where we begin to develop records—because it would be folly to say okay we want this thing finished in a few months so we can wind it up. And then in the meantime the whole picture changes because of medicare. We have wasted our time and money on the first phase of the project. In a way I think that the project is about 6 months premature ... we have got all this spade work behind us, and there is no reason why it can't continue, but I think I am going to have to make it clearer to A and B that I don't think that we ought to attempt to wind it up in the next few months. [Tape 9.]

The initial funding period of the project was coming to a close (there had been a two-month extension beyond the first five months planned), and an upcoming conference with the state health department group who had funded the project was, in essence, a request by the health officer for consultation on "where do we go from here?" The uncertainty about what could be done for a program in cardiovascular disease control had become manifest in the discussions held with various expert consultants. One consultant had suggested doing a household survey, but when this suggestion was offered by the health officer in the conference with the state health representatives, it was not picked up by the state health department consultants. During that meeting one person suggested to the health officer that the next step should be for the health officer to arrange data in a cohesive and comprehensive fashion and to come up with some kind of presentation. Although a great deal of verbal support was given to the efforts of the health officer at this meeting, suggestions were left vague and concrete and explicit ideas about project directions were not made. Toward the end of the conference both of the consultants emphasized closure of the data analysis that was in process. In many ways this conference reinforced all the uncertainties with regard to the usefulness of data for program development and evaluation. It was two weeks following this meeting with the state health department that the health officer, in reviewing what had happened, said:

> Oh, I want to sit down and take stock of where I am. I just want to summarize what we have got. Take a look at what we have got as data. And then see where we go from there. In other words, a sort of stock taking of one's self... a self-inventory. This is going to take a fairly large block of uninterrupted time and a large space on which to lay everything out and look and see what I've got. [Tape 11.]

Another two weeks went by, and this time had not been available, although the project had been extended until June 30. The health officer was still contemplating a mailing to internists and general practioners in the area to see whether physician-reporting was feasible. Much of the interview time was taken up with a review of a checklist in preparation to closing off this stage of the project.

An opportunity came up unexpectedly to talk with a group of physicians in a hospital in the county, and this provided the extra stimulus for sending out a questionnaire to physicians. At the same time there was still a great deal of search activity in relation to potential program activities a health department might undertake. Again the etiology of the disease was uppermost in the thinking about project activities.

> We are trying to stay out of epidemiology, but it is terribly hard to because once you have got this information it is just terrible not to be able to see what it is. If we decide this is a feasible method for getting information... and it may not be if the return is poor, unless we are willing to accept something as low as 10, 15, or 20 % return... we may want to repeat the survey, say, next January when the morbidity will be high... if we don't use this method again, by gosh, I'm stuck, I don't know where to go and try to get information... at this point, I feel that what this study is turning into is a study of negative results. We know how bad death certificates are; we know you can't get anything out of emergency room records; we know that you can't get anything out of physician reporting; we know that you can't get anything out of hospitals; so where do you get your information? And what possible use can you make out of whatever you get, considering it is incomplete, both in quantity and quality. [Tape 14.]

Even though there was still a great deal of work to be done on finishing up what had been started in regard to data sources, the general conclusions had been drawn before the final pulling together and report-writing.

A conference in June with another consultant about a feasible health department program once again reinforced the uncertainty about etiology of disease and its control. By late June, in answer to a question by the interviewer as to what had been gotten out of the project, the health officer said:

> I might not have anything to show really on paper; I don't have a lot of fancy statistics; I really don't know what are worthwhile methods of collection of data to look at, at this point; the whole thing is just a jumble. This is good here, and this is there, but nothing adds up to any one good solid method you can use... and in relation to where I ought to be going, I had the feeling that he (one of the consultants) thought the whole thing was kind of futile... in terms of altering human behavior. Probably by the time you get one damaging pattern of living altered something else will come along to take its place.... How do you control or prevent a disease in the early years of life when it is something that you would be perfectly willing to have them die of in later life... in contrast to something else. How can you prevent the premature ones in this and yet try to foster its occurrence in later life? It may be expecting too much. We may increase cancer deaths or accidents because people will be living longer, giving them a greater time in which to act and play their mischief, however they do it. Maybe we can't have our cake and eat it too. [Tape 16.]

This explicit recognition of the value problems inherent in the medical model ideal of preserving life seemed to be the stimulus to end the search for a feasible program. The idea of preventing a premature death implies that some deaths are acceptable while others are not. This opposes the emphasis on preservation of life, which is the medical ideal.

By August there only remained the final preparation of the report. At that stage there was still some thought of action—a feeling that perhaps the information might be presented to the advisory committee for discussion of what might be done in the county regarding the problem. However, there also was real discouragement as to what might be feasible:

> I think that one of the problems is that the things we know have to be done to make any headway are not the things that people like to do or would willingly do readily.... Just the simple problem of diet or more exercise or no smoking or something else. [Tape 17.]

At this point the project was drawing to a close, and other activities began to take precedence. By December, when the final report was completed and submitted to the funding agency, no further action had been taken.

FINDINGS FROM THE STUDY

The decision-maker in this study held a rather general, diffuse model of a possible outcome at the beginning of his project. This was an image of a changing community profile of cardiovascular disease experience from which health department programs and activities would evolve. It was assumed that a cardiovascular disease control program involved prevention of heart disease. With this image in mind the health officer concentrated on means problems as the figure against this large and diffuse area in which the problem solution lay. At first information about means was collected and analyzed in terms of its logic in relation to this first general image. The image, in turn, was revised in relation to the reality of each new bit of information. Concurrently, this information became the stimulus for new kinds of problems to which possible solutions were conjectured: for example, new strategies for dealing with death certificates to solve certain legal problems, epidemiologic studies, and new services that might be developed within the community. Gradually, as the initial image began to deteriorate and become less and less tenable as a feasible outcome, search activity began to focus on new outcome images.

As logical, feasible outcomes became delineated more specifically, the criteria used for assessing the value of means shifted. At the beginning the sources of data had been assessed on their usefulness for creating a "community profile," but later in the project assessment was made on the utility of data sources for demonstrating effectiveness of specific program activities designed to reduce cardiovascular disease.

Throughout the process there was a continual reduction and specification of both the means and end problem spaces to the point where other problems stimulated by the new information brought forth became more salient.

In many ways the over-all problem-solving process that occurred in this case study was not so much one of finding and assessing strategies for solving a problem as one of having solutions or means that are searching for problems they can solve.

In this case the health officer held certain program strategies that related to a particular model of reality, stemming from past actions used to control the spread of communicable disease: The model is that of intervening to alter the host's behavior or that of his environment to change factors "known to cause" the disease. Thus attention was placed on the disease process rather than elsewhere—for example, on the individual having these biologically or medically defined symptoms.

Even the term cardiovascular disease control is a structure for a certain set of strategies.

If—as Newell, Shaw, and Simon suggest—the "stimulus determines what strategy or strategies will be evoked, [and] the content of these strategies is largely determined by the previous experience of the system,"[5] it appears that, at least in this case, the most immediate "stored programs" may be means strategies rather than strategies for developing feasible ends. It suggests also that strategies for defining or identifying the problem to be solved may be quite different from those described by these authors. Evoking stimuli enter into the cognition by way of some model of reality stored in the system; this model structures what is and what is not stimulated as a problem. The heuristic problem-solving process perhaps best describes the process reported here. It involved testing models of reality and finding a feasible problem to which available solutions can be applied.

At the completion of the health officer's project, no feasible problem had been defined. The decision to defer action was really a negative decision, because it probably served as a strategy for dealing with the uncertainties of the environment as well as with the conflict in values that had been made explicit during the learning process. Perhaps much of the time and effort involved in dealing with means problems could have been reduced if the stimulus had not occurred as it did. If the state health department group had hoped to stimulate health department activities around problems of cardiovascular disease in the community through involvement of the health officer in looking at data about the disease, the strategy was unsuccessful. The evoking stimulus set a pattern of problem-solving in a way that called forth strategies on means before the ends problem was adequately clarified.

References

1. Allen Newell, J. C. Shaw, and Herbert A. Simon, "Elements of a Theory of Human Problem-Solving," *Psychological Review*, 65:3 (1958), 159, 163.
2. Richard M. Cyert and James G. March. *A Behavioral Theory of the Firm*, Englewood Cliffs, N.J.: Prentice-Hall, 1963, p. 99.
3. William J. Gore, *Administrative Decision-Making: A Heuristic Model*, New York: Wiley, 1964, p. 21.
4. Herbert A. Simon, *The Shape of Automation for Men and Management*, New York: Harper & Row (Harper Torchbooks), 1965, pp. 53–56.
5. Allen Newell, J. C. Shaw, and Herbert A. Simon, "Elements of a Theory of Human Problem-Solving."

~23~

Health Agency Decision-Making: An Operations Research Perspective

David H. Stimson

Much of the current literature on operations research deals with extensions of theory without reference to their actual use in organizational analysis. The study reported here, however, is an attempt to analyze through the method of operations research the actual decision-making process of a large state health department (hereinafter called Department) in its administration and allocation of the Chronically Ill and Aged Services (CI&A) federal formula grant. This grant resulted from Congressional legislation designed to "increase the availability, scope and quality of outside-the-hospital services for the chronically ill and aged." The study should be regarded as an exploratory study in the use of operations research to evaluate a decision-making process in a public agency.

THE OPERATIONS RESEARCH APPROACH

The approach used in this study* was that of operations research.[1, 2, 3, 4, 5] Operations research may be defined as the application

* The study was supported in part by a Ford Foundation Fellowship, by the National Aeronautics and Space Administration under General Grant #NSG-243, and by a Community Health Services Project Grant from the United States Public Health Service.

The author wishes to express his appreciation to Professors C. West Churchman and C. Bartlett McGuire for their assistance, and to the director and other members of the public health agency for the opportunity to conduct a study in their organization.

of scientific methods, techniques, and tools to problems involving the operations of systems in order to provide those in control of the operations with optimum solutions to their problems. Although operations research has been used successfully in solving many organizational problems, persons writing about operations research have been careful to point out some of its limitations and shortcomings. In addition to the literature cited elsewhere in this section, Koopman,[6] Drucker,[7] and Arrow[8] have warned that operations research is not a panacea for management problems.

Churchman, Ackoff, and Arnoff[1] believe that most practitioners would agree that the following are the major phases of an operations research project:

1. Formulating the problem. (The components of a problem are the decision maker(s), his (or their) relevant objectives, the possible courses of action, and the environment or context within which the problem occurs.)
2. Constructing a model to represent the system under study.
3. Deriving a solution from the model and testing it.
4. Establishing controls over the solution.
5. Putting the solution to work: implementation.

Dorfman has pointed out the difficulty in defining operations research:

> The proper way to begin an inquiry into this movement operations research would be to define it. But this is difficult; for operations research is not a subject-matter field but an approach or method. And, even after a study of hundreds of examples of work classified as operations research, it is by no means clear just what the method is other than that it is scientific (like all respectable methods), because operations analysts are typically resourceful and ingenious men who tackle their problems with no holds barred.[9, p. 575]

After considering various definitions Ackoff elected to define operations research by a discussion of its scope and methods.[3] In his discussion he cited three characteristics of operations research studies: a "holistic" approach to problems, use of an interdisciplinary team, and construction of a model.

"Holistic" Approach

The operations researcher wants to study the system as a whole. Thus the researcher says that he is going to try to solve an organizational problem in which, for example, resource allocation plays an important part, rather than that he is going to solve a resource allocation problem. Analysis within an organizational context is helpful in more ways than one. It aids in determining problems that are important from the viewpoint of the organization as a whole. In addition, it leads to solving a problem in a manner consistent with the organizational goals rather than with the goals of some subunit of the organization.

Because every system is part of a larger system, the difficulty becomes one of what can be left out of the statement of an organizational problem. In addition, operations research has not reached the point where it can study a complex organization as an entity and tell the manager how to rearrange his organization for optimal performance. Thus in practice the operations researcher first looks at the over-all functioning of the organization and then divides the organization into subunits for detailed analysis. (In the author's study of a public health agency he first looked at all the Department's programs before focusing on one particular program.) The hope is that these subunits are relatively independent of each other. If the researcher is successful in partitioning the organization, the solution to a problem in one part of the organization helps to achieve the over-all goals of the organization. If not, he is faced with the likelihood that improvement in the performance of a part of the organization may lead to poorer performance of the organization as a whole. This problem is referred to as "suboptimization."[10, 11]

For example, the performance of a warehouse, a subunit of an organization, might be measured by the number of orders that could not be filled during the month. Given this criterion a solution to improve the performance rating of the warehouse would be to increase the inventory of all items carried by the warehouse. This solution, however, would result in increased inventory carrying costs and might cause a decrease in profits for the organization as a whole.

Interdisciplinary Team

Complex organizations contain aspects that fall into the domain of many disciplines. Solutions to problems in such organizations may require knowledge of economics, engineering, physics, sociology, statistics, and psychology. But the increased specialization in the sciences makes it impossible for one person to have the relevant knowledge of such a variety of disciplines. Through an interdisciplinary research team, knowledge from a variety of fields is brought to bear on a problem.*

Although the study in the health agency was not conducted by an interdisciplinary team, the author consulted with persons from a variety of disciplines during the course of his research. These persons included several agency members as well as persons outside the agency who were familiar with its operations. In this manner the interdisciplinary team characteristic of operations research was brought into the study.

Model

Perhaps the most striking feature of the operations research approach to organizational analysis is the explicit use of a model to represent the system under study.

The complexity of the real world forces the researcher to construct a model that simplifies reality and focuses attention on those aspects of the real world relevant to the problem to be solved. Because parts of reality are omitted the solution to the model may not be a solution to the real world problem represented by the model. If it is not, the model must be changed and another solution derived and tested in the real world. This iterative process is a common feature of operations research studies.

The great advantage of a model is that it is much easier to manipulate a model than the system it represents. Indeed, in many cases it is not possible to manipulate the system or it is too costly to do so. Dorfman stated the value of the model-building approach in the following manner.

> Much of the value of the model-building approach resides in disclosing and defining... gaps [in substantive knowledge]. There is much testimony to indicate that the most valuable results of operations research are by-products. Again and again businessmen have stated gratefully that they learned more about their business by answering an analyst's questions, supplying data for his model, and checking over the model with him than they did from his final report.[9, pp. 614–615]

A good discussion of model construction is contained in Chapter 3 of Ackoff and Sasieni.[4] Ackoff[12] defined three types of models:

* Persons who have worked in interdisciplinary research teams have pointed out some drawbacks to this kind of research. A discussion of problems that may be encountered is found in Ackoff[12, pp. 191ff] and Candill and Roberts.[13]

iconic, analogue, and symbolic. Iconic models look like what they represent. Photographs or model airplanes are examples.

Analogue models employ one set of properties to represent another. Thus a rising line on a graph may represent an increase in sales. The communication model of the Department shown in Table 2 is an analogue model.

Symbolic models, which include mathematical models, express the properties of the thing represented through the use of symbols. (The effectiveness model used in this study is a mathematical model.) A mathematical model describes what the operations researcher has decided are the relevant features of the system he is analyzing, states the relations among the variables, and related the variables to some measure of system performance.

In summary, an operations research study is unlike many of the research studies listed in *An Inventory of Social and Economic Research in Health.*[14] In these studies a dependent variable such as heart disease is related to independent variables such as age, race, sex, and occupation; or the various scaling techniques of psychology and sociology are used; or sample survey techniques are used to collect information about a particular population. An operations research study, in contrast, is a method of problem-solving that may use any of these as well as other techniques.

In industry, operations research has been used to solve a wide variety of problems.[15] Understandably, most of the studies have dealt with the technological aspects of production and distribution processes and have concentrated on price and quantity variables rather than on the more difficult to measure psychological, sociological, and political variables. Thus linear programming and computer simulation—two operations research techniques that are convenient to represent technological variables—have been widely used in industrial studies.[16, 17] The result has been increased efficiency in the operation of petroleum refineries, chemical plants, and steel mills. The technologies of these systems are well known. Engineers have studied them for years. Thus when operations researchers began studying these systems they were investigating well-structured and explored areas. Even so it takes several man-years to simulate or to build linear programming models of such systems.

In contrast, the public sector is a largely unexplored area whose 'technology" is not well known. Certainly this is true of the systems for the delivery of medical care services. Hence the emphasis in this article is on the exploratory aspects of an operations research study in the public health field.

The industrial applications of operations research cited above often lead to a narrow view of the field as being merely a continuation of the scientific management movement of the 1920s with computers substituted for stop watches. The definition of operations research used in this study is a much broader one. However, many persons do hold the narrow view.[18, 19, 20]

Applications of operations research to the health field have been surveyed by Flagle,[21, 22] Gue,[23] and Horvath.[24] In general, the hospital has been the organizational unit investigated. For example, staffing requirements of outpatient departments and demand for hospital beds have been studied through the use of queuing theory.[25, 26] Computer simulation models have assisted hospital administrators in solving policy problems dealing with a maternity suite, an outpatient clinic, and a surgical pavilion.[27] A stochastic model of the flow of patients through a hospital system was constructed, and three alternative organizational structures for handling the patients were evaluated.[28] The size and importance of the nursing staffs in hospitals have led to several studies of this group of health personnel. One investigator developed a Markov model to predict the demand for nursing services while another used multivariate regression analysis to estimate the hours needed for various categories of nursing activities.[29, 30] The Oxford nursing studies reflect the pioneering work in operations research carried out by the Oxford Regional Hospital Board.[31]

Other health agencies and alternative systems for the delivery of medical care have not received much attention. Thus there are not many operations research studies dealing directly with problems faced by public health administrators.

Economists and statisticians have contributed to studies of the health field. Economists have used cost–benefit analysis to calculate the economic costs of various diseases.[32, 33, 34, 35] Significant advances both conceptually and computationally have been made in the measurement of these costs. Critics have pointed out, however, that these studies did not compare alternative possible programs and omitted the institutional arrangements through which disease identification, control, or eradication programs would have to be carried out.[36, 37, 38, 39]

Statistical applications to the health field have been made in several areas. Dozens of articles have been written about multiphasic screening, medical diagnosis, drug screening, sequential medical trials, and choice among medical treatments. As an example of the size of the literature, Federer's bibliography of articles on screening procedures runs to 23 pages.[40] The same general statement previously made about the economic literature can also be made here, i.e., typically the problems facing public health administrators are not dealt with in these articles.

Thus it seemed to the author that an operations research study of decision-making and resource allocation in a health agency would be a test of the usefulness of this approach to problem-solving in the public sector. In addition a demonstration that other than technological and economic variables could be included in a mathematical model would be of interest.

SELECTION OF THE PROBLEM

The Department was first visualized as a black box with inputs of state and federal money and outputs of services and allocations of funds to local health agencies.* A black box is any system "whose detailed internal nature one willfully ignores" and "whose input and output characteristics alone are of interest."[41, p. 32; 42, p. 26] A black box was made for each of the post-World War II years. The black boxes formed a gross picture of the Department's growth and resource allocation activities. The changes in dollar amounts and the addition and deletion of inputs and outputs displayed by the black boxes proved an effective means for the author to orient himself to the organization. This method of depicting the organization facilitated further analysis of the inputs and outputs for the purpose of selecting some part of the Department for detailed study.

Table 1 is the black box for the 1963–1964 fiscal year. The black box shows the flow of state and federal funds into the Department and the division of these funds into money retained at the state level to support operations and services of the Department and money allocated to local health departments for use at the local level.

Federal formula grants seemed a more feasible area for study than state appropriations because the Department has much more discretion in the use of federal funds than in the use of state funds and because, from a systems analysis point of view, a federal formula grant can be thought of as an exogenous-variable in the system encompassing the Department's administration of the grant.

* By law the Department is responsible for the administration of the state and federal appropriations for public health programs. Even though most of these appropriations are passed on to local health departments and to other local agencies which provide most of the direct public health services, the Department must account for the use of the money to the state legislature and to the United States Public Health Service.

TABLE 1. *Black Box of the State Department of Public Health: 1963–1964 (in thousands of dollars)*

State funds	39,902		State level operations[a]	13,906
			State funds	10,975
Federal funds	19,442		Federal funds	2,931
Chronically ill and aged	937			
General health	947		Assistance to local agencies[b]	45,440
Cancer control	254		State funds	28,927
Heart disease control	410	State	Federal funds	16,513
Maternal and child health	1,322	Department		
Crippled children	1,159	of		
Tuberculosis control	207			
Venereal disease control	—	Public		
Radiological health	172			
Neurological and sensory disease	42	Health		
Hospital construction under Hill–Burton Act	11,394			
Medical facilities construction under Wolverton Act	2,598			
Special projects activities[c]	2,970	Total flow: 64,013	Special projects activities[c]	2,970
Reimbursements[d]	931		Reimbursements[d]	931
Capital outlay	766[e]		Capital outlay	766[e]

[a] *State level operations* refers to the operations carried out by the Department. Salaries and expenses of departmental employees are in this category. Some funds classified here reach the local level through Department contracts with hospitals, universities, voluntary agencies, and local health departments. For example, the CI&A contract program is included in this category.

[b] *Assistance to local agencies* consists of funds earmarked for the following categories:
- Assistance to counties for care of crippled children
- Assistance to counties for tuberculosis sanatoria
- Assistance to counties without local health departments
- Assistance to local health departments
- Assistance to local agencies for gnat control
- Assistance to local agencies for mosquito control
- Assistance to local agencies for the treatment of physically handicapped children
- Assistance to local and nonprofit agencies for hospital construction

[c] *Special projects activities* consists primarily of grants from NIH and the Bureau of State Services of the Public Health Service for specific research projects.

[d] *Reimbursements* are activities carried out by the Department for other agencies of the state government for which the Department is reimbursed by these agencies.

[e] Includes $150,000 in federal funds not included in "Federal funds" above.

There were several reasons for choosing to study the CI&A grant from among the various federal formula grants. Because it was new the individuals who made the initial decisions about the program in 1961 were all available for interviews. In addition, although the CI&A grant is a categorical grant, i.e., the money must be used in the category for which the money is appropriated, "chronically ill and aged" is a sufficiently broad category to place a heavy responsibility on the Department to decide how the funds should be used. Finally, the grant was controversial because it involved public health in medical care programs.

ANALYSIS OF THE CI&A PROGRAM

Even though the CI&A program was a new program there was much material to analyze. Within two years after the passage of the federal legislation, the Department had provided funds to support sixty-two local programs in the state.

The information needed for this study was obtained from the following sources: interviews with more than fifty members of the Department; attendance at many meetings, which provided opportunities for direct observation of the decision-making process; analysis of letters, memoranda, documents, and other material in various departmental files; and discussions with persons outside the Department who had knowledge of its operations. The author was furnished a desk in the Department, where he did most of his work. His association with the Department over a period of eighteen months hopefully minimized the "observer effects."

Initially a communications flow chart of the CI&A program in the state (Table 2) was used as a framework within which to gather information. Although the chart proved useful in understanding organizational behavior, it did not prove to be as useful as communications flow charts have been in other operations research studies. A comparison of the communication flow chart (Table 2) with the formal organization chart (Table 3) demonstrates how important the informal organization was for the operation of the CI&A program.

TABLE 2. *Communication Flow Chart. Allocation of the CI&A Formula Grant: A Cross-Sectional View*

Exhibit L

ALLOCATION OF THE CI&A FORMULA GRANT
(FY 1963-64 - $937,000)

A CROSS SECTIONAL VIEW

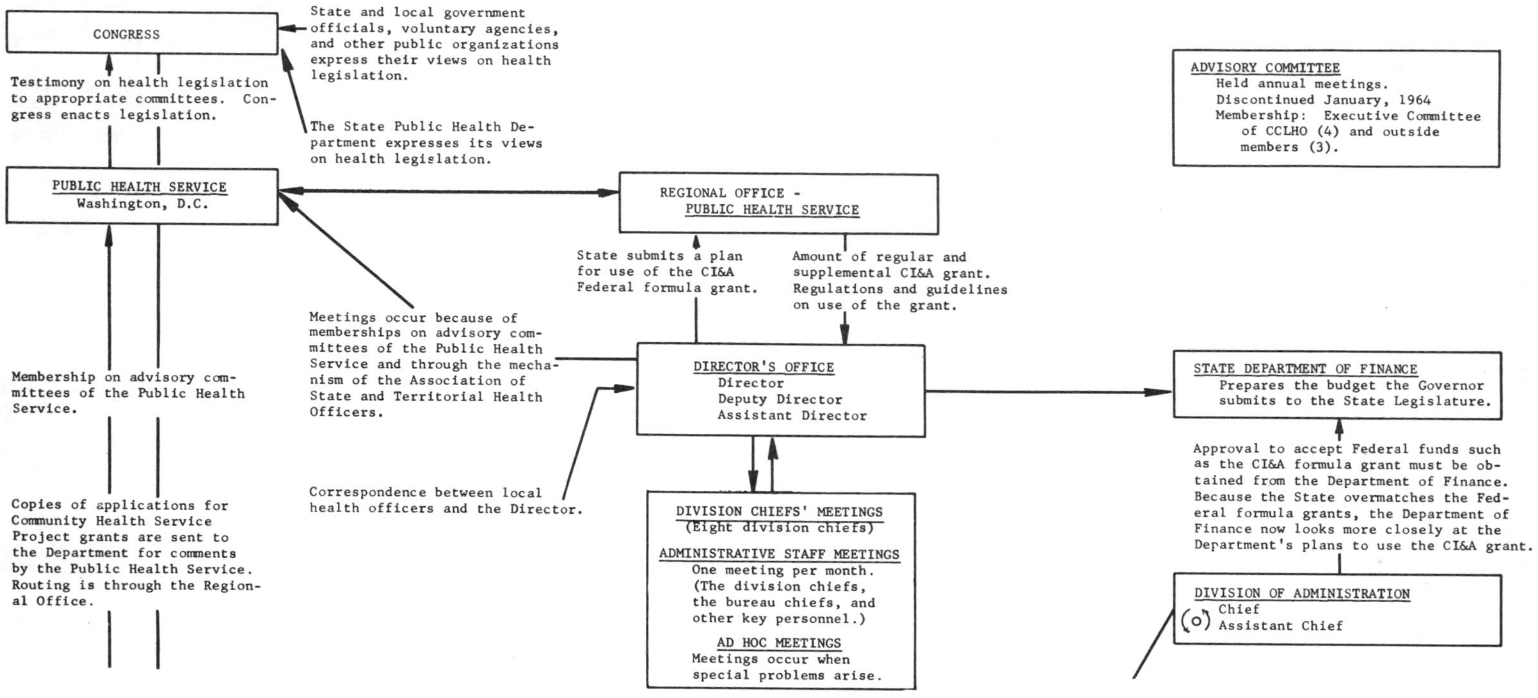

TABLE 2. *Communication Flow Chart. Allocation of the CI&A Formula Grant: A Cross-Sectional View (Cont'd.)*

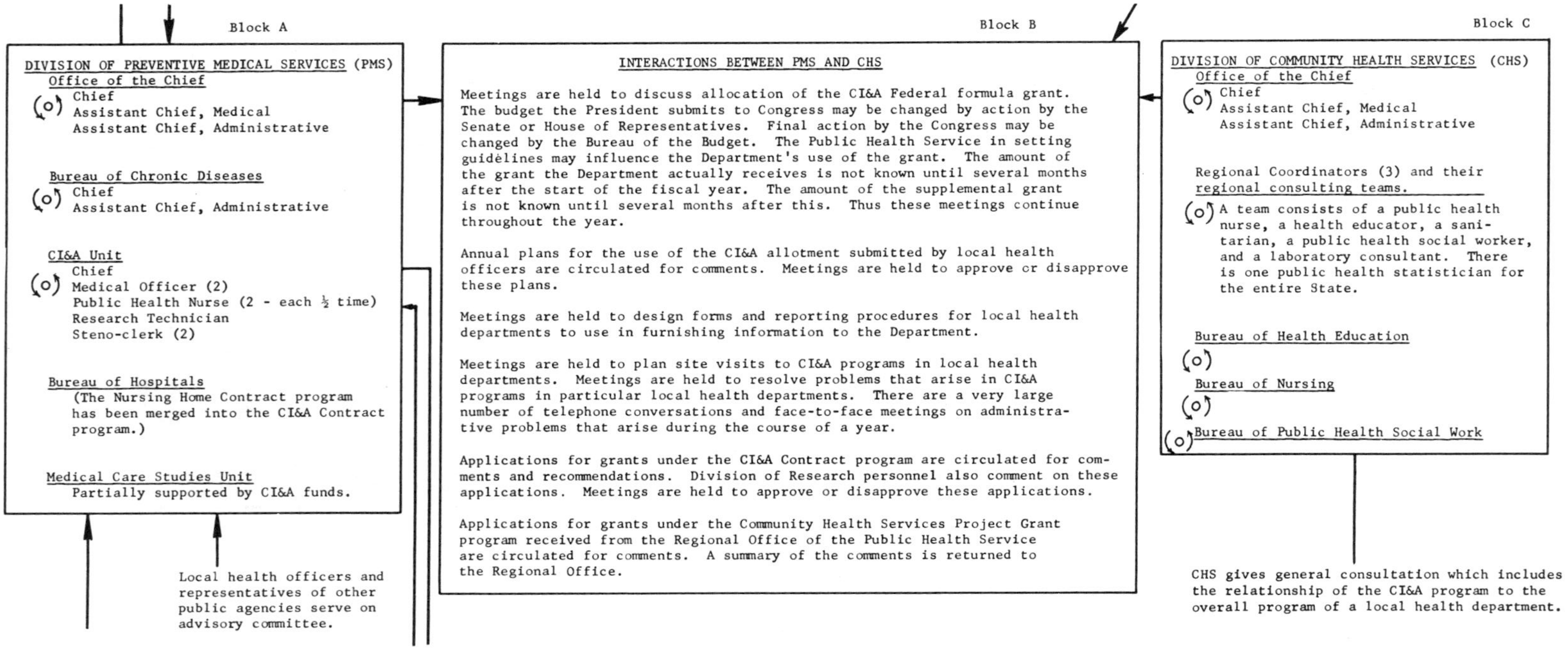

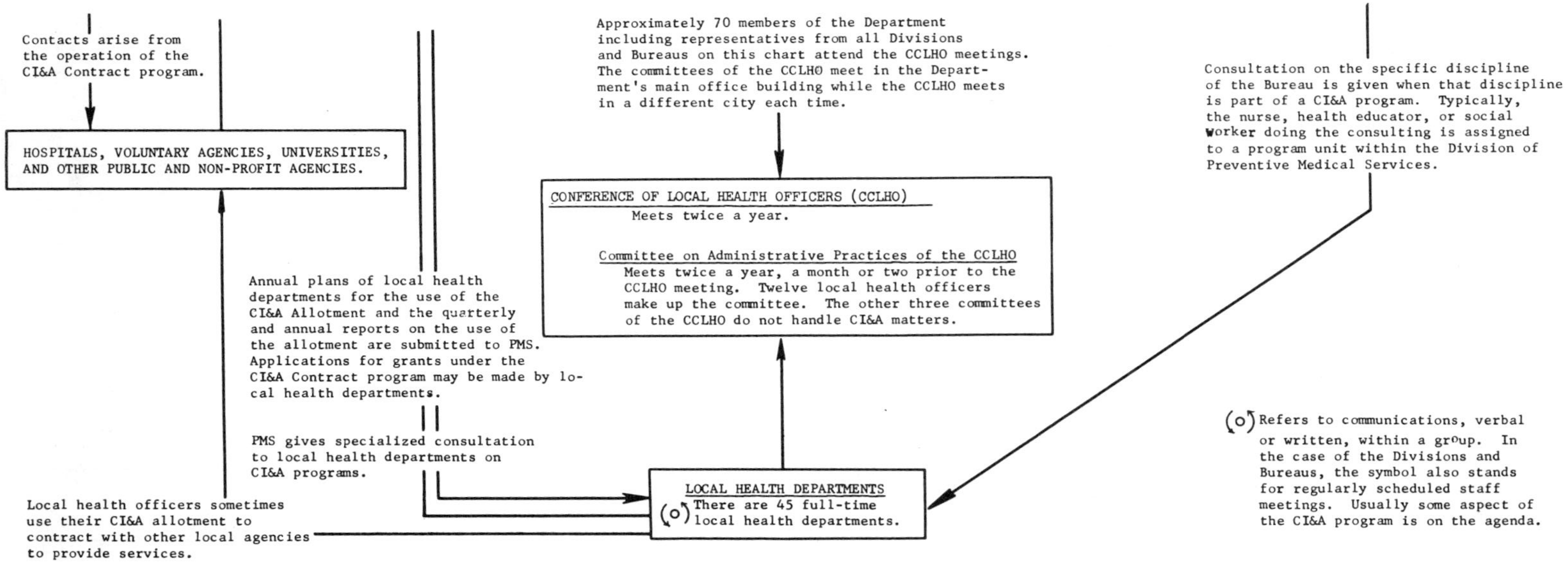

Contacts arise from the operation of the CI&A Contract program.
HOSPITALS, VOLUNTARY AGENCIES, UNIVERSITIES, AND OTHER PUBLIC AND NON-PROFIT AGENCIES.
Approximately 70 members of the Department including representatives from all Divisions and Bureaus on this chart attend the CCLHO meetings. The committees of the CCLHO meet in the Department's main office building while the CCLHO meets in a different city each time.
CONFERENCE OF LOCAL HEALTH OFFICERS (CCLHO)
Meets twice a year.
Committee on Administrative Practices of the CCLHO
Meets twice a year, a month or two prior to the CCLHO meeting. Twelve local health officers make up the committee. The other three committees of the CCLHO do not handle CI&A matters.
Consultation on the specific discipline of the Bureau is given when that discipline is part of a CI&A program. Typically, the nurse, health educator, or social worker doing the consulting is assigned to a program unit within the Division of Preventive Medical Services.
Annual plans of local health departments for the use of the CI&A Allotment and the quarterly and annual reports on the use of the allotment are submitted to PMS. Applications for grants under the CI&A Contract program may be made by local health departments.
PMS gives specialized consultation to local health departments on CI&A programs.
LOCAL HEALTH DEPARTMENTS
There are 45 full-time local health departments.
Local health officers sometimes use their CI&A allotment to contract with other local agencies to provide services.
Refers to communications, verbal or written, within a group. In the case of the Divisions and Bureaus, the symbol also stands for regularly scheduled staff meetings. Usually some aspect of the CI&A program is on the agenda.

TABLE 3. *Formal Organization Chart: State Department of Public Health*

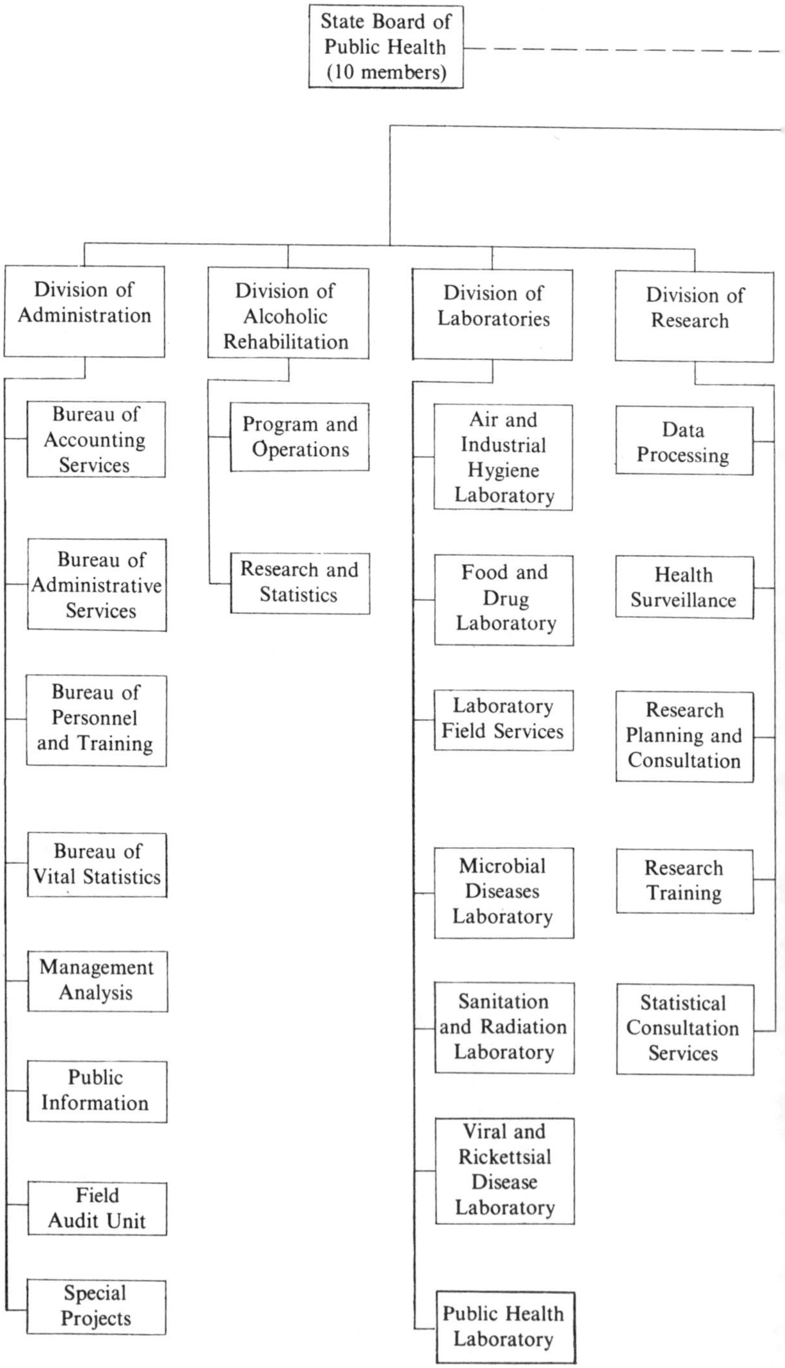

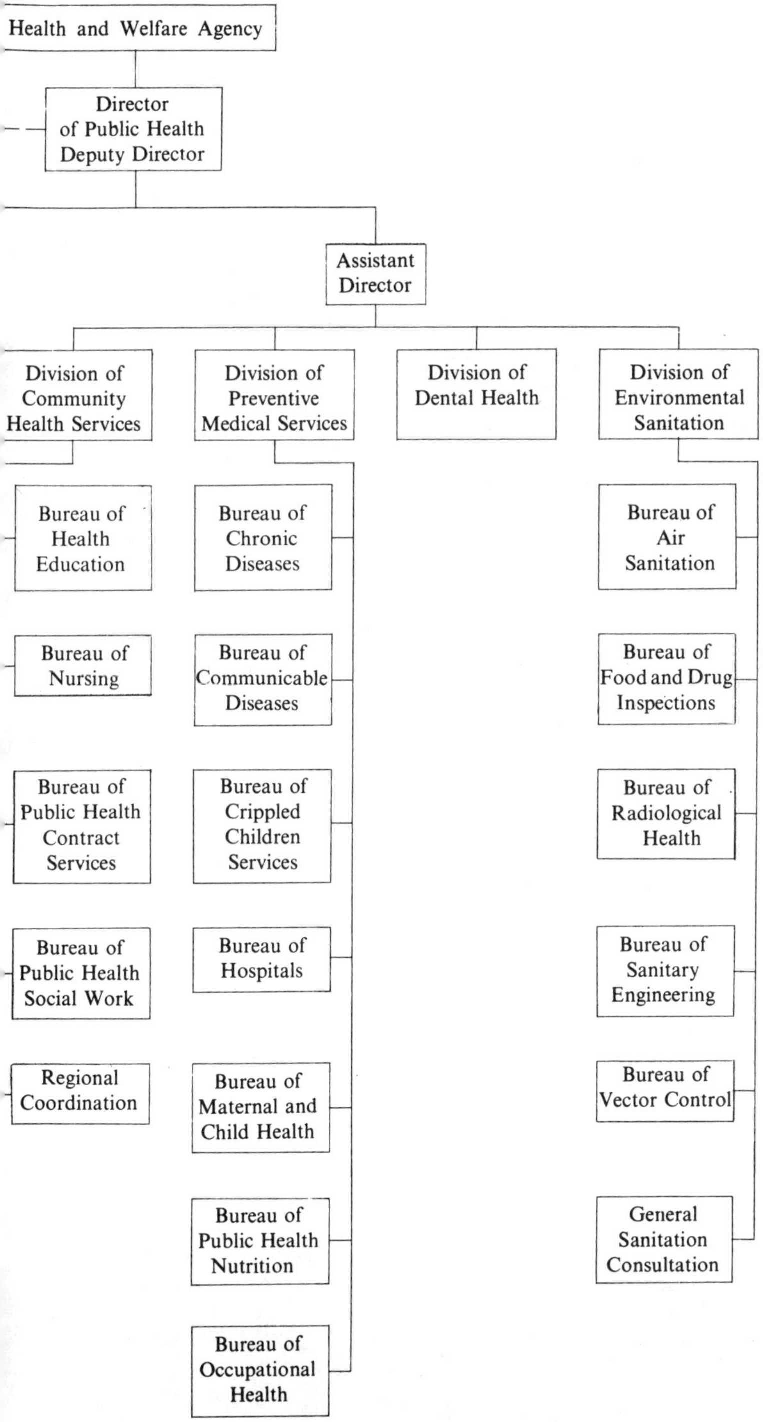
Health and Welfare Agency
Director of Public Health Deputy Director
Assistant Director
Division of Community Health Services
Division of Preventive Medical Services
Division of Dental Health
Division of Environmental Sanitation
Bureau of Health Education
Bureau of Nursing
Bureau of Public Health Contract Services
Bureau of Public Health Social Work
Regional Coordination
Bureau of Chronic Diseases
Bureau of Communicable Diseases
Bureau of Crippled Children Services
Bureau of Hospitals
Bureau of Maternal and Child Health
Bureau of Public Health Nutrition
Bureau of Occupational Health
Bureau of Air Sanitation
Bureau of Food and Drug Inspections
Bureau of Radiological Health
Bureau of Sanitary Engineering
Bureau of Vector Control
General Sanitation Consultation

The communications flow chart seems to work well in a stable environment where there is a repetitiveness in the operations studied (such as weekly or monthly schedules) and where changes in the routines occur infrequently. It did not work well in the study of the CI&A program, however, because of the lack of repetitiveness—the Department's CI&A program made annual allocations, and only three allocations had been made when the study started—and because of significant changes made each year in the Department's allocation process.

A more effective way of analyzing the Department's CI&A program was to develop a chronology of events in connection with the establishment and implementation of the CI&A program. Another set of black boxes (Table 4) was made in which the outputs were the different programs supported by each annual CI&A grant. Changes and additions in the allocations to the output categories served as indicators of what to look for in departmental files and what questions to ask

TABLE 4. *Input–Output Tables for CI&A Federal Formula Grants to State (in dollars)*

Output	*1961–1962* (*Input*: *356,300*)	*1962–1963* (*Input*: *911,390*)	*1963–1964* (*Input*: *937,188*)	*Totals* (*Input*: *2,204,878*)
Allocated to local health departments (services at local level)	280,052	584,736	593,849	1,458,637
State level support (Administrative overhead —program development)	26,248	105,694	114,143	246,085
Bureau of chronic diseases	7,647	45,697	61,754	115,098
Bureau of hospitals	18,000	18,000	18,000	54,000
Division of community health services	601	12,655	10,800	24,056
Division of administration	0	24,150	11,801	35,951
Division of laboratories	0	0	6,000	6,000
Bureau of health education	0	0	1,000	1,000
Retirement, health, and welfare	0	5,192	4,788	9,980
Studies, experiments, and demonstrations	50,000	220,960	229,197	500,157
CI&A contract program	0	170,960	133,931	304,891
Nursing home contract program	50,000	50,000	45,266	145,266
Medical care studies unit	0	0	50,000	50,000

departmental members. Copies were made of several hundred pieces of pertinent material from files throughout the Department. These pieces, when placed in chronological order, formed the basic file on the CI&A program. This chronology focused upon key decisions, the discussions preceding the decisions, and the results of the decisions as shown by the actual allocations of the CI&A funds.

COMPONENTS OF THE CI&A RESOURCE ALLOCATION PROBLEM

The Decision-Maker

The analysis of the CI&A program revealed that the basic decisions were made by the director. In the first two years of the program's operation the Department made three major decisions about the allocation of the CI&A grant. A careful study of each decision led to the conclusion that the director was the decision-maker. Details of this analysis and of the study in general are given in Stimson.[51]

However, it is at a certain point in time that the director is the decision-maker—after he has received recommendations from departmental members, after he has received suggestions from other individuals and organizations that form the environment in which the Department exists, after he has evaluated the information directed to him by the divisions and bureaus of his Department, and after he has considered the implications of the decision to be made upon the internal workings of the Department and upon the Department's relation with its environment.

The Objectives

Although there are general objectives that guide all the activities of the Department, these objectives are stated in such broad terms that it was necessary as part of this study to determine a set of objectives pertinent to the Department's allocation of the CI&A grant. (The general objectives are "the prevention of disease and the provision of a healthful environment for the people of [the state].")

It was important for the experiment described later in this chapter that the meaning of each objective for the allocation of the CI&A grant was the same for the departmental members as for the researcher.

Therefore the language of the objectives was edited several times in order to insure agreement on meaning. Successive drafts of the set of objectives were read by the persons who would participate in the experiment, and revisions were based upon their comments.

Seven objectives were used in the model to encompass medical and scientific goals, the relationship of the Department with its environment, and the psychological needs of departmental members. The behavior of those connected with the CI&A program and the decision reached were consistent with the pursuit of one or more of these seven goals.

THE SEVEN OBJECTIVES

1. To strengthen and support local health departments by providing funds for new or improved services in chronic disease. This objective includes the maintenance of good relations with the local health departments.

2. To increase the availability, scope, and quality of out-of-hospital community health services for the chronically ill and aged. This is a personal health care objective.

3. To achieve self-fulfillment and enhance the prestige of those who administer the CI&A program in the Department. This objective includes the natural desire to be identified with a good, well-respected program.

4. To conduct the CI&A program in such a manner that the Department of Finance is satisfied with the Department's administration of this federal grant. This objective also covers the influence of the state government acting through the Department of Finance on the CI&A program.

5. To show the Public Health Service that the states can do a good job with federal formula grant funds so that the trend toward centralizing the funding of individual projects in Washington does not continue. This objective also includes the maintenance of good relations with the Public Health Service.

6. To get the support of various community and voluntary agencies in carrying out the Department's CI&A program. This objective includes the maintenance of good relations with the state medical association, the county medical societies, and other voluntary agencies.

7. To add to knowledge in the field of chronic illness and aging by doing and supporting significant demonstrations and specific investigations aimed at improving and extending out-of-hospital services for the chronically ill and aged.

The Alternatives

There was an extremely large number of alternative ways in which the CI&A grant for the following year (1964–1965) might have been allocated by the Department. Merely shifting a few dollars from one category to another would have resulted in a different allocation. It therefore became necessary to select from this large number of alternatives. Because members of the Department had different opinions about which means would best achieve certain goals, the alternatives were chosen to see if differing evaluations of these means would be reflected in the experiments reported on later in this chapter.

In this study eight alternatives were selected. These alternatives do not reflect radical changes from past practices because the commitments made by the Department's allocation of the CI&A grant in the three previous fiscal years precluded radical changes. The alternatives cover a wide range of feasible departmental programs, yet the number is small enough for a decision-maker to evaluate in terms of the seven objectives.

The eight alternatives for allocating the 1964–1965 CI&A grant deal with the allocation of funds among three major categories: (1) allocations to local health departments to provide services, (2) funds retained at the state level to support studies and demonstrations under three programs (the CI&A contract program, the nursing home contract program, and the medical care studies unit program), and (3) funds used to pay the Department's costs of administering the CI&A grant. The last category is called administrative overhead, but it includes the program development and promotion activities of the members of the CI&A Unit and others in the Department.

All alternatives for allocating the 1964–1965 CI&A grant contain a reduction of $75,000 compared to the previous year's grant. President Johnson's budget message to Congress in January 1964 recommended such a reduction. Because the allocation decision had to be made by the Department prior to Congressional action on the President's budget, the sum used in planning for 1964–1965 was the amount that would come to the state if Congress approved the recommended reduction.

THE EIGHT ALTERNATIVES

1. The first alternative for allocating the 1964–1965 CI&A formula grant keeps the tentative allotment to local health departments the same as in 1963–1964. The formula for allocating funds to local health departments remains the same, as do all the other administrative regulations. (The formula is essentially a per capita allotment.) The first alternative also keeps the funds for the Department's administrative overhead and for the medical care studies unit the same. The CI&A contract program is to bear the brunt of the proposed $75,000 cut. The supplemental CI&A grant from the Public Health Service is to be used for the CI&A contract program. Procedures for obtaining CI&A funds remain the same, i.e., local health departments will continue to fulfill the current reporting requirements. Applicants for the CI&A contracts will have to submit their applications in the present manner.

2. The second alternative is the same as the first except that support for a particular CI&A program in a local health department would be restricted to a fixed period of time. The first alternative does not restrict support for a particular CI&A program in a local health department to a fixed period of time.

3. The third alternative is the same as the first except that all CI&A contract program funds and supplemental CI&A grant funds would be used for a single large demonstration, or at most a few, arranged by the Department. The first alternative uses the CI&A contract program to support many small projects.

4. The fourth alternative is the same as the first except that all CI&A contract program funds and supplemental CI&A grant funds would be used to run a service program at the state level. The first alternative has no service program at the state level.

5. The fifth alternative is the same as the first except that the number and length of reports submitted by local health departments would be greatly reduced. The first alternative requires a local health department to submit an acceptable plan for its intended use of its CI&A allotment and to submit quarterly reports on the use of the CI&A funds if its plan is approved.

6. The sixth alternative is the same as the first except that the local health departments' share of the CI&A grant is allocated by the project

grants rather than by per capita allotments based on submission of acceptable plans. There is no guarantee that a particular local health department will receive any CI&A funds from the State Department as there is in the first alternative.

7. In the seventh alternative the proposed cut of $75,000 in the CI&A formula grant is absorbed by reducing each of the three major categories—allocation to local health departments for services at the local level; state administrative overhead costs which include program development activities; and studies, experiments, and demonstrations—by approximately 9% of the 1963–1964 levels. All departmental rules, regulations, and administrative procedures remain the same in 1964–1965 as in 1963–1964.

8. In the eighth alternative the proposed cut of $75,000 in the CI&A formula grant is absorbed by reducing the allocations to local health departments $75,000 and leaving allocations to other categories the same as in 1963–1964. All departmental rules, regulations, and administrative procedures remain the same in 1964–1965 as in 1963–1964.

The Environment

The Department lives in a highly political environment. It must get its funds and support from the state and federal governments. It also must get the cooperation of many different groups in order to achieve its over-all objectives. Decisions made by the Department have far-reaching effects. The relationship of the Department with its environment entered into this study through the set of objectives for the CI&A program. In particular, objectives 1, 4, 5, and 6 relate the environment to the CI&A program.

A MODEL FOR ALLOCATION OF THE CI&A GRANT

The model developed for the Department's allocation of the CI&A grant attempts to measure the effectiveness of alternative courses of action under consideration by a decision-maker. It is based on the Churchman–Ackoff approximate measure of value.[52] The procedure for measuring effectiveness requires two component measures: the relative importance (value or utility) of each objective and the efficiency of each alternative in achieving each objective, i.e., the probability that the selection of a particular alternative will achieve a particular objective.

Reasons for Selecting the Effectiveness Model

Although the Department's records showed to what agencies and to what programs the past allocations of CI&A money went, they did not show in detail what the money bought in new and increased services for the chronically ill and aged. In addition, the goals of the CI&A program were difficult to measure in terms of a common scale. Because of these considerations and because of the obvious difficulties in program evaluation, the director and others in the Department were uncertain about the effectiveness of the present method, let alone of alternative methods, of allocating the forthcoming 1964–1965 CI&A formula grant. The model selected to represent the allocation of the CI&A grant is well adapted to situations having these features. Also the information required by the model could be obtained in a reasonable amount of time.

Published reports indicate that the effectiveness model has been used successfully to solve problems in private industry.[1, pp. 145-152; 43] Also, there is some evidence that two of the basic assumptions of the model, additivity of values[44, 45, 46, 47] and the use of maximization of expected utility[48, 49, 50] as an indication of rational behavior, are useful in studies of decision-making.

In the effectiveness model described in the next section, the allocation of the CI&A grant is limited to three major categories:

Services: Allocations to local health departments to support a wide variety of service programs.

Research: Allocations to health agencies to support demonstration or research projects. Some departmental studies also were supported.

Administration overhead: That portion of the grant retained at the state level to pay for the administration of the grant. The cost of maintaining records required by the Public Health Service and the salaries of those engaged in program development activities for the CI&A program are included here.

Had other data been available or easily obtained, other models could have been used to represent the allocation of the CI&A grant. For example, the information needed to apply classical economic theory—allocate the CI&A funds to alternative uses until the marginal benefit from the last dollar in each category is equal to the marginal benefit from the last dollar in all other categories—was not available. Also, it was not possible to do a cost-benefit analysis of each health program supported by CI&A funds. An attempt at such an analysis would have been an entire study in itself. Finally, a linear programming model was not used to obtain the optimal allocation of the grant because of the lack of information and the difficulty of formulating the CI&A allocation problem in that way.

Description of the Effectiveness Model

Briefly, in the experimental procedure used in this study, to obtain a measure of effectiveness the subject ranks the set of objectives in order of importance to him and then indicates his preference between pairs of subsets of the set of objectives. From these choices a numerical value (v_j) may be associated with each objective. Then the subject is asked to evaluate the efficiency (the e_{ij}'s) of each alternative in achieving each objective. A schematic representation of the effectiveness model is shown in Figure 1.

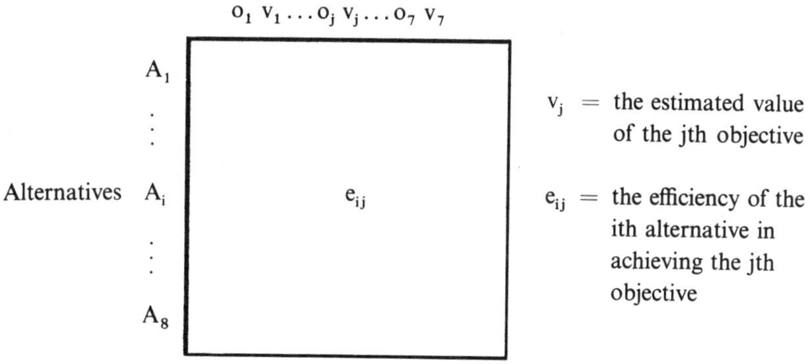

FIGURE 1. *The Effectiveness Model*

The criterion used in this study to select the "best" alternative calls for the calculation of the effectiveness, i.e., the weighted sum of the efficiencies ($\Sigma_j e_{ij} v_j$) of each alternative, and for the selection of the alternative with the highest weighted sum.

The model to measure effectiveness described above depends on the verbal judgments of individuals. There is no estimate of the accuracy or the bias of the judgments. This defect, however, is shared by the other methods of estimating preference. In addition, the model assumes that persons choose actions (in this study the actions are the alternative allocations) in terms of the importance of goals and of the probabilities that actions will achieve goals.

EXPERIMENTAL METHOD

Twelve key departmental members closely involved with the federal grant program were interviewed individually. The interviews lasted from 75 to 90 minutes. During that time each participant was asked to complete three tasks. These tasks were based on the Churchman–Ackoff approximate measure of value method previously described. The purpose of the first two tasks was to assign numerical utilities to the seven objectives. The purpose of the third task was to obtain the probabilities that alternatives would achieve objectives.

The procedure for obtaining the utilities of the objectives consisted of several steps. In the first task the subject ranked the seven objectives in order of their importance to him. Then the author divided the objectives into two groups. The objective the subject had ranked as most inportant (O1) was placed in both groups. One group contained the objectives ranked first, second, third, and sixth (O1, O2, O3, and O6). The other group contained the objectives ranked first, fourth, fifth, and seventh (O1, O4, O5, and O7). The subject was asked to consider the group containing O1, O2, O3, and O6 and to state which he would prefer to achieve, the objective he had ranked as most important (O1), or the combination of O2, O3, and O6. If the combination was preferred, the subject was asked to indicate his preference between O1 and the combination of O2 and O3. The final question about the subset of objectives was whether the subject would prefer to achieve O2 or the combination of O3 and O6. The same series of questions was repeated with the other subset of objectives (O1, O4, O5, and O7).

The choices involving the two subsets of objectives were checked to see whether they were compatible. If they were not, the author pointed out the inconsistency to the subject and asked him to reconsider his choices and make adjustments to achieve consistency. An example of an inconsistency between the two subsets of objectives would be if the subject responded that he preferred O1 to the combination of O2, O3, and O6 and that he also preferred the combination of O4, O5, and O7 to O1.

Finally the choices involving the two subsets of objectives were checked with the original ranking of the seven objectives. Again any inconsistencies were pointed out, and the subject was asked to reconsider and to make adjustments to achieve consistency. Procedures to be used for handling different numbers of objectives are given in Churchman and Ackoff.[52]

In the second task (Figure 2) a unique set of values for the objectives was obtained by asking the subjects to rate the objectives on a ratio scale. The ratio scale in the second task was presented as an extension of the ranking the subjects had done in the first task. The objective that the subject had ranked as most important was arbitrarily given a value of 100. A vertical scale marked off from 0 to 100 was placed in front of the subject, and an arrow marked 1 was placed opposite 100. The subject then placed the remaining six arrows numbered 2 through

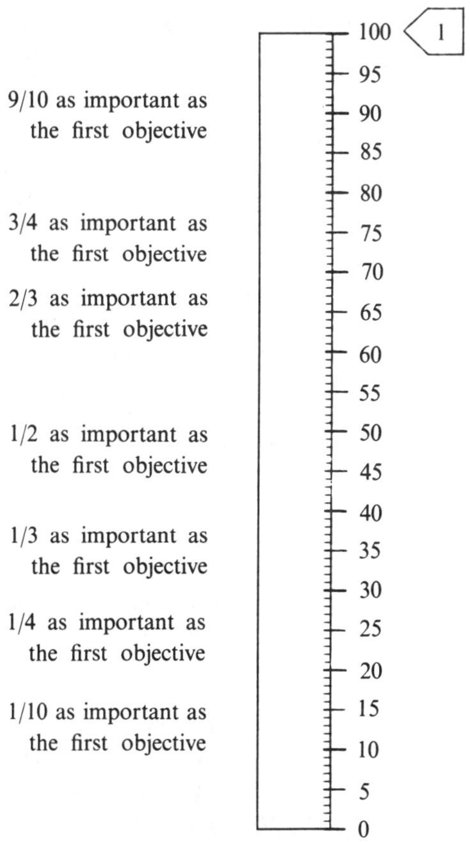

FIGURE 2. *Second Task*

7 on the scale to indicate the ratio he believed each objective had to the value of 100 assigned to the first objective. For example, an objective considered by a subject to be one-half as important as his top-ranked objective would receive a value of 50.

After the subjects had indicated a value on the ratio scale for each objective, their number assignments on this scale were compared with their verbal choices of the task to arrive at a final numerical value for each objective. For example, if a subject had stated in the first (verbal) task that he would rather achieve the objective he had ranked as most important than achieve the combination of objectives he had ranked second and third in importance, the numerical value he had assigned on the ratio scale to the first objective would have to be greater than the sum of values assigned to the second and third objectives. If not, the subject was asked to change his verbal choice or to change his number assignment to achieve consistency.

The third task (Figure 3) was a complex one that asked the subjects to evaluate the efficiency of each alternative to achieve each objective.

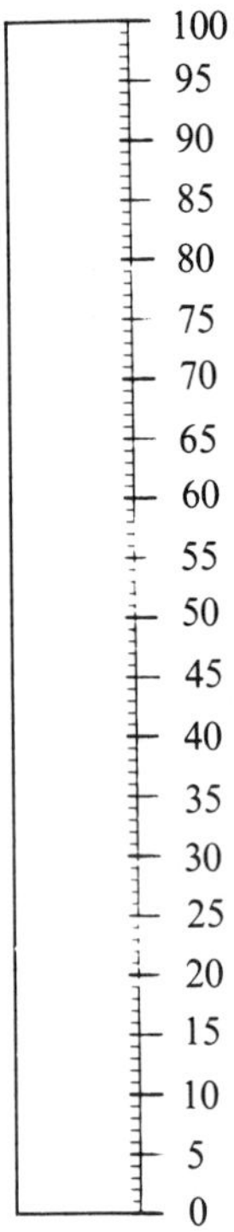

A rating of 100 means that you think the selection of the alternative is virtually sure to achieve the objective (the probability of attainment is practically 100%).

A rating of 80 means that you think the selection of the alternative is four times as likely to achieve the objective as not to achieve it.

A rating of 50 means that you think the selection of the alternative is equally likely to achieve or not to achieve the objective (or that you don't know if the selection of the alternative will help or hurt the achievement of the objective).

A rating of 20 means that you think the selection of the alternative is four times as likely not to achieve the objective as to achieve it.

A rating of O means that you think the selection of the alternative is practically certain not to achieve the objective (the probability of attainment is practically zero).

FIGURE 3. *Third Task*

The subject had to consider seven cards with the objectives on them, eight cards of a different color with the alternatives on them, and a scale with probabilities marked off from 0 to 100. The author went over the scale with the subject to familiarize him with the responses required for the task. Then the subject was given the card with the first alternative on it and the seven cards with the objectives on them. He was asked to give the probability that the selection of the first alternative would achieve each of the seven objectives. He responded with a number ranging from 0 to 100. A 0 meant that the selection of the alternative was practically certain not to achieve the objective; a 100 meant that the selection of the alternative was practically certain to achieve a particular objective.

The author recorded each probability on a score card that was kept where the subject could see it at all times. The procedure was repeated with the second alternative, and so on through all eight alternatives.

After the probabilities were recorded for all alternatives, the subject was asked to reread the cards with the alternatives on them and to indicate which alternative he thought would be the best way to allocate the federal grant and which would be the second best way.

Later the author calculated the effectiveness of each alternative. If the alternative with the highest effectiveness had not been rated by the subject as his first or second choice, the subject was reinterviewed and asked to comment on why he had not chosen that alternative.

RESULTS AND DISCUSSION

First Task

The first task, assigning values to the seven objectives, was the easiest for the subjects because the concept of ranking was familiar to them. Nevertheless, there were some problems.

The first choice among the subsets of objectives caused most of the subjects some difficulty and caused considerable difficulty in two cases. This was the choice between the objective the subjects had ranked as most important and the combination of the second, third, and sixth ranked objectives. It was hard for the subject to conceive of the value of an objective alone. The tendency was to think of these objectives as a cluster. One subject commented that there was "some overlap" in the choice situation. Another said, "Choices are never this absolute, not all black or all white." The additivity assumption used in the experiment implies the objectives are independent, but most persons are not used to valuing an objective by itself. It was the first choice that was hard to make; the rest of the choices caused no trouble.

The two subjects who had the most difficulty with the task both ranked the objective concerning the provision of new or improved services first and the adding-to-knowledge-by-demonstrations objective second. One of these subjects said it was impossible for him to separate the two objectives because he would never agree to a "service only" program: "If the feds said to me, here is $900,000 for a service program to put VNA-type [Visiting Nurse Association] activities everywhere in the state but you can't use any of the money for demonstrations, I would reject it." The other subject said that the requirement to choose between his first ranked objective and the combination of his second, third, and sixth ranked objectives forced him to make "an unrealistic choice" because the second objective would always lead to the first. After some discussion with the author about demonstrations funded by the CI&A Contract program, this subject said that in his opinion results of demonstrations were always translated into practice.

Practically all the subjects ranked the objectives dealing with services, local health departments, and adding to knowledge by demonstrations in the top three. The objectives dealing with the Public Health Service, the Department of Finance, and the psychological needs of departmental members tended to be ranked toward the bottom of the order. The general agreement among subjects in the rankings of the objectives was borne out by calculating the Spearman rank correlation coefficient for several pairs of rankings. The correlation coefficients ranged from .62 to .93. Such coefficients would occur by chance only between 1% and 10% of the time. The limitation imposed by the small number of objectives in the model prevents more precise statements about the correlation coefficients.

Second Task

The purpose of the second task was to compare the assignment of numerical values to objectives implicit in the choices of the first task with the ratings of the objectives in the second task in order to get a unique set of values for the objectives. Of the eleven subjects who completed the experiment, only one had no inconsistencies between the first and second tasks. Of the remaining ten who had inconsistencies, six changed their numerical ratings only, three changed their verbal choices and numerical ratings, and one changed the rank order of his three lowest ranked objectives and also changed his numerical ratings.

In general the second task went smoothly. Two subjects had trouble with the additivity assumption. In his verbal choice one subject preferred the first objective to the combination of the second, third, and sixth. But his ratings on the numerical scale for the combination of the three objectives added up to well over 100. When the inconsistency was pointed out, the subject argued that the average of the three objectives should be considered rather than their sum. The choices of the second subject showed the same inconsistency. Moreover, he had considerable difficulty in recognizing the inconsistency.

The number of shifts in numerical ratings made it doubtful whether the subjects' original ratings on the ratio scale expressed their actual values of the objectives. Nevertheless, the second task provided a good check on the number assignment implicit in the first task. Faced with a numerical scale and their verbal choices, the subjects had to reconsider whether they really preferred one subset of objectives to another. The use of the ratio scale also made the additivity assumption explicit and permitted the subjects to react to it. With the two exceptions already noted the idea of additive values was readily grasped by the subjects and they were able to adjust their values and choices to achieve consistency.

Third Task

Although the third task was a complex one, the subjects, for the most part, were able to do it successfully.* The subjects had to keep several things in mind: the alternatives, the objectives, and a scale of probabilities. First, each was to estimate the probability that each alternative would achieve each objective. Eight alternatives and seven objectives required a total of fifty-six estimates from each subject. Second, each was asked to select the alternative he believed was the best way to allocate the 1964–1965 CI&A grant. Finally, each was asked to select the second best alternative for allocating the grant.

* One subject was unable to respond to the tasks in the experiment. He thought it was artificial to separate the objectives because all of the things mentioned in the objectives were needed for a good program. In the third task, after he read the first alternative and was asked the probability that the selection of the first alternative would achieve the various objectives, he said, "I'm getting a headache trying to think out these possibilities. This is like a crossword puzzle." He went on to say, "I don't think of these things in relation to each other [the probability that an alternative would achieve an objective], and I don't think of them in numerical terms." Referring to the scale of probabilities he said, "When you start talking about 90 or 50 or 75, I just don't think that way."

The comments made by the subjects during this task showed that they thought seriously about the consequences of each alternative before arriving at their estimates of probabilities. Usually the subjects commented briefly before estimating the probability that an alternative would achieve an objective. They made such statements as these:

> The Department of Finance would think that the state might have to pick up support of state level programs if federal funds were withdrawn, so they wouldn't like it.
>
> The big local health departments would like it; the little, local health departments wouldn't.
>
> I think it is good for the local health departments to do some thinking and planning. It pushes them a little.
>
> The Public Health Service would accept it, but they wouldn't be so happy so [the rating] would go down to 65.

Everyone agreed that the eighth alternative was less likely to achieve the objective of strengthening and supporting local health departments than was the first alternative. The eighth alternative was the one that would cut $75,000 from the amount available to local health departments, while the first alternative would not affect the amount of money allotted to local health departments but would cut $75,000 from the CI&A contract program. The agreement on such an "obvious" point supports the belief that the subjects were responding to the task and discriminating among the objectives and alternatives.

ANALYSIS USING THE MODEL

The criterion for the selection of one alternative from the eight alternatives in the model was the maximization of effectiveness. This criterion is essentially the same as the criterion of the maximization of expected utility. Rational behavior in terms of this study is defined as selecting the alternative with the highest effectiveness.

The experimental procedure used to obtain the utilities and the probabilities was such that it would have been very difficult for the director and other departmental members to see how the answers they gave in the three tasks would be put together to make a measure of effectiveness, Thus it is doubtful that the subjects in this experiment deliberately tried to give answers that would make the measure of effectiveness of alternatives (when calculated later by the author) coincide with their choice of the two alternatives they really preferred. In addition, the subjects did not know in advance the tasks they would be asked to do during the interview.

Because the study identified the director as the decision-maker, a comparison of his choices of alternatives with the rankings by the model is given first. The director selected the first alternative as his first choice. This is the choice he had actually made for the CI&A program a few months before. In this experiment he picked the third alternative as his second choice. Calculations using the model showed that the first alternative had the highest effectiveness and the third alternative had the second highest effectiveness. Thus, in terms of the model for allocating the CI&A grant, the director was a "rational" decision-maker, i.e., his behavior was consistent with the hypothesis that he chose his alternatives as if he were maximizing expected utility.

Of the 11 participants who completed the tasks in the experiment, 7 selected as their first or second choice the alternative that the model ranked first. Of these 7, there were 4 whose first and second choices were also ranked first and second by the model. The complete results are shown in Table 5.

TABLE 5. *Results of Experimental Tasks*

Subjects	*Model Ranking of Subject's 1st Choice*	*Model Ranking of Subject's 2nd Choice*
A	2	3
B	1	2
C	1	2
D	1	6
E	3	1
F	n.a.	n.a.
G	6	1
H	2	3
I	5	2
J	1	2
K	1	2
L	2	3

Of the 22 first and second choices made by the 11 subjects who completed the tasks in the experiment, the model ranked 19 of them as first, second, or third in effectiveness. A test which supports the hypothesis that the subjects chose alternatives as if they were maximizing expected utility is to calculate the probability that 4 of the 11 subjects would have made "perfect choices" by chance. (A perfect choice is one in which the subject's first and second choices of alternatives are the same as the alternatives ranked first and second in effectiveness by the model.) The probability of 4 perfect choices among the 11 subjects is .0000545.*

The use of departmental members as sources for data required by the effectiveness model warrants some discussion. As previously mentioned, the lack of knowledge of the consequences of the allocation of the CI&A grant precluded the use of other models that required service statistics from field programs. The use of members of an organization as experts to provide rankings and ratings in organizational studies is a well-recognized research technique. It has been used to assign electronic equipment to naval ships[53] and to evaluate defects in product packaging.[54] A short discussion of this technique and other examples of its use are given in Scott.[55]

The analysis and evaluation of the CI&A program showed that the departmental information gathering and processing system did not generate all the data needed to judge whether more effective use could have been made of the CI&A grant by changes in its allocation. Arrow has called attention to this aspect of operations research studies:

> In many cases, the improvements in performance attendant upon operations research is caused not so much by the formal optimization procedure, but by the fact that it calls attention to the proper data to be collected. It stresses the information upon which any rational decision must be made, and by so doing improves the value of the decision as much as or more than the exact attainment of the optimum solution of the problem, once properly formulated.[8, p. 772]

The investigation of the CI&A program helped generate support for two studies designed to give the departmental management better knowledge of the effects of its CI&A grant allocation. These were studies of home care nursing and disease detection programs, the two most popular chronic disease service programs in local health departments.[56, 57] If another study of the CI&A program is made, it might

* The probability of a subject selecting by chance as his first and second choices from the eight alternatives the two alternatives the model ranked first and second is 1/56. Because λ [$=np$] is a small number in this study ($11 \times 1/56 = .196$), the Poisson approximation of the binomial distribution was used to calculate P (4 out of 11 "perfect choices" $| \ p = 1/56$). For $\lambda = .20$, the probability of four or more perfect choices is .0000568 and the probability of five or more is .0000023. The difference, .0000545, is the probability of getting four perfect choices out of eleven by chance.

well be that a different model will be used because additional information is now available.

One member of the Department questioned whether the possible improvement in the operation of the CI&A program would be worth the expense involved in specifying the data requirements. changing the method of data collection, improving program evaluation, and so on. It is true that the acquisition of the information required by the effectiveness model is a costly and time-consuming process. However, the method adopted by the Department for decision-making in the CI&A program also was costly. In evaluating alternative methods of decision-making, comparisons need to be made in terms of the cost of a decision-making process in relation to its effectiveness in achieving organizational goals. The point in question is not whether more information would result in better decisions—the problem lies in deciding what information should be collected. To increase the effectiveness of the administration of the CI&A program, different information was needed but not more information. There is no reason to believe that the cost of a new decision-making process to generate the needed information would exceed the cost of the existing process.

CONCLUSIONS

The study of the CI&A program demonstrated to departmental members that some of their problems could be analyzed in a systematic way through the use of operations research. Their increased awareness of operations research concepts and techniques was no doubt the main benefit, because if operations research is accepted in the Department it may be used in many contexts.

Early skepticism had been voiced in the Department regarding the feasibility of a study of values in public health decision-making. At the time the study was proposed one division chief remarked to the author, "There is such utter confusion with respect to aims in public health that no study like this can possibly succeed." At the conclusion of the study the same division chief said the study reinforced his belief that program evaluation should be done and that decisions could be looked at objectively.

The effectiveness model described in this chapter is a very general decision model. It was used because the information required for other models was not available. In other studies different models would likely be needed. It is not the intention of this essay to recommend that other health agencies start measuring the values of objectives using the Churchman–Ackoff method. However, the effectiveness model is a good framework for thinking about any problem because it leads the administrator to examine his present decision-making procedure in terms of its effectiveness in achieving organizational goals. In particular, it causes the administrator to check his management information system to see whether it provides him with the consequences of his present decision-making procedure.

The use of operations research in organizational analysis requires time, money, and professionally trained personnel. Many of the limitations of operations research cited in the literature exist at this stage of development. However, the field is growing in its ability to handle complex problems. Realizing that it still required a "tremendous amount of faith" on the part of an executive to introduce operations research into his company, Ackoff and Rivett[58] wrote a book in 1963 aimed at explaining operations research to such executives and reducing the amount of faith required. Developments since that time have reduced the amount of faith required still further. Now health administrators may well find operations research of value to them in the solution to managerial problems.

References

1. C. West Churchman, R. L. Ackoff, and E. L. Arnoff, *Introduction to Operations Research*, New York: Wiley, 1957.
2. R. N. McKean, *Efficiency in Government Through Systems Analysis*, New York: Wiley, 1958.
3. R. L. Ackoff, "The Meaning, Scope, and Methods of Operations Research," in R. L. Ackoff (ed.), *Progress in Operations Research*, New York: Wiley, 1961, pp. 1–34.
4. R. L. Ackoff and M. Sasieni, *Fundamentals of Operations Research*, New York: Wiley, 1968.
5. H. J. Miser, "Operations Research in Perspective," *Operations Research*, 11 (1963), 669–677.
6. B. Koopman, "Fallacies in Operations Research," *Operations Research*, 4 (August 1956), 422–426.
7. P. R. Drucker, "'Management Science' and the Manager," *Management Science*, 1 (January 1955), 115–126.

8. K. J. Arrow, "Decision Theory and Operations Research," *Operations Research*, 5 (December 1957), 765–774.
9. R. Dorfman, "Operations Research," *American Economic Review*, 50 (September 1960), 575–623.
10. C. Hitch and R. McKean, "Suboptimization in Operations Problems," in J. F. McCloskey and F. N. Trefethen (eds.), *Operations Research for Management*, Baltimore, Md.: Johns Hopkins Press, 1954, pp. 168–186.
11. C. Hitch, "Suboptimization in Operations Problems," *Operations Research*, 1 (May 1953), 87–99.
12. R. L. Ackoff with the collaboration of S. K. Gupta and J. S. Minas, *Scientific Method: Optimizing Applied Research Decisions*, New York: Wiley, 1962.
13. W. Candill and B. H. Roberts, "Pitfalls in the Organization of Interdisciplinary Research," in R. N. Adams and J. J. Preiss (eds.), *Human Organization Research*, Homewood, Ill.: Dorsey Press, 1960, pp. 11–18.
14. Health Information Foundation, *An Inventory of Social and Economic Research in Health*, 14th ed., Chicago: Health Information Foundation, 1965.
15. D. B. Hertz and R. T. Eddison (eds.), *Progress in Operations Research*, New York: Wiley, 1964, Vol. II.
16. G. Hadley, "Applications of Linear Programming to Industrial Problems," *Linear Programming*, Reading, Mass.: Addison-Wesley, 1962, Chapter 12.
17. D. G. Malcolm, "Bibliography on the Use of Simulation in Management Analysis," *Operations Research*, 8 (March–April 1960), 169–177.
18. H. Simon, *The New Science of Management Decision*, New York: Harper & Row, 1960.
19. S. Beer, *Cybernetics and Management*, New York: Wiley, 1964.
20. D. Katz and R. L. Kahn, *The Social Psychology of Organizations*, New York: Wiley, 1966.
21. C. D. Flagle, "Operations Research in the Health Services," *Operations Research*, 10 (September–October 1962), 591–603.
22. C. D. Flagle, "Operations Research in Community Services," in D. B. Hertz and R. T. Eddison (eds.), *Progress in Operations Research*, New York: Wiley, 1964, Vol. II, pp. 329–344.
23. R. L. Gue, "Operations Research in Health and Hospital Administration," *Hospital Administration*, 10 (Fall 1965), 6–25.
24. W. J. Horvath, "Operations Research in Medical and Hospital Practice," in P. M. Morse (ed.), *Operations Research for Public Systems*, Cambridge, Mass.: The MIT Press, 1967, pp. 127–157.
25. N. T. J. Bailey, "A Study of Queues and Appointment Systems in Hospital Outpatient Departments, with Special Reference to Waiting Times," *Journal of the Royal Statistical Society, Ser. B*, 14 (1952), 185–199.
26. N. T. J. Bailey, "Calculating the Scale of Inpatient Accommodation," in

Nuffield Provincial Hospital Trust, *Towards a Measure of Medical Care: Operational Research in the Health Services*, London: Oxford University Press, 1962, pp. 55–65.

27. R. B. Fetter and J. D. Thompson, "The Simulation of Hospital Systems," *Operations Research*, 13 (September–October 1965), 689–711.
28. C. D. Flagle, "The Problem of Organization for Hospital Inpatient Care," in The Institute of Management Sciences, *Management Sciences: Models and Techniques*, New York: Pergamon Press, 1960, Vol. 2, pp. 275–287.
29. W. H. Thomas, "A Model for the Prediction of Demand for Nursing Services," paper presented at the 27th National Meeting of the Operations Research Society of America, May 6–7, 1965.
30. R. C. Jelinek, "A Structural Model for the Patient Care Operation," *Health Services Research*, 2 (Fall–Winter 1967), 226–242.
31. I. James, A. Barr, C. Butler, M. J. Tobin, and J. O. F. Davis, "Operational Research in Nursing," a series of short papers in G. McLachlan (ed.), *Problems and Progress in Medical Care*, London: Oxford University Press, 1964, pp. 73–114.
32. B. A. Weisbrod, *Economics of Public Health*, Philadelphia: University of Pennsylvania Press, 1961.
33. R. Fein, *Economics of Mental Illness*, New York: Basic Books, 1958.
34. H. E. Klarman, "Syphilis Control Programs," in R. Dorfman (ed.), *Measuring Benefits of Government Investments*, Washington, D.C.: The Brookings Institution, 1965, pp. 367–410.
35. I. S. Blumenthal, *Research and the Ulcer Problem*, Santa Monica, Calif.: The RAND Corporation, Report R-336-RC, 1960.
36. M. S. Feldstein, review of B. A. Weisbrod, *Economics of Public Health*, in *Economic Journal*, 73 (March 1963), 129–130.
37. S. J. Mushkin, "Comments," in Robert Dorfman (ed.), *Measuring Benefits of Government Investments*, Washington, D.C.: The Brookings Institution, 1965, pp. 410–414.
38. M. S. Feldstein, "Economic Analysis, Operational Research and the National Health Service," *Oxford Economic Papers* (1963), 19–31.
39. J. Wiseman, "Cost–Benefit Analysis and Health Service Policy," in A. T. Peacock and D. J. Robertson (eds.), *Public Expenditure: Appraisal and Control*, London: Oliver & Boyd, 1963, pp. 128–145.
40. W. T. Federer, "Procedures and Designs Useful for Screening Material in Selection and Allocation, with a Bibliography," *Biometrics*, 19 (December 1963), 553–587.
41. G. B. Dantzig, *Linear Programming and Extensions*, Princeton: Princeton University Press, 1963.
42. R. L. Ackoff (ed.), *Progress in Operations Research*, New York: Wiley, 1961, Vol. 1.
43. P. Stillson, "A Method for Defect Evaluation," *Industrial Quality Control*, 11 (1954), 9–12.

44. H. H. Gulliksen, "Measurement of Subjective Values," *Psychometrika*, 21 (1956), 229–244.
45. S. Stouffer, "The Point System for Redeployment and Discharge," in S. Stouffer et al. (eds.), *The American Soldier*, Princeton: Princeton University Press, 1949, Vol. 2, pp. 520–548.
46. G. Suzuki, "Procurement and Allocation of Naval Electronic Equipment," *Naval Research Logistics Quarterly*, 4 (1957), 1–7.
47. E. Adams and R. Fagot, "A Model of Riskless Choice," *Behavioral Science*, 4 (1959), 1–10.
48. O. G. Brim, Jr., et al., *Personality and Decision Processes*, Stanford, Calif.: Stanford University Press, 1962.
49. J. Marschak, "Actual Versus Consistent Decision Behavior," *Behavioral Science*, 9 (1964), 103–110.
50. S. Siegel, A. E. Siegel, and J. M. Andrews, *Choice, Strategy, and Utility*, New York: McGraw-Hill, 1964.
51. D. Stimson, *Decision Making and Resource Allocation in a Public Health Agency*, Internal Working Paper No. 18, Social Sciences Project, Berkeley: Space Sciences Laboratory, University of California, rev. 1967.
52. C. West Churchman and R. L. Ackoff, "An Approximate Measure of Value," *Operations Research*, 2 (1954), 172–181.
53. R. J. Aumann and J. B. Kruskal, "Assigning Quantitative Values to Qualitative Factors in the Naval Electronics Problem," *Naval Research Logistics Quarterly*, 6 (1959), 1–16.
54. P. Stillson, "A Method for Defect Evaluation," *Industrial Quality Control*, 11 (1954), 9–12.
55. W. R. Scott, "Field Methods in the Study of Organizations," in J. G. March (ed.), *Handbook of Organizations*, Chicago: Rand McNally, 1965, pp. 293–294.
56. *Bedside Nursing Program Pretest*, Internal Department document, mimeographed, n.d.
57. A. F. Nunez, "Model for the Evaluation of Disease Detection Programs," in C. E. Weber and G. Peters (eds.), *Management Action: Models of Administrative Decision*, Scranton: International Textbook Company, 1969.
58. R. L. Ackoff and P. Rivett, *A Manager's Guide to Operations Research*, New York: Wiley, 1963.

Index